HUMAN FETAL ENDOCRINES

DEVELOPMENTS IN OBSTETRICS AND GYNECOLOGY

VOLUME 1

1. J. E. Jirásek, Human fetal endocrines, 1980. ISBN 90-247-2325-6.
2. P. M. Motta, E. S. E. Hafez, eds., Biology of the ovary, 1980. ISBN 90-247-2316-7.
3. J. Horský, J. Presl, eds., Ovarian function and its disorders, 1980. ISBN 90-247-2326-4.
4. D. W. Richardson, D. Joyce, E. M. Symonds, eds., Frozen human semen, 1980. ISBN 90-247-2370-1.
5. E. S. E. Hafez, W. A. A. van Os, eds., Medicated intrauterine devices, 1980. ISBN 90-247-2371-X.

Series ISBN 90−247−2334−5

Human Fetal Endocrines

JAN E. JIRÁSEK, M. D., D. Sc.

Institute for the Care of Mother and Child,
Prague

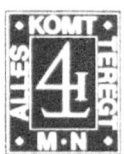

1980

SPRINGER-SCIENCE+BUSINESS MEDIA, B.V.

ISBN 978-94-009-8194-2   ISBN 978-94-009-8192-8 (eBook)
DOI 10.1007/978-94-009-8192-8

© translation: J. E. Jirásek, 1980

Copyright © by Springer Science+Business Media Dordrecht
Originally published by Martinus Nijhoff Publishers bv, The Hague, in 1980
Softcover reprint of the hardcover 1st edition 1980

This book is published with an arrangement of Avicenum, Czechoslovak Medical Press, Prague

To my wife Věra
in appreciation of all her support.

CONTENTS

VII

PREFACE

The study of prenatal development provides many clues for understanding the physiology as well as the pathogeny of malformations and many diseases. I became interested in the analysis of human development as a young medical student more than 30 years ago, and I have stayed in this field all my life. In my studies, I always tried to compare the events of different disciplines such as genetics, anatomy, biochemistry and physiology. I learned that the development of a structure is, under normal circumstances, strictly determined and that the development of structures always precedes their proper function. There are no changes in function without changes in structure. The life of every cell is genetically preprogrammed and the program may be modified by complicated interactions with environment. Recent progress in our knowledge is basicly related to technology. However, using all the tools of today's technology, we are still unable to understand the basic normal development.

After almost thirty years of work, I am trying to present a subjective review of the development of the human endocrine glands. I am presenting an image emerging from my experience. I personally studied several hundred human embryos using mostly anatomical, histochemical and some biochemical techniques. I found much additional information in the literature. However, there is so much different information available today that, using the limited brain capacity, I did not try to register all observations and discoveries, but I selected some which seemed to me to be the most important. The following books were the valuable sources of my information:

In genetics and congenital anomalies:

McKusick V. A.: Mendelian inheritance in man; catalogs of autosomal dominat, autosomal recessive and X-linked phenotypes. Baltimore, Johns Hopkins Press, 1975.
Bergsma D. (Ed.) Birth defects, atlas and compendium. The National Foundation March of Dimes, Baltimore, Williams and Wilkins Co., 1973.

In embryology:

Keibel F. and Mall. F. P. (Eds.) Manual of human embryology. Philadelphia London, J. B. Lippincott Co., Vol. I, 1910, Vol. II, 1912.
Streeter G. L.: Developmental horizons in human embryos. Contrib. Embryol. Carnegie Inst., Washington, 1951.
O'Rahilly R.: Developmental stages in human embryos, including a survey of the Carnegie Collection. Carnegie Inst., Washington, 1973.
Willis R. A.: The borderland of embryology and pathology. London, Butterworth, 1958.

In comparative anatomy and phylogenesis:

Kent G. C. Jr.: Comparative anatomy of the vertebrates. St. Louis, *C. V. Mosby Co.* 1969.
Romer A. S. Parson T. S.: The vertebrate body. Philadelphia, London, Toronto, W. B. Saunders Co., 1977.

In biochemistry:

Harper H. A.: Review of physiological chemistry. 15th ed., Los Altos, California, Lange Med. Pub., 1975.

These references will generally not be mentioned in the text.

The first version of Human Fetal Endocrines appeared in Czech in 1977. Since then, much new information has emerged. I completely revised and rewrite the manuscript for the English edition during my stay in Minneapolis as Visiting Professor in the Department of Obstetrics and Gynecology, University of Minnesota Medical School.

I am deeply grateful to Dr. K. A. Prem for his kind invitation to join the Department of Obstetrics and Gynecology, University of Minnesota. I also wish to express many thanks to Mrs. Blanka Faltinová, Miss Donna Lidstad and Mrs. Rachel Roverud for their linguistic and secretarial help.

CHAPTER I

GENERAL IDEAS

Endocrinology could be defined in the broadest context as a field dealing with chemical integrations in individuals. The integrating substances may act within the same cell they originate from, in the neighborhood of this cell passing through the cellular membranes from one cell to the other, or in some remote cells where the substance is transported by blood or by another extracellular fluid. The exchange of substances between adjacent cells represents, phylogenetically, the oldest system of intercellular communication. All the cellular functions are strictly genetically determined. At the beginning of ontogenic development, after fertilization of a highly specialized cell known as the oocyte, all the genes are in a repressed stage. During the oocyte cleavage, only some basic genes involved in the mitosis are operating, and most of the genes are repressed. The differentiation is a process based on the differential switching on and off of genes. The early differentiation (during blastomere formation) is influenced by intracellular cytoplasmic gradients and intercellular contacts. Later on, organizing centers develop; organizers are released and morphogenetic movements take place producing the basic embryonal layers: ectoderm, endoderm, mesoderm and notochord. Organizers of a higher degree (secondary, tertiary, etc.), inducing and repressing substances are involved in the differentiation of the primordia of different organs. Differentiation based on specific genes is related to the synthesis of specific peptides, proteins, glycoproteins or lipids and to their recognition. In morphological and physical terms, differentiation means the build-up of complicated systems of membranes keeping the chemical substances apart to prevent them from mixing freely.

HORMONES

The term, hormone, was first used by *Starling* (1905) in his study of gastrin secretion. The term is used for substances catalysing different metabolic reactions. Most of the hormones are produced by the ductless gland and most of them are transported to the target tissue by blood. In contrast to organizers, the action of hormones is bilateral, even if produced unilaterally.

Phylogenetically, most of the endocrine cells were originally in an exocrine position. This feature is repeated during embryogenesis. A special kind of integration between the CNS and the organism as a whole represents the neurosecretion and neurotransmission.

1

There are some chemical messengers which are closely related to hormones but do not satisfactorily fit the definition of hormone. Among those are prostaglandins, histamin, etc. Chemically, the hormones may be classified as (1) aromatic aminoacid derivatives, (2) oligopeptides, (3) polypeptides, (4) pure large proteins, (5) glycoproteins and (6) hormonal steroids.

(1) In the group of aromatic aminoacid derivatives, DOPA, norepinephrine and epinephrine originate from phenylalanine. Thyroxin and triiodothyronine are derived from tyrosine. Serotonine and melatonine represent tryptophan derivatives.

(2) The oligopeptidic hormones (less than 21 aminoacids) include the hypothalamic-releasing factors such as TRF, LHRH, SRIF and some others such as vaso-pressin, oxytocin, gastrin, etc.

(3) The polypeptidic hormone group (more than 20 aminoacids) includes: glucagon, calcitonin and ACTH.

(4) Large pure proteins are the growth hormone, the prolactin and the chorionic somatomammotropin.

(5) The glycoproteins are the folliculostimulating hormone, the luteinizing hormone the thyreostimulating hormone and the chorionic gonadotropin.

(6) Hormonal steroids are subdivided into three subroups: C-21 steroids, C-19 steroids and C-18 steroids. Among the C-21 steroids, the progesterone is known as a gesta-gen, cortisol as a glucocorticoid, and aldosterone as a mineralocorticoid. The C-19 steroids are androgens, testosterone being the most important. The C-18 steroids are estrogens: estrone, estradiol and estriol.

The hormone-producing cells originate from all embryonal layers. However, some general rules may be stressed. The cells synthesizing phenylalanine derivatives, tryptophan derivatives and oligopeptides are usually neuroectodermal in origin. The cells involved in the formation of polypeptides might be derived from a specific clone of cells already present in the embryoblastic pool. Cells involved in the synthesis of hormonal glycoproteins are ectodermal. The steroid-producing cells (with the exception of the trophoblast) are coelomic, either mesodermal or mesenchymal, in origin. The cells synthesizing "big" and "big-big" hormonal precursors (which consequently become hydrolyzed and split into smaller active hormones, such as prolactin, insulin, gastrin, or thyroxin), originate embryologically from derivatives evaginating from, or closely related to the digestive tube. This reinforces the statement that big prohormones in phylogenesis were sometimes secreted by the exocrine glands into the digestive tube where they were digested, transformed into a biologically active form and absorbed into the blood.

The intracellular synthesis of hormones is closely related to their chemical structure. The proteosynthetic process, by which polypeptidic chains are formed, is relatively well known and includes DNA-RNA transcription by which at least three character-istic forms RNA are formed: transfer RNA, ribosomal RNA and messenger RNA. The transfer RNA's specific for each aminoacid, bind the corresponding aminoacids within the cytoplasm of the cell and bind them to the ribosomes.

Ribosomal RNA, together with some necessary proteins, constitutes the ribosomes. Each ribosome has two components: a smaller on (30 s) and a bigger one (50 s). The one messenger RNA determines the sequence of the aminoacids in the polypeptide chain formed at the ribosomes. The small component of the ribosome binds the messenger RNA with the corresponding transfer RNA carrying the aminoacid. The big component of the ribosome binds aminoacids into the polypeptidic chain. The operating genetic mechanisms are: (1) removing of the nucleohistone blocking the DNA-RNA transcription, (2) transcription of RNA catalyzed by RNA polymerase (The DNA unit coding one polypeptidic chain is known as the cistron. Several cistrons coding closely related proteins form operons) and (3) translation of messenger RNA at the ribosomes and formation of the polypeptidic chain.

From the site of their origin, the polypeptides and proteins are transported through the cisternae of the rough endoplasmic reticulum into the Golgi complex, and from the Golgi complex the product is released into the cytoplasm in the form of membrane-coated granules. The hydrolysis of the product occurs within these granules by the hydrolases bound to the membrane, or by hydrolases provided by lysosomes fusing with the granules. After synthesis has been accomplished, the product may be stored within the granules for a considerable time. The release of the product occurs by exocytosis. In neuroendocrine cells, the neurohormone is synthesized in the peri-karyone, then is transported along the axon and is released at the axon terminals into the blood or to another cell across the cytoplasmic membranes.

Within the blood, the hormones are transported either in a free form or bound to specific proteins of the blood plasma. The free unbound hormone usually represents the metabolically active form. Energy required for the synthesis of the hormone is liberated by oxidations (and reductions). The energy is generated by the respiratory chains. In the chain, electrons are transported from the more electronegative components to the more electropositive, ending with oxygen. The main chain proceeds from the NAD-linked dehydrogenase system through the flavoproteins and cyto-chromes to molecular oxygen. Electron transfer from dehydrogenases such a hydroxy-butyrate, glutamate, malate and isocitrate couple directly with NAD. NADH is oxidized by NADH dehydrogenase. Co-enzyme Q (Co Q, ubiquinone), collects reducing equivalents from different substances, such as the tricarbonic acids, pyru-vate, succinate, or glycerophosphate and acyl-CoA, and transports them through cytochromes to oxygen.

During NAD-linked dehydrogenase oxidation, three moles of inorganic phosphate are incorporated into three moles of ADP to form three moles of ATP, and a half mole of O_2 is consumed. An alternative process, oxidation by flavoprotein-linked dehydro-genase yields only two moles of ATP per half mole of O_2. These reactions by which ATP is generated are known as the oxidative phosphorylation. ATP originates from glycolysis. In the mitochondria, respiration cannot occur without phosphorylation of ADP.

NADH is produced by the 3-phosphoglyceraldehyde dehydrogenase and cannot cross the mitochondrial membrane. (The amount of NAD available to the mesenchymal cell regulates its differentiation such as, either to become a chondrocyte or a muscle cell). Under anaerobic conditions, however, NADH is oxidized in mitochondria. Mitochondria have an outer membrane (containing monoaminooxidase) which is permeable to most metabolites, and a cristae-forming selective inner membrane. The inner membrane is permeable to water, acetate, acetoacetate, pyruvate, CO_2 and O_2. Inorganic phosphate penetrates into the mitochondria as undissociated acid. Respirating mitochondria accumulate K^+, Na^+, Ca^{2+} and Mg^{2+}. Over 50% of the energy released from ATP is used for active ionic transport across the cellular and mitochondrial membranes. Regulation of the energy supply may limit the synthesis and release of hormones.

ACTION OF HORMONES

The specific action of hormones in target tissue requires their peripheral recognition. Most of the hormones bind to specific receptor proteins. The hormones may regulate (1) the proteosynthesis, (2) the intracellular cyclic nucleotides level, (3) the membrane permeability or the enzyme activity.

(1) All steroids influence proteosynthesis in the target cells. Steroids bind to specific cytoplasmic receptors, such as aldosterone binding, glucocorticoid binding, progesterone binding, testosterone binding and estrogen binding proteins. The hormone. or its metabolite, forms a combination with the receptor. The combination is transported, into the nucleus of the cell, acts on the DNA chromatin removing the repressor from the specific site. Increase in a specific RNA synthesis occurs involving t-, m- and rRNA. RNA's are transported into the cytoplasm, mRNA is transported to the ribosomes resulting in a specific steroid-dependent proteosynthesis.

(2) Cyclic 3.5-AMP level in different cells may increase or decrease in response to a hormonal stimulation. Hormones involved in such a mechanism are bound to a specific receptor located at the cellular membranes in the target tissues such as liver (glucagon), distal renal tubule (parathormone), adrenergic receptors (epinephrine stimulating both receptors alpha and beta, norepinephrine stimulating primarily alpha receptors), etc. The cAMP system represents a phylogenetically-old mediator involved in the effects of other non-hormonal substances, such as the prostaglandins, or in reactions leading to lipolysis. In addition, cAMP also stimulates protein kinases which phosphorylate nuclear histones regulating RNA transcription. Some membrane phenomena and cAMP regulation may be related since the adenylcyclase is localized in the cell membranes. Cyclic AMP is formed from ATP by adenylate cyclase. Cyclic AMP is destroyed by conversion to AMP by phosphodiesterase.

(3) Membrane transport and enzyme activation are difficult to distinguish. Thyroxin increases the Na^+, K^+ ATPase. The permeability of the cellular and mitochondrial membranes to calcium modifies most effects of protein hormones. In the absence of calcium, the elevated or decreased level of cAMP are without any metabolic effects. Protein hormones increase the uptake of extracellular calcium. Cyclic AMP mobilizes bound intracellular calcium. Secretion of all hormones stored in granules requires calcium.

There is no "ahormonal" state in human development. From the beginning, the fertilized oocyte, cleaving embryo, or free blastocyst is under the influence of the hormones contained in the maternal environment. After implantation, as soon as the chorionic (early placental) barrier becomes established, the trophoblast produces fetal hormones. The fetal endocrine glands develop in a highly balanced environment, where the changes in temperature, glucose, sodium, potassium, calcium, magnesium and other cation concentrations are very limited under normal circumstances.

In the prenatal development of most endocrine glands, the primary stage, the stage of an increasing secretion, the stage of a decreasing secretion and the stage of a balanced secretion may be distinguished.

1. The primary stage includes formation of the glandular primordium. The formation of anlage of any endocrine gland is hormone independent. The basal secretion of the gland is very low without the proper stimulation resembling the secretion in tissue culture "under basal conditions".

4

2. The stage of increasing secretion is related to the specific stimulation, usually the development of the hypothalamic-releasing hormone neurons. At the beginning, the secretion of hypothalamic-releasing hormone-producing neurons is increasing. A similar increase in secretion follows in their target cells in the adenohypophysis.

3. The decrease in hypothalamic hormonal secretion is a consequence of the developed sensitivity of hypothalamic neurons to the proper peripheral metabolic hormone. As the sensitivity of the neuroendocrine neuron increases, the secretion of the releasing hormone falls, followed by the decrease of the tropic hormone.

4. As the stage of a balanced secretion is reached and the sensitivity of the hypothalamic neurosecretory neuron becomes stabilized, the corresponding amount of a tropic hormone and the level of the "metabolic hormone" remains stable. In the stabilized system, if the level of the "metabolic hormone" falls, the increased secretion of the releasing hormone stimulates the secretion of a tropic hormone.

FEED-BACK MECHANISM

The essential role of many hormones is to maintain a stable level of "metabolic" substances such as glucose, aminoacids, or calcium. The role of "tropic" hormones is to stabilize the levels of other "metabolic" hormones, such as glucocorticoids, androgens, estrogens and thyroxin. The "releasing" hormones regulate production of tropic hormones.

In the developing fetus, the energy comes primarily from glucose. The fetal glucose leve depends on the maternal blood level. The levels in the umbilical vein are higher than in the umbilical artery. Amniotic fluid glucose decreases and insulin content increases with gestational age. The mother and the fetus (fetoplacental unit) do not share their regulatory mechanisms. The regulation of glycemia is primarily related to the secretion of insulin. Insulin antagonists are glucagon, epinephrine, thyroxine, glucocorticoids and growth hormone. The main feed-back mechanism exists directly between B-cells of the pancreatic islets and blood glucose. A similar direct feed-back mechanism exists between ionized calcium and parathormone secretion. The main antagonist of parathormone is calcitonin. The antagonist helps to correct glycemia or calcemia in exaggerated situation which may happen at birth, but which are very rare during intrauterine life.

The feed-back systems regulating the levels of aminoacids, hormonal steroids and thyroxin involve, in addition to direct regulations (short loop feed-backs), one or more of several steps (long loop feed-backs). In those systems, there is usually an adenohypophyseal tropic hormone-producing cell in a central position whose function is regulated by one or more hypothalamic-releasing hormones. The adenohypophyseal tropic hormone regulates synthesis of another "metabolic" hormone-producing cell in a peripheral endocrine gland. The hormone produced by the peripheral gland regulates the secretion of the hypothalamic-releasing hormones (long loop feed-back) and simultaneously influences the production of the tropics hormone in the adenohypophysis (short loop). The hypothalamic-releasing hormones are sometimes paired, one stimulating and one enhancing the secretion. Such antagonists are: SRIF-TRH, SRIF-gastrin, LHRH-melatonin. One hypothalamic hormone may regulate two hypophyseal hormones (SRIF→GH and TSH; LHRH→FSH, LH).

The prenatal sensitivity of hypothalamic neuroendocrine neurons is reduced by steroids (DHA, progesterone?). There are differences in the sensitivity between males and females. The testosterone present in males from the beginning of the third month of development (week 9) makes the hypothalamic neurons and the whole feedback system more sensitive. In several steps including feedbacks, the sensitivity of every cell is to be considered separately (sensitivity of the endocrine neurons, adenohypophyseal cells and endocrine cells in the peripheral gland).

In males, the balanced secretion of LHRH, FSH and the LH-involving system is reached around week 25 of gestation, whereas in females it is around week 32 when a sufficient amount of androgen is formed in the ovaries and adrenals. The free androgens seem to be the decisive factor because estrogens do not pass the blood-brain barrier (rats; *Naftolin et al.*, 1975; *Lieberburg and McEven*, 1975) and cannot reach the hypothalamic neurons. After birth, when the placental influence is passed, the hypothalamic steroid sensitivity increases tremendously. In childhood, minimal levels of androgens and estrogens suppress the secretory activity of LHRH neurons. The fetal hypothalamic "tuning" remains preserved in the memory of the cells in the postnatal ontogenesis and is probably responsible for the differences in the timing of puberty between males and females. Postnatally, the sensitivity of the hypothalamic neurosecretory neurons diminishes with the advancing age and is influenced by the DHA and DHAS produced by the adrenals. The diminishing sensitivity triggers puberty (and induces menopause in women). As the hypothalamic sensitivity to sexual steroids decreases, the gonadal steroidogenesis becomes reactivated and puberty starts.

The neuroendocrine regulations involving the cerebral cortex are completed after birth. The electrical activity of the brain is not detected during the second month of gestation. The asynchronous stage of EEG activity begins in mid-gestation, and the asynchronous activity persists postnatally. Diencephalic electrical activity may be detected by the fifth gestational month. EEG changes consistent with sleep are found postnatally in two month-old babies. Circadian rhythms, expressed in the secretory pattern of many hormones, are related to the light-dark cycles and the sleeping cycle. The early postnatal period is decisive for the tonic or cyclic secretion of LH and for sexual behavior in rats. A similar short decisive prenatal period for LH secretory patterns and sexual behavior was found in the monkey and guinea pig.

The fetal endocrinology remains a fascinating field with many unsolved problems.

CHAPTER 2

BASIC SURVEY OF HUMAN PRENATAL DEVELOPMENT

EMBRYONAL PERIOD

1. UNICELLULAR STAGE (48 HOURS)

Development of a new human being results from an oocyte fertilization, taking place normally in the ampulla of the uterine tube. The sperm penetrates into the oocyte shortly after ovulation, around day 14 of a normal menstrual cycle. Within the cytoplasm of the oocyte the sperm head breaks from the tail and transfoms into the male pronucleus.

At the time of ovulation the oocyte completed its first meiotic division (whose prophase had begin many years ago, sometimes in the prenatal period), expelling the first polar body (Fig. 1). During the formation of the male pronecleus, the so-called secondary oocyte undergoes the second meiotic division, which results in the formation of the second polar body and the female pronucleus.

The female pronucleus is constituted from a haploid set of chromosomes remaining in the oocyte after the second meiotic division. The oocyte with both male and female pronuclei is known as the ootid. The male and female pronuclei approach, paternal and maternal chromosomes reappear, homologous chromosomes of maternal and paternal origin pair at the equatorial level, and establish a new individual genome. The chromosomes become attached to the fibres of the meiotic spindle of the oocyte at the end of the prophase of the first mitotic division. The impregnated oocyte at the stage of the first mitosis is properly named the zygote. The zygote contains a new combination of maternal and paternal genes.

From the genetic point of view, the zygote formation represents the most important period in the individual life.

2. BLASTOMERIC STAGE (DAYS 3 AND 4)

The first mitosis triggers the process of cleavage. The oocyte splits into blastomeres approximately 24—36 hours after sperm penetration. Subsequent cleavage divisions give rise to equally-sized smaller and smaller blastomeres. A solid aggregate of blastomeres enclosed in the zona pellucida is called morula.

3. BLASTODERMIC STAGE (DAYS 4—6)

At approximately 16—20 blastomere stage ($3—3^1/_2$ days), desmosomes appear between adjacent outer blastomeres and the morula becomes converted into a blastocyst.

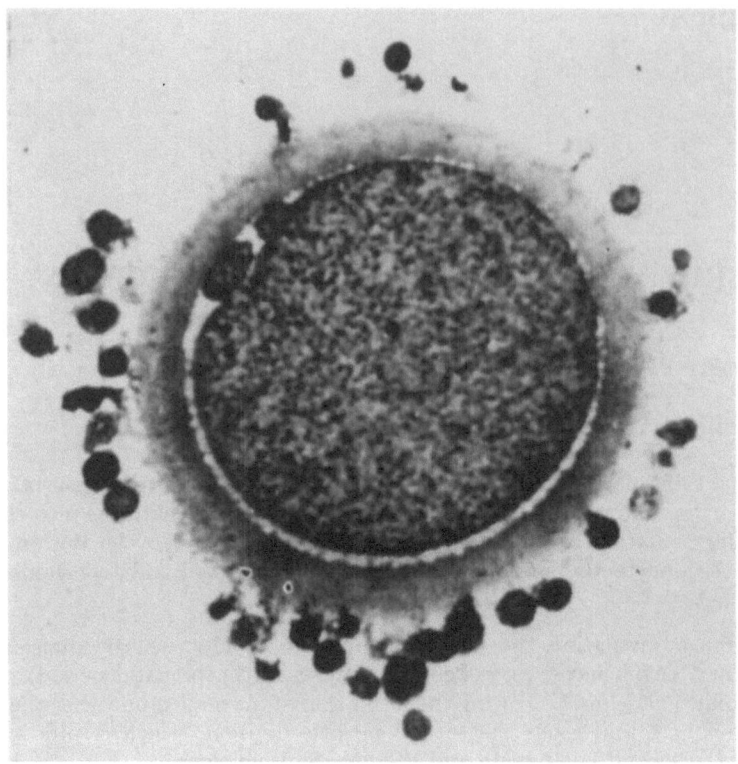

Fig. 1. Hnman oocyte with a detaching second polar body. Zona pellucida with some attached granulosa cells is present.

The desmosomes formation, followed subsequently by tight junctions between adjacent blastomeres, indicates the differentiation of the blastocystic trophoblast. The blastocyst (Fig. 2) represents a hollow sphere formed by two components:
(a) singlelayered trophoblast lining the cavity
(b) an excentrically-located aggregate of blastomeres representing the embryoblast (inner cell mass).

The blastocystic cavity is filled with blastocystic fluid. In a human blastocyst formed by 107 cells, 8 cells represent the inner cell mass, 30 cells the polar trophoblast (covering the inner cell mass), and 69 cells the mural trophoblast (lining the blastocystic cavity). These blastocysts enter the uterine cavity ($3^1/_2$ days after fertilization) still enclosed in the zona pellucida of the oocyte from which they developed. The blastocyst remains unimplanted within the uterine cavity for an additional 48—60 hours. At the end of this period, covering approximately day 21 of a normal menstrual cycle, the zona pellucida is shed and implantation begins (*Hertig, Rock, Adams*, 1956).

During *in vitro* experiments, rhythmic pulsation of the human blastocyst similar to that of the mouse (*Cole*, 1967), expelling of blastocystic fluid and hatching from the zona pellucida, were not observed.

In several species, steroid transformations were documented in preimplantation stages (rabbit — *Huff and Eik-Nes*, 1966; pig — *Perry et al.* 1976; rat — *Dey and*

Fig. 2. Advanced unimplanted human blastocyst (Hertig, Rock specimen, Carnegie Inst. No 8663). PT — polar trophoblast covering the embryoblast, MT — mural trophoblast.

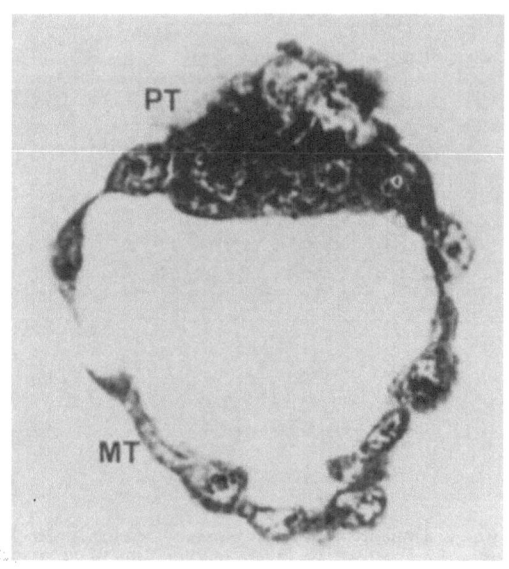

Dickman, 1974), and were considered with the pathways leading to estrogens. Gonadotropins, or at least immunocompetent hCG-like material was found in rabbit blastocysts (*Haour and Saxena,* 1974).

Neither hCG, nor steroids were found in tissue culture media used for human blastocysts for 2—3 days (*Edwards,* 1973). The addition of prostaglandin E, estradiol-17β and LH to the culture medium increased the number of human oocytes undergoing maturation (*Jagiello et al.,* 1975).

In preimplantation embryo, the first period of DNA synthesis appears in ootids (mouse, *Barlow et al.* 1972). All classes of RNA are synthesized beginning with the 2-cell stage (mouse, *Woodland and Graham,* 1969). About 50 percent of protein synthesis in early morulas is suppressed by actinomycin D suggesting that at this stage, the amount of RNA was translated from the embryonic RNA and the rest from maternal RNA (*Monesi et al.,* 1970). The types of protein synthesized in a mouse 8-cell embryo are basically the same as in blastocysts (*Epstein,* 1975).

Regarding energy, glucose is probably used in human oocytes via pentose shunt as the oocytes are rich in glucose-6-phosphate dehydrogenase. Glycogen is synthesized from glucose during cleavage (*Wales,* 1975). Lactate concentration within blastomeres reflects the concentration of the surrounding medium. The blastocyst represents a system of two cellular compartments: trophoblast and embryoblast (inner cell mass). The embryoblast of a late blastocyst is a pool of cells providing stem cells destined to become components of different organs (melanocytes, haemocytoblasts, primordial germ cells).

4. BILAMINAR EMBRYO (DAYS 6—14)

The inner cell mass differentiates shortly before implantation into an embryo consisting of adjacent ectoderm and endoderm (Fig. 3). Both primary germ layers are

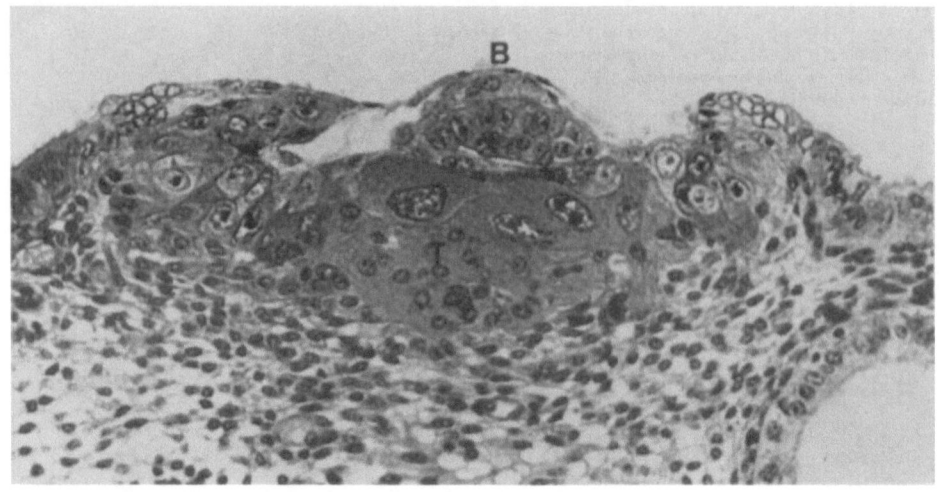

Fig. 3. Implanting human blastocyst (Hertig, Rock specimen, Carnegie No 8020) 7 1/2 days old. B — remnant of the blastocystic trophoblast. T — trophoblast of the developing trophoblastic shell.

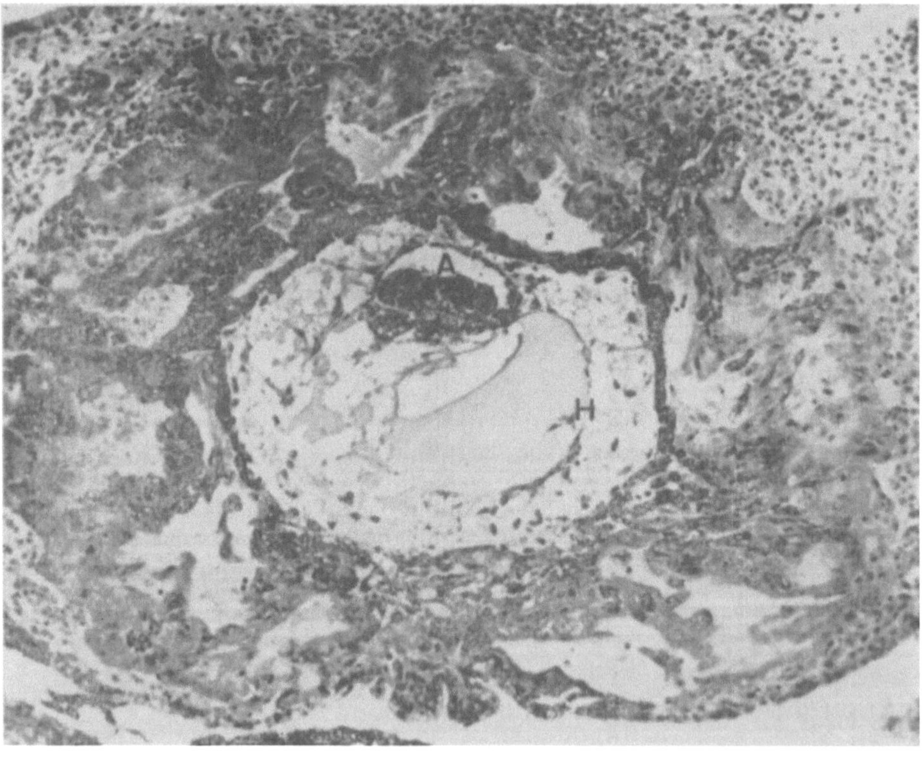

Fig. 4. Bilaminar implanted ca 13 days old human embryo with a disrupting Heuser's membrane (primary yolk sac). A — amnionic vesicle, H — remnant of Heuser's membrane.

arranged into a circular bilaminar embryonic disc. Simultaneously, as the primary mesoderm delaminates from the implanted trophoblast, the amnionic sac and the primary yolk sac become evident (Fig. 4). The proper embryo at this stage is formed by two vesicles, the amnionic sac and the yolk sac. The ectoblast of the embryonic disc forms the floor of the cavity of the amniotic sac. The adjacent endoblast of the disc forms the ceiling of the primary yolk sac. The wall of the primary yolk sac formed

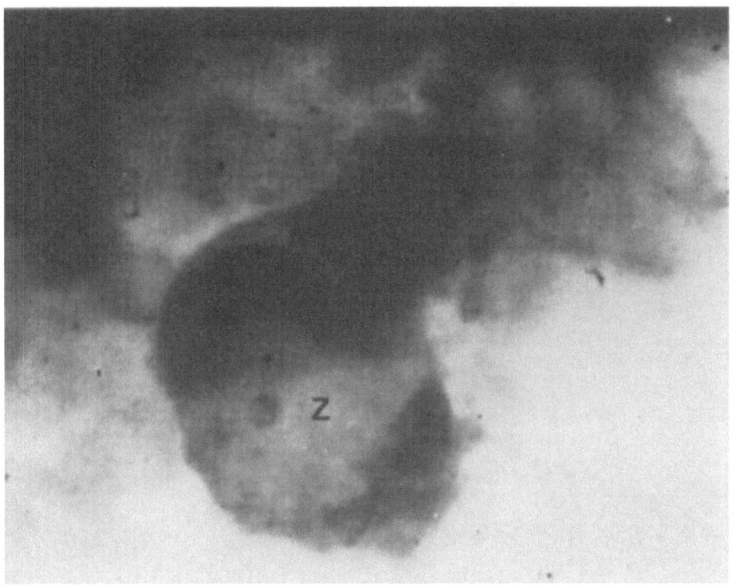

Fig. 5. Very early trilaminar human embryo (16—17 days old) after the chorion has been opened. The amnionic vesicle (A) and the yolk sac (Z) are attached to the chorion by the connecting stalk. The embryonal disc is dorsally convex.

by flattened cells is known as Heuser's membrane. The development of the bilaminar embryo until the primary yolk sac stage covers days 6—13. As the chorionic sac of an implanted embryo grows much faster than the primary yolk sac, the primary yolk sac ruptures. The part of the ruptured yolk sac adjacent to the embryonic disc closes again and becomes the secondary yolk sac. The abembryonal part of the ruptured primary yolk sac transforms into an endodermal cyst adjacent to the chorion. The spaces formed in the extraembryonic mesoderm between the yolk sac and chorion fuse to a single extraembryonic coelom. At this stage there are three fluid-filled compartments within the conceptus: amnionic cavity, yolk sac cavity and the extraembryonic coelom. The amnionic and yolk sac vesicles enclosed in a unicellular layer of cells of the primary mesoderm are attached to the chorionic mesoderm by a mesodermal connecting stalk. The connecting stalk joins the caudal part of the embryonal disc (Fig. 5, 6).

The stage of a bilaminar embryo with a secondary yolk sac covers days 13—14 after conception.

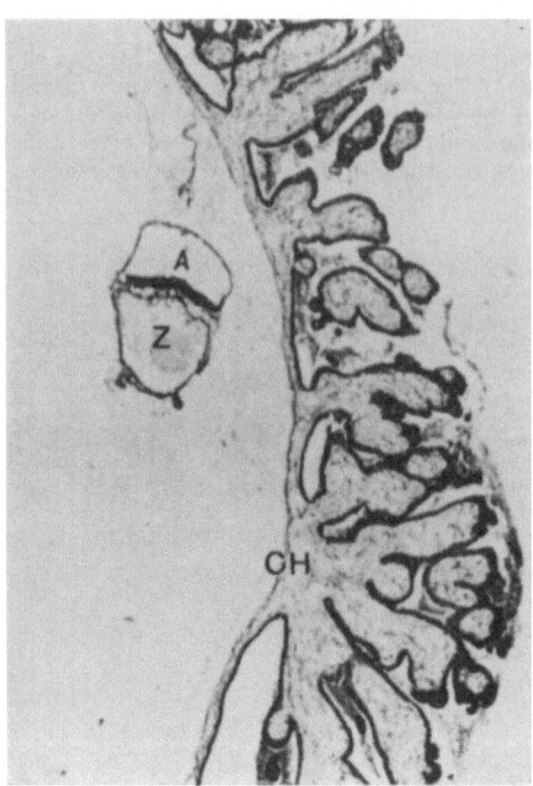

Fig. 6. Transverse section of the embryo depicted on fig. 5. A — amnionic sac, Z — secondary yolk sac, CH — chorion consisting of chorionic plate and villi.

5. TRILAMINAR EMBRYO (DAYS 15—20)

Formation of the intraembryonal mesoderm turns the round-shaped embryonal disc of the bilaminar embryo into a pear-shaped trilaminar embryo. The primitive streak is formed on the embryonal disc (extending rostrally from the primitive knot to the anal membrane caudally) representing the center of the intraembryonal mesodermal proliferation (Figs. 7, 8). The primitive streak is a midline thickening on the caudal portion of the embryonic disc. A cellular condensation on the cranial end of the primitive streak is known as a primitive (Hensen's) node. Apposition of ectoderm and endoderm on the caudal end of the primitive streak forms the anal membrane and is located just in front of the allantois — a narrow endoblastic canal growing into the connecting stalk. The mesoderm proliferates as a cellular layer spreading from the primitive streak in all direction between ectoderm and endoderm of the embryonal disc reaching its margin and joining the primary mesoderm of extraembryonal origin. The primitive groove in the primitive streak appears as a consequence of mesodermal proliferation. Cells growing from the primitive node form a narrow midline tubule known as the chordomesodermal canal (Lieberkuhn's canal, head process). The amnionic opening of the chordomesodermal canal is known as the primitive pit. The chordomesodermal process is incorporated into the ceiling of the yolk sac and ends at the area of thickened endoblast known as the prechordal plate. The prechordal plate contributes to the oral membrane, a small area of an interim contact between ectoblast and endoblast. As the ventral part of the chordomeso-

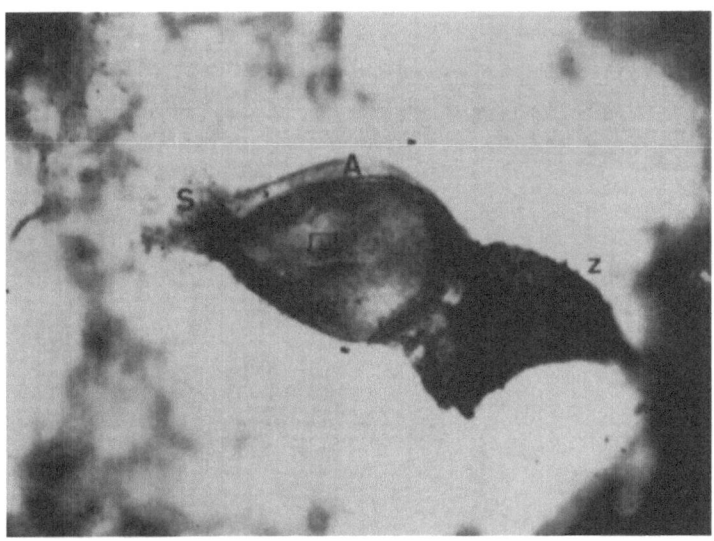

Fig. 7. Trilaminar human embryo (ca 19 days old) photographed after opening of the chorion. The yolk sac was dissected and removed to the right side. The embryonal disc is pear shaped. A — amnionic vesicle, Z — remnant of the yolk sac, S — connecting stalk.

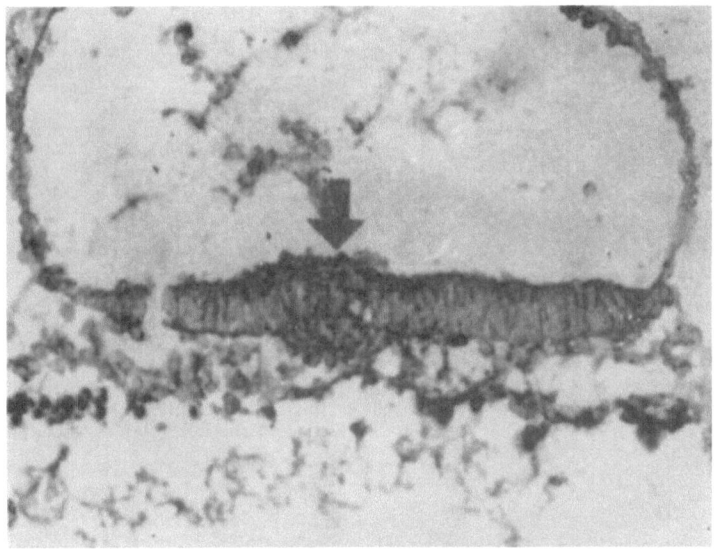

Fig. 8. Mesodermal proliferation (arrow) suggesting the development of the primitive streak.

dermal process desintegrates, a temporary communication — the neurenteric canal — leading through the primitive node connects the amniotic and yolk sac cavities (Fig. 10). The chordomesodermal process induces the development of ectoderm

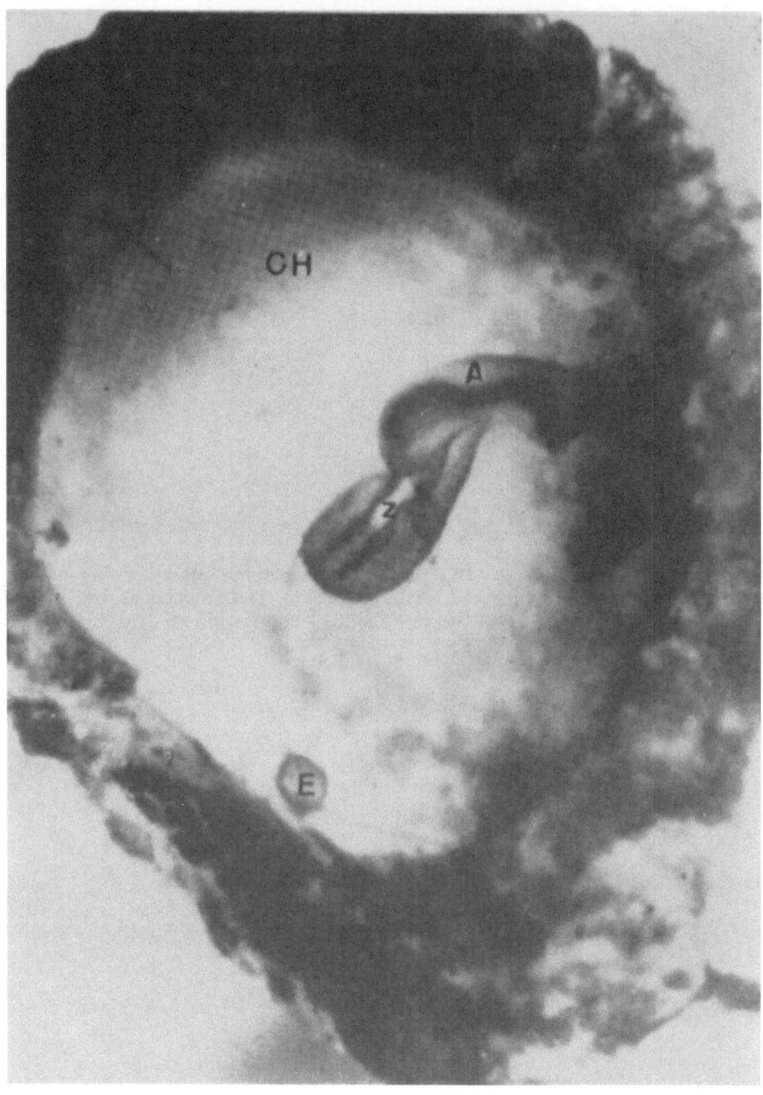

Fig. 9. Trilaminar human embryo (ca 20 days old) photographed from the lateral side. A — amnionic vesicle, Z — yolk sac (arteficially pushed to the left side), S — connecting stalk, E — endodermal cyst, CH — chorion.

into the neural plate, which consequently changes in interaction with the adjacent mesoderm into a neural groove.

At this time the first haematopoetic islands appear in the mesoderm (extraembryonal splanchnopleura) of the yolk sac. The stage of a trilaminar presomite embryo represents day 15—20 after conception ("true age").

During this period (approximately three weeks), known as blastogenesis, all three germinal layers, ectoderm, endoderm and mesoderm make their appearance.

14

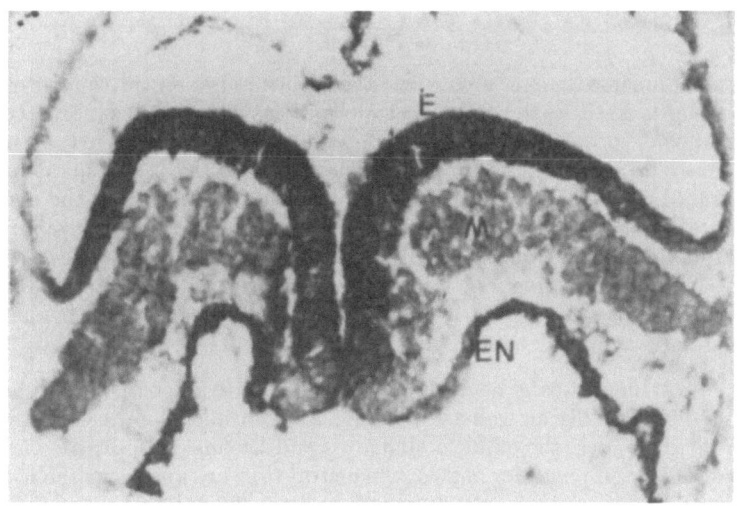

Fig. 10. Transverse section through the neurenteric canal in an embryo showing mesodermal proliferation. E — ectoderm, EN — endoderm, M — mesoderm.

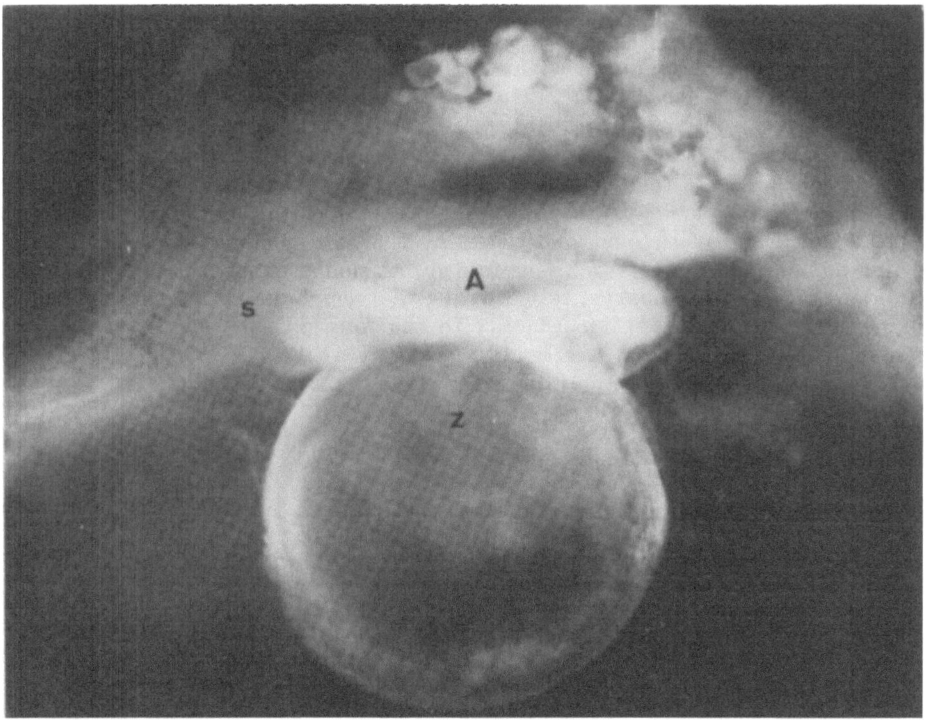

Fig. 11. Human embryo with 10 somite pairs (lateral view, age ca 24 days). A — amnionic vesicle, Z — yolk sac, S — connecting stalk.

6. EARLY SOMITE EMBRYO (DAYS 20—30)

The next developmental stage is characterized by the differentitation of mesoderm. The paraaxially-located part of the mesodermal layer on each side of the neural groove transforms into vesicles known as somites, the lateral part of mesoderm splits into a parietal layer — somatopleura — and a visceral layer — splanchnopleura. At the margin of the embryonal area, the somatopleura continues as the mesodermal layer of the amnion, and the splanchnopleura continues extraembryonally as the mesodermal layer of the yolk sac. Groups of mesodermal cells located between the somites medially and pleuras laterally are known as the intermediate meso- derm. Seven pairs of somites are formed, before the neural groove begins to close transforming into a neural tube. This stage (somite 1—7) covers days 20—23.

The closure of the neural tube begins at the seven-somite stage at the level of somite four and extends cranially as well as caudally. As additional somites are formed and as the neural tube closes, the embryo elongates and become cylindrical. The tempor- arily open anterior and posterior ends of the neural tube are known as the neuropores. The anterior neuropore closes at the 20 somite embryo (26 day), where as the posterior neuropore obliterates at the 28—29 somite embryo (approximately 30 days). Some neuroectodermal cells become detached from the posterior margin of neural tube, before the neural tube closes, forming a neural crest. The neural crest is the main source of the head and neck mesenchyme, provides neurons for spinal and vegetative ganglia, pheochromocytes, melanoblasts, C-cells of the thyroid and some peptide-producing cells of the mucosa of the digestive tract and pancreatic islets.

At the early somite stage the shape of the embryo is more or less cylindrical (Fig. 11). The head with open cerebral vesicles and distinct eye primordia bulges over the yolk sac. The two otic placodes, and later grooves are present laterally to rhomben- cephalon. The medullary tube with paired somites laterally and open posterior neuropore represent the body of the embryo. The relatively huge spheroid endodermal yolk sac is attached to the ventral side of the embryo. The dorsal part of the yolk sac incorporated in the body of the embryo represents primordium of the alimentary canal. A blind endodermal pocket (closed by the oral membrane) in the anterior portion of the embryo is known as the fore gut. A similar endodermal pocket in the posterior portion of the embryo, closed by the anal membrane, is known as the hind gut. In the pharyngeal region, laterally to the fore gut, pharyngeal arches and pouches make their appearance (Fig. 12). Ventrally to the fore gut there is a peri- cardial cavity with primordium of the heart.

7. STAGE OF LIMB DEVELOPMENT (DAYS 28—53)

After the neuropores have closed, the embryo becomes C-shaped. The pharyngeal arches and pouches are very distinct and unsegmented primordia of the extremities appear (32—36 days, Figs. 13, 14).

In later stages of embryonal development extremities become segmented (Fig. 15). The nasal placodes and different facial and nasal growth centra contribute to the development of the face (35—50 days). The pharyngeal arches disappear becoming partially involved in the formation of pinna, middle ear ossicles and laryngeal cartilages. During the late embryonal period the segmentation related to somites become lost, and the distinct tail of the embryo is gradually incorporated into the

Fig. 12. Somite embryo (ca 28 days old). First (I), second (II) and third (III) pharyngeal arches are very distinct. P — the eminence of the heart.

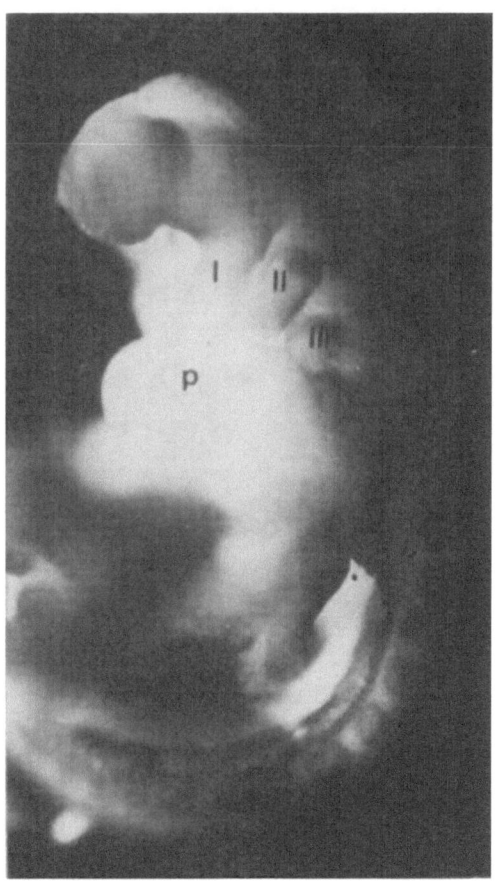

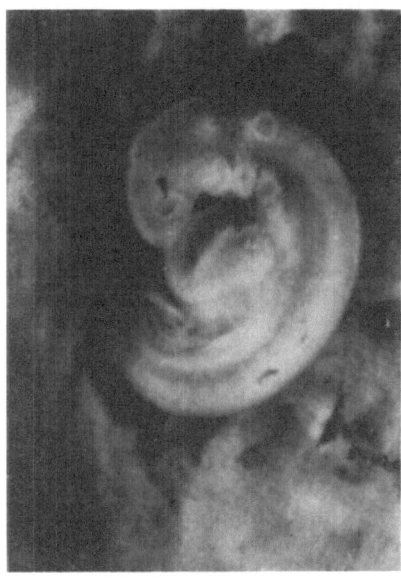

Fig. 13. Embryo with closed otocyst and invaginating lens placode (ca 35 days old).

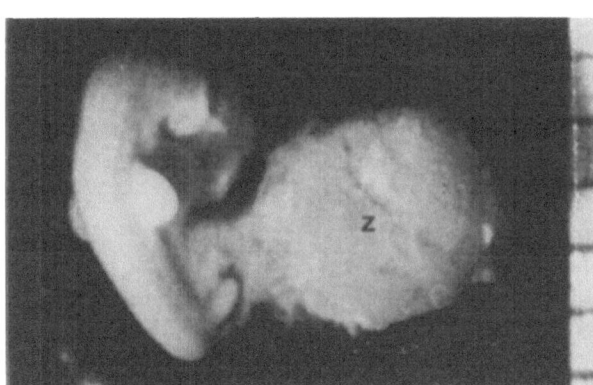

Fig. 14. Embryo attached to the yolk sac (Z), (ca 36 days old). Developing extremities are evident.

coccys (Fig. 16). The connecting stalk containing the allantois and the ductus omphaloentericus (with their accompanying vessels) are pushed together as the amnion expands, and form the umbilical cord.

17

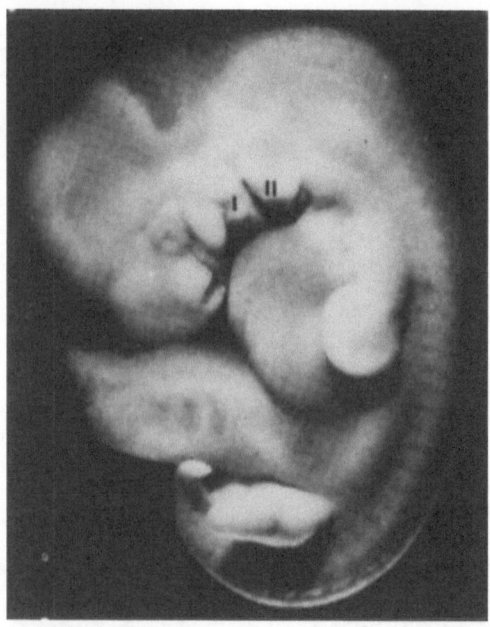

Fig. 15. Somite embryo with extremities divided into segments. (ca 40 days old.) No digital rays evident. In the face, eyes, olphactory grooves, nasal and maxillary centres are present. First (I) and second (II) pharyngeal arch contribute the primordium of the external ear.

8. LATE EMBRYONAL STAGE (DAYS 52—60)

At the end of the embryonal period (56—60 days), the digits and toes are developed, the hands cross the midline (digits overlapping) and the legs reach the midline.

The face has a distinct human character, the rims of the eyelids fuse. The fusion of the eyelids is arbitrarily regarded as the end of the embryonal period.

Primordia of all organs become evident during embryonal period and are highly sensitive to all kinds of teratogens.

9. FETAL PERIOD (WEEKS 9—26)

The fused eyelids are characteristic for the fetal period (Fig. 17). Many fetal organs are becoming functional. The sensitivity to teratogens is less expressed.

10. PERINATAL PERIOD (WEEKS 27—40)

The eyes reopen (weeks 26—28) and eyelashes are present. The fetus, if born prenataly (during weeks 26—36) may survive.

Endocrine glands of the conceptus are of different embryological origin. Endocrine tissues of the placenta are derived from the trophoblast of the blastocyst (trophoectoderm).

Surface ectoderm of the primitive oral cavity provides material for the Rathke's pouch which is the anlage of the anterior hypophysis. Neuroectoderm of the mesencephalon evaginates forming the posterior hypophysis, neuroectoderm of the neck

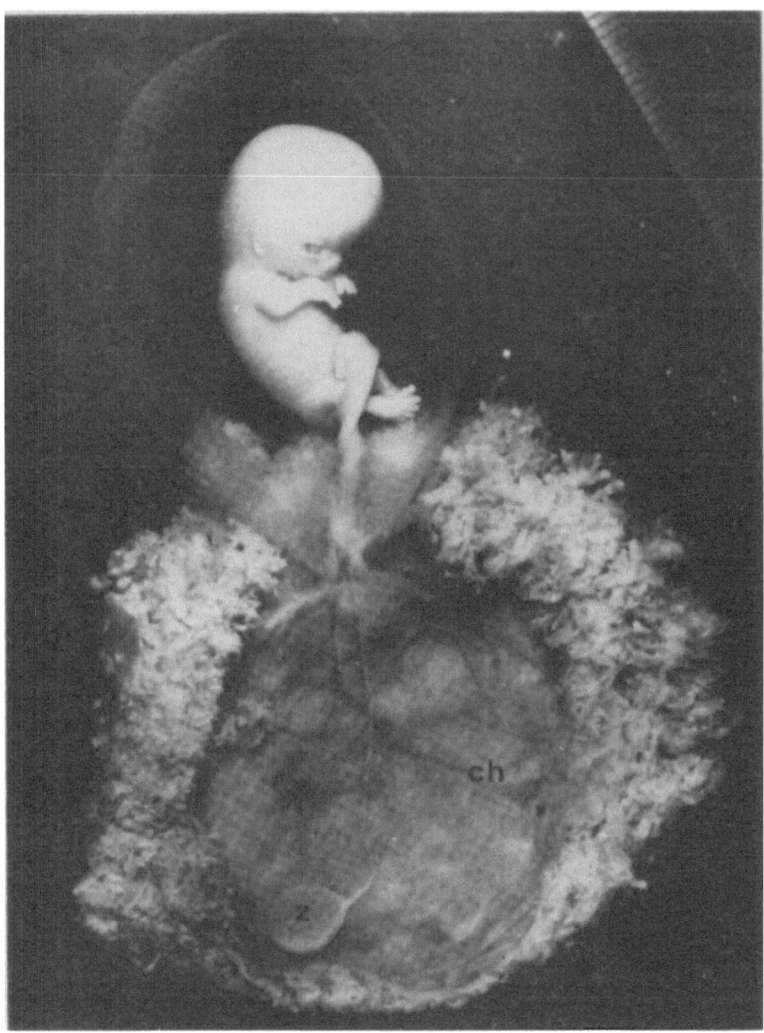

Fig. 16. Embryo with differentiated extremities and open eyes (ca 54 days old) enclosed in the amnionic sac and connected with the chorion (CH) and the yolk sac (Z).

(neural crest) contributes cells which become incorporated into the pharyngeal endoderm and subsequently give rise to the C-cells in the thyroid. Neuroectoderm of the thoracal and lumbal crest contributes adrenergic cells inducing medulla of the adrenal. Thyroid (except C-cells), parathyroid and endocrine pancreas (except somatostatin producing D-cells) are considered as endodermal derivatives. Steroidogenic tissues, adrenal cortex and endocrine tissues of gonads, are mesodermal from the coelomic epithelium. Basic data regarding embryonal development and the appearance of the primordia of the human endocrine glands are summarized in Table 1, 2 and Graph 1.

To make the interpretation of the results from animal prenatal experiments easier, a table comparing human, macaccus, rat and mouse development is added (Table 3).

3

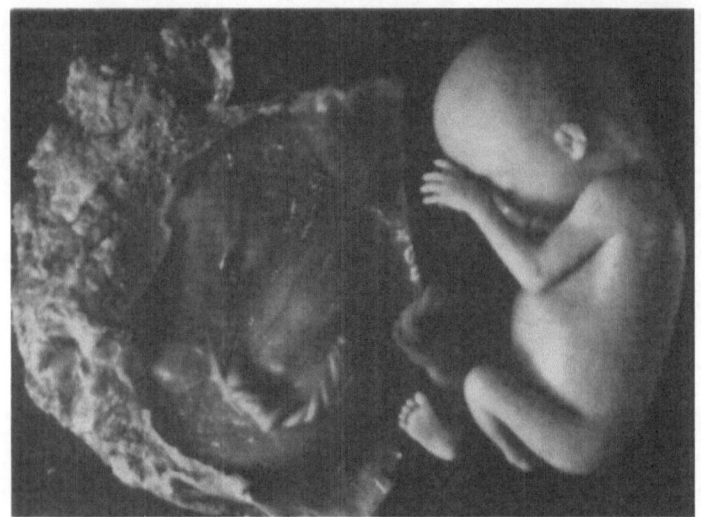

Fig. 17. 14 weeks old fetus with fused eyelids attached by the umbilical cord to the placenta.

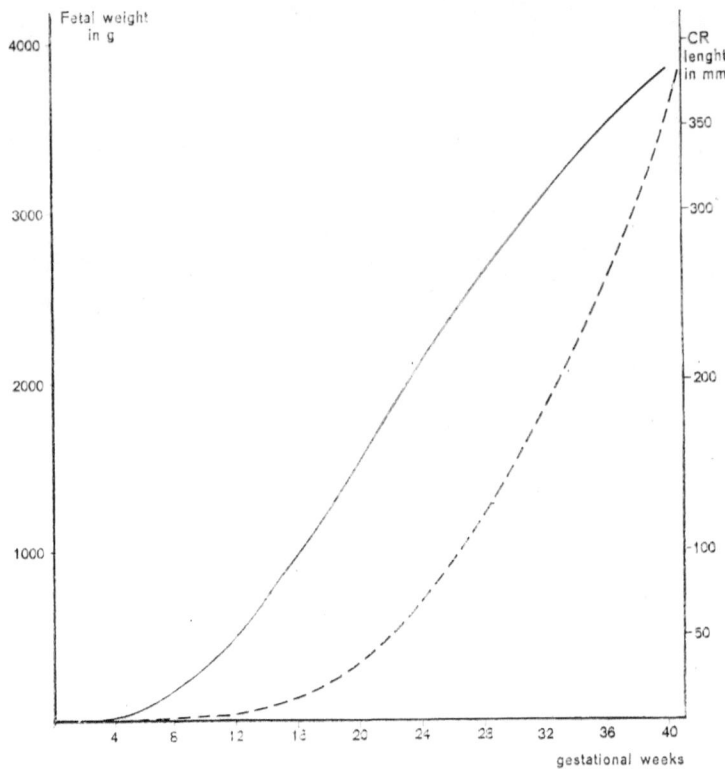

Graph 1. Fetal weight (dashed line) and crown-rumph length (CR, solid line).

Table 1.: Survey of the early development of human endocrine glands.

Weeks	Stage	Placenta	Adrenal	Testis	Ovary	Hypophysis	Pineal	Thyroid	Parathyroid	Pancreas
1	1									
	2	Blastocystic trophoblast								
	3	Tropho-blastic shell hCG, 3βHSD								
2	4	Early chorion								
3	5			Primordial germ cells migration of primordial germ cells				medial primordium		
4	6					Rathke's pouch	pineal evagination	lateral primordia	primordia	ventral and dorsal evagination
5	7—1	Late chorion (fetal circulation)								
6	7—2		Coelomic migration; blastema blastematous and central zones 3βHSD	indifferent stage						
	7—3									
7	7—4			testicular cords (embryonal testis)						
	7—5									
	7—6		capillaries present							
8	7—7				embryonal ovary		cords of neuroblasts	lamellae	parathyroid III	
9	8—1	hCG peak								
	8—2									
	9	chorion laeve and frondosum	blastematous and fetal (intermedial central) zones	Leydig cells (fetal testis) 3βHSD	meiosis begins (aerly fetal ovary)	ACTH		follicles with colloid	parathyroid IV	
10	9		subcapsular (defin.) and fetal zones			TSH GH FSH LH				islets; A, B-cells

Table 2.: Stages of human embryonal development
Comparison of the Carnegie classification (Streeter's horizons, roman numerals, and O'Rahilly's stages) and Jirásek's classification.

	Carnegie stages and horizons	Comparative stages (*Jirásek*)		Length of embryo in mm	Age in days (C)
Horizon	External characteristics	External characteristics	Stage		
	BLASTOGENESIS				
1	Unicellular	Unicellular	1	0,2	0—2
2	Segmentation	Blastomeric	2	0,2	2—4
3	Free blastocyst	Blastodermic	3	0,4	4—6
4	Implantation	Bilaminar embryo	4	0,1	6—14
5	Avillous implanted ovum	Bilaminar plate primary yolk sac	4—1 4—2		
6	Secondary yolk sac	secondary yolk sac	4—3	0,2—0,4	
6b	Primitive streak	Trilaminar embryo with primitive streak	5 5—1	0,4—1,0	15—17
7 8	Notochordal process Neurenteric canal	with notochordal process	5—2	1,0—2,0	17—20
	ORGANOGENESIS				
IX	Somites 1—3	Early somite stage completely-open neural groove	6 6—1	1,5—2,0	20—21
X XI	Somites 4—12 Somites 13—20, otic groove	Neural tube closing, both ends open	6—2	1,5—4,0	21—26
XII	Somites 21—29 closing post neuropore	One or both neuropores closed	6—3	3—5	26—30
XIII	Buds of extremities	Bud of proximal extremity	7—1	4—6	28—32
XIV	Lens pit	Buds of proximal and distal extremities	7—2	5—8	31—35

			ORGANOGENESIS		
XV	Lens vesicles closed, anterior extremity two segments	Proximal extremity two segments	7–3	7–10	35–38
XVI	Retinal pigment	Proximal and distal extremity two segments	7–4	8–12	37–42
XVII	Digital rays	Digital rays, foot plates	7–5	10–14	42–44
XVIII	Digital tubercles,	Digital tubercles	7–6	13–21	44–51
XIX	Deflection of the head toe rays				
XX	Digits, toe rays	Digits, toe tubercles	7–7	19–24	51–53
XXI	Feet reach the midline		8–1	22–28	52–56
XXII	Overlapping digits	Differentiated extremities			
XXIII	Fusing eyelids	Fusing eyelids	8–2	27–35	56–60

For the Streeter's classification, histological examination of specimens is necessary. That makes difficulties, if a large number of specimens is to be staged. To overcome this complication, Jirásek's classification is based entirely on external characteristics.

Table 3.: Comparison of prenatal development of human, macaccus, rat and mouse.
Classification is based on Jirásek's staging. Comparable stages have the same numbers.

Comparative Stages (Jirásek)		Human		Macaccus		Rat		Mouse	
Characteristic	Stage	Length in mm	Age (C) in days	Length in mm	Age (C) in days	Length in mm	Age (C) in days	Length in mm	Age (C) in days
Unicellular	1	0.2	0—2	0.15	1		1		1
Blastomeric (16—20 blastomeres)	2	0.2	2—4	0.15	2—4		2—3		2—3
Blastodermic	3	0.4	4—6	0.2—0.3	7—9		4—5		4—4½
Bilaminar embryo stage: bilaminar plate	4—1	0.1	6—14	0.3	10—13		6—7		5
primary yolk sac	4—2								6½
secondary yolk sac	4—3	0.2—0.4							
Trilaminar embryo stage: with primitive streak	5—1	0.4—1.0	15—17	0.5	17—19				7
with a notochordal process	5—2	1.0—2.0	17—20	1.5			8—9		
Early somite stage: completely open neural groove	6—1	1.5—2.0	20—21	1.9	21—24		9½		8
neural tube closing, both ends open	6—2	1.5—4.0	21—26	2.0—4.0	24	1.3—3.0	10—10¾	1.8—3	9½
one or both neuropores closed	6—3	3—5	26—30	4.0—6.0	24—26	3—4.1	11		
Stage of limb development: bud of proximal extremity	7—1	4—6	28—32	6.0	26	4—4.5	11	2—3.3	9½—10
buds of proximal and distal extremities	7—2	5—8	31—35	8.0	27	4—6	11.5	7.9	10½
proximal extremity two segments	7—3	7—10	35—38			5.8—8	13		11
proximal and distal extremity two segments	7—4	8—12	37—42	7—9		8—9.5	13½		
digital rays, foot plates	7—5	10—14	42—44	10	34	10	14	11.5	13
digital tubercles	7—6	13—21	44—51	9—11	36	12.5	15½	13	14
digits, toe tubercles	7—7	19—24	51—53	19	41	16	17	14	

Late embryonal stage: differentiated extremities, eyes open fusing eyelids	8—1 8—2	22—23 27—35	52—56 56—60	22 39—44	44 52	19 22	17½ 19½	14—17 22	16 16—18
Fetal period	9	31— 200	60— 182+	40— 260	53— 170	25	19—21	22—25	18—19
Perinatal period	10	201— 450	170— 266+	postnatal			postnatal		postnatal

In this classification corresponding stages are marked with the same numbers Using this classification, the interpretation of teratogenic experiments is very easy.

CHAPTER 3

THE PLACENTA

A survey of placental development is presented in Table 4.

Table 4. Survey of placental development.

Days	Structures	Comment
4—6	trophoblast of the blastocyst	
7—12	trophoblastic shell: cytotrophoblast, syncytium	implantation, hCG production, 3β HSD present
13—30	early chorion: primary, secondary, tertiary villi: anchoring-free	uterochorionic circulation established
31 ca. 110	late chorion: chorion laeve, chorion frondonum, chorionic stems, branches, terminal villi	fetoplacental circulation established
ca. 110—265	placenta: lobules, cotyledons fetal part — amniochorionic plate, "villi" intervillous space maternal part — basal plate, septae fetal membranes: extraplacental amniochorion, decidua capsularis and parietalis	

a) TROPHOBLAST OF THE BLASTOCYST AND TROPHOBLASTIC SHELL

Two different components become evident as the morula differentiates during the third day of development. The external layer of cells connected by tight junctions and desmosomes is known as the trophoblast, whereas the aggregate of inside blastomeres forms the embryoblast, or inner cell mass. The trophoblast of the blastocyst (trophoectoderm) consists of a single layer of cuboidal cells which become flattened as the blastocyst extends. The trophoblast covering the inner cell mass is considered as polar, the trophoblast lining the cavity of the blastocyst as mural. Implantation begins after the zona pellucida has been shed during day seven after fertilization. During implantation, the polar trophoblast becomes first attached to the uterine epithelium. The blastocyst collapses, losing fluid, and penetrates into the lamina propria of the endometrium. The trophoblast of the blastocyst differentiates in contact with the endometrium into the syncytiotrophoblast and the cytotrophoblast. The mechanism of trophoblastic penetration is poorly understood. Endocytosis, phagocytosis and enzymatic digestion were observed during implantation in different species of animals (*Denker*, 1972; *Kirchner*, 1972).

In humans, the invading trophoblast is formed by multinucleated giant cells with big anaplastic nuclei and unusually big basophil nucleoli (Fig. 3). Among the trophoblastic giant cells, irregular cytotrophoblastic cells are present. As implantation proceeds, the blastocystic trophoblast transforms into trophoblastic giant cells (syncytium) and cytotrophoblasts. At the end of implantation, all the blastocystic trophoblasts become transformed into the syncytiotrophoblast and the cytotropho-

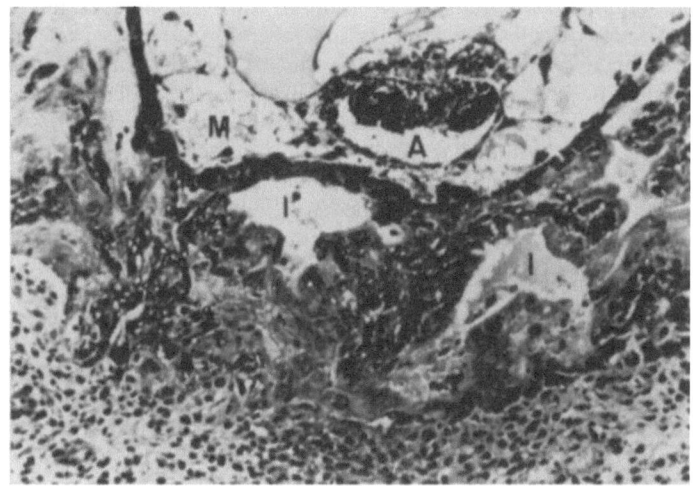

Fig. 18. Formation of the intervillous space, chorionic plate and primary chorionic villi in a 13 days old embryo. A — amnionic vesicle, M — primary mesoderm, I — primordium of the intervillous space.

blast of the trophoblastic shell. After penetration of the blastocyst into the compact layer of endometrial lamina propria (days 7—8), the blastocyst re-expands. The blastocyst is implanted within endometrium (uterine wall) outside of the uterine cavity. This type of implantation is considered as interstitital. Within the syncytiotrophoblast (represented at this stage by the giant cells) fusing vacuoles with striated borders are formed, giving rise to intercellular spaces called lacunae. The syncytiotrophoblast lining of the lacunae becomes lamellar in character. As the trophoblast grows, the syncytiotrophoblast penetrates into the maternal vessels of the endometrium and maternal blood enters the lacunae. The lacunae of the trophoblastic shell interconnect into a primitive intervillous space (days 9—12, Fig. 18). Before the uterotrophoblastic circulation appears, some accumulation of maternal leucocytes within the lacunae is observed. The blood comes into the lacunar system of the trophoblastic shell from the spiral arterioles of the endometrium and drains into the dilated veins. Most of the vessels are perpendicular to the surface of the endometrium. The circulation begins within the lacunar system of the trophoblastic shell (uteroplacental circulation) at days 12—13. At this time a fibrin-filled defect in the surface epithelium and propria of the endometrium where the penetration of the blastocyst took place may still be present, and is called operculum. As uteroplacental circulation begins, there may be some leakage of blood through the operculum, and vaginal bleeding may occur. This bleeding is scanty, mostly spotting, coming at the time of the expected menstruation and represents the "placental sign" (sign of implantation). The bleeding is often mistaken for a scanty menstruation.

DECIDUA

Four to five days after implantation (at days 25 and 26 of the menstrual cycle in which the conception took place) the decidual transformation of the endometrium becomes evident.

Stimulated by estrogens and gestagens, the fibroblasts of the compact layer of the propria of the endometrial functionalis undergo an epithelioid transformation and are known as decidual cells. Decidualization is preceeded by an edema. Reticular fibers are present between decidual cells, and the intercellular spaces are filled with a fluid rich in proteoglycans. Decidualization of the endometrium is fully developed approximately two weeks after implantation. The endometrial glands of the early decidua in the first and second month of pregnancy are dilatated, wide and lined with a columnar epithelium of clear cells. Their character is hypersecretory. In the later months of pregnancy, they become "exhausted" and undergo degeneration being compressed by the expanding product of conception. According to the localization related to the implanted ovum, decidua capsularis, decidua marginalis, decidua basalis and decidua parietalis are distinguished.

The decidua capsularis covers the implanted ovum, the decidua basalis is interposed between the ovum and basal endometrial layer over the myometrium. The decidua marginalis connects the decidua capsularis and basalis (Fig. 20). The decidua parietalis covers the rest of the uterine cavity. The decidua prevents penetration of the trophoblast into the basal layer of endometrium or even the myometrium. As the product of conception increases in size, decidua capsularis becomes apposed to the decidua parietalis. As the uterine surface epithelium degenerates, the uterine cavity disappears. A layer of detritus and fibrinoid material is evident at the contact between decidua capsularis and parietalis in the second half of pregnancy.

b) CHORION

EARLY CHORION (PERIOD PRECEEDING EMBRYOCHORIONIC CIRCULATION)

The chorion is characterized by the presence of villi. Primary chorionic villi are formed within the trophoblastic shell. They represent cords of cytotrophoblastic cells penetrating radially through the trophoblastic shell between the lacunar spaces (Fig. 18). The surface of the primary, or epithelial, villi is incompletely covered by the syncytiotrophoblast. Primary chorionic villi are present in 13 day-old embryos exhibiting the primary yolk sac (stage 5, *O'Rahilly*, 1973). At the stage when the bilaminar embryo exhibits the secondary yolk sac, (*Streeter h. VI, O'Rahilly* 6a) days 13—14 post-conception, the mesenchyme penetrates into the core of primary chorionic villi, and the primary chorionic villi become converted into the secondary chorionic villi. Secondary villi branch (at the stage of the presomite trilaminar embryo VII; VIII S. H.: stage 7,8 O'Rahilly). In 15—20 day-old ova, some mesenchymal cells within the stroma of the villi become arranged into the cords, providing endothelial cells for the future vascular net. Vascularized villi are called tertiary. Anchoring and free villi are distinguished. Anchoring villi connect the chorionic plate with the peripheral trophoblast and the decidua. The free villi branch within the intervillous space. Chorionic villi form all over the implanted blastocyst.

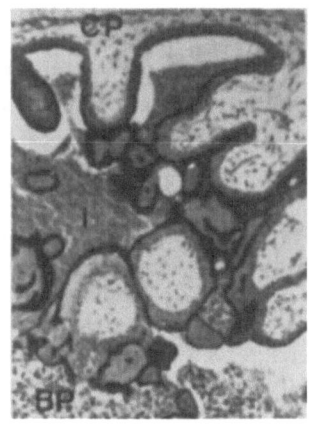

Fig. 19. Chorion of a 22 days old embryo. CP — chorionic plate, BP — basal plate, I — intervillous space. The brush border of the trophoblastic syncytium (dark) is stained for the alkaline phosphatase.

Neither erythroblasts nor other blood cells are present within chorionic vessels, for the next ten days, until days 28—30 (S. H. XIII). During formation of secondary and tertiary chorionic villi, the peripheral parts of the trophoblastic shell contribute to the peripheral trophoblast. Those parts of the trophoblastic shell which do not contribute either to the trophoblast of chorionic villi or to the peripheral trophoblast, become the trophoblastic islands found between the villi (Fig. 19). After being detached from the trophoblastic shell, some of the multinuclear cells penetrate into the decidua and decidual vessels in the vicinity of the implant (mostly basal decidua), but some are present even in myometrium. They are called "placental" site cells, or giant cells.

Regarding histological differentiation, the following should be mentioned. First, syncytial elements are present as the implantation begins. Within the trophoblastic shell, syncytium is formed by fusing cytotrophoblastic cells. The poorly differentiated cytotrophoblastic and syncytiotrophoblastic elements become organized in contact with the mesenchyme and the maternal blood. In the collapsed implanted blastocyst, some cells of the cytotrophoblast detach into the blastocystic cavity, giving rise to the primary mesoderm (chorionic mesenchyme). As the blastocyst re-expands and as the primary yolk sac expands, the cytotrophoblast lining the former blastocystic cavity becomes arranged into a cuboidal epithelium contributing the lining of the chorionic plate.

The chorion gradually replacing the trophoblastic shell, is formed by three components: chorionic plate, chorionic villi — anchoring and free — and peripheral trophoblast contacting the decidua. The decidua basalis covered by the peripheral trophoblast (derived from the trophoblastic shell) is known as the basal plate. The chorionic plate is formed by the mesenchyme and bilaminar trophoblasts consisting of cytotrophoblasts arranged like a single-layered cuboidal epithelium (Langhans cells), covered by trophoblastic syncytium. The free villi have a mesenchymal stroma and are covered by the bilaminar trophoblasts similar to that of the trophoblastic plate.

The anchoring portions of the villi are formed by cytotrophoblastic columns covered only partially by a lamellar syncytiotrophoblast. Syncytial trophoblastic giant cells may be present among the cytotrophoblasts of the columns.

29

The peripheral trophoblast contains both cytotrophoblastic elements and syncytium. Syncytium lines the intervillous space. The trophoblastic cells (fetal in origin) intermingle with the decidual (maternal) cells forming a so-called deciduotrophoblastic complex. Decidual cells may be recognized by the presence of reticular fibers around them.

Trophoblastic syncytium and its derivatives (syncytiotrophoblast of the chorionic plate, of the free parts of villi, of trophoblastic islands and of anchoring parts of the villi, of the peripheral trophoblast, and the trophoblastic giant cells) share the following common futures: microvilli on the surface containing heat-resistant alkaline phosphatase, smooth endoplasmic reticulum, rough endoplasmic reticulum, activity of 3β-hydroxysteroid dehydrogenase, mitochondria with both lamellar and tubular cristae. Using immuno-histochemical techniques, both placental proteohormones hCG and hCS were localized within the syncytium. There is evidence that as soon as the syncytiotrophoblast becomes differentiated during implantation on day seven, hCG and progesterone are formed. Wherever the syncytiotrophoblast becomes exposed to the maternal blood, a thin layer of sialomucin covers the microvilli. The early cytotrophoblast (Langhans cells of secondary and tertiary villi, cytotrophoblastic columns of anchoring villi, cytotrophoblast of islands and of peripheral trophoblast) is rich in glycogen. The cytoplasm of the early cytotrophoblast is basophilic, and there is a well-developed, rough endoplasmic reticulum. These features suggest that the early cytotrophoblast is a proliferating tissue contributing to the syncytium and to the growing anchoring villi. Basophilia and rough endoplasmic reticulum become lost during the second month in the cytotrophoblast of the villi (Langhans layer), but remain preserved in the cytotrophoblast of the anchoring villi.

THE LATE CHORION. DEVELOPMENT OF THE EMBRYOCHORIONIC CIRCULATION. CHORION FRONDOSUM AND CHORION LAEVE

At days 28—30 the embryonal heart begins to beat, pushing the blood from the yolk-sac haematopoetic islands into the circulation. The chorionic vessels become filled with blood, mostly erythroblasts. The blood comes into the chorion by the umbilical arteries. At the beginning, only the chorionic villi near the insertion of the umbilical arteries are supplied. The circulation within the villi oriented toward the basal decidua is preferential (Fig. 20). With the improving embryonal circulation, the blooed supplied area expands but never reaches the entire chorion. In most of the chorionic villi oriented against decidua capsularis circulation never develops. Consequently, the area of the chorion exhibiting the intravillous circulation becomes the chorion frondosum, and that part of the chorion not supplied by fetal blood turns into the chorion laeve (Fig. 21). The chorion frondosum is the main constituent of the fetal part of the placenta. Chorion laeve together with amnion and decidua constitute the placental membranes.

As the chorionic vessels within the branching chorionic villi are filled with blood, the cotyledons become evident and the nomenclature of the villi changes.

Each umbilical artery splits into 30—40 branches entering the primary chorionic stems extending from the chorionic plate. There are about 60—70 primary chorionic stems. Each stem branches into several secondary and tertiary stems which are arranged in a bell shaped fashion and are anchored to the basal plate (Wilkin, 1958). Other branches of the chorionic stems extending free into the intervillous space

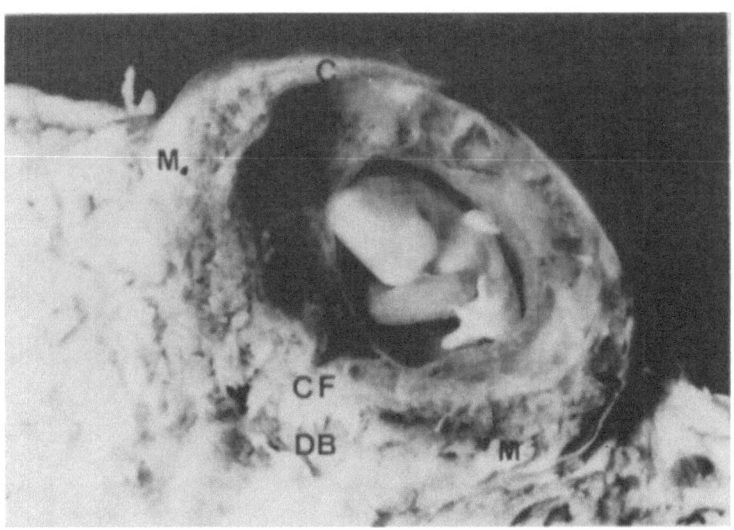

Fig. 20. 43 days old embryo with its envelopes embedded within the uterine wall. A — amnionic cavity, CF — chorion frondosum, DB — basal decidua, M — marginal area between decidua basalis and decidua capsularis, C — capsular decidua,

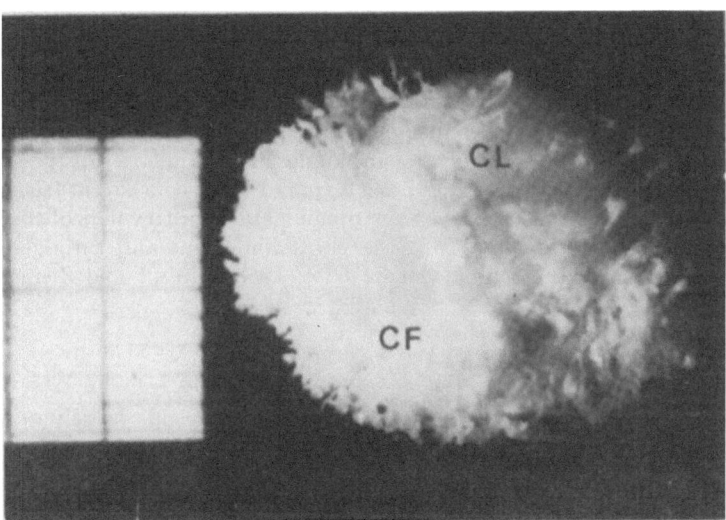

Fig. 21. Early differentiation of the chorion laeve (CL) and the chorion frondosum (CF) in a superfiacially implanted prodnct of conception ca 30 days old.

are known as the chorionic branches. They divide into numerous terminal villi. The chorinic stems, branches and villi are improperly called the "placental villi". Para-axial arteries and veins run within the chorionic stemps and branches. Only capillary nets are present within the terminal villi. The system of chorionic secondary stems, branches and terminal villi supplied by arteries from a primary chorionic stem constitute the fetal cotyledon. The cotyledons are arranged in lobules, separated by placental (decidual) septa. There are about 15—30 placental lobules, most of them

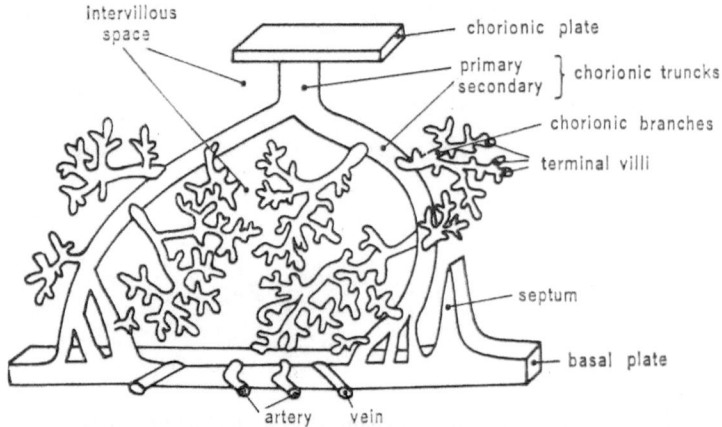

Fig. 22. Drowing suggesting the organization of the fetal cotyledon.

including two or three cotyledons (Fig. 22). The two main umbilical arteries split into several arteries and veins present within the chorionic stems. The main chorionic arteries split into the para-axial arteries of the primary and secondary chorionic branches. There is only one para-axial artery and vein within the terminal chorionic branches. Arteries and veins are connected with the subtrophoblastic capillary net by numerous short connections coming at right angles. The capillaries of the subtropho-blastic net extend to the terminal villi. Each terminal villus contains at term 2 - 8 capil-laries in loops. Blood coming from the subtrophoblastic capillary nets of the chorionic branches and terminal villi flows into the para-axial veins and through the veins of chorionic stems into the umbilical vein (*Boe*, 1953; *Jirásek and Zwinger*, 1972).

c) STRUCTURE OF THE PLACENTA

As already stressed, the arrangement of the placenta depends largely on the feto-placental circulation.

As the fetal part of the placenta develops from chorion frondosum, which covers the basal plate (mostly maternal decidua basalis), the human placenta is considered to be discoidal, cotyledonic, haemochorial and deciduate in type. The fetal part of the placenta is formed by the chorionic plate covered by the amnion and by the "pla-cental villi". The maternal part of the placenta is formed by the decidua basalis. Decidua basalis, together with the basal trophoblasts, is known as the placental basal plate. In the space between the chorionic plate and basal plate, the chorionic stems and branches and terminal villi ("placental villi") are found. The intervillous space between the villi is filled with maternal blood. "Placental villi" are arranged in cotyledons. Two or three cotyledons are enclosed in a placental lobule. The lobules are incompletely separated by decidual septa coming from the basal plate. The full-term placenta may be round, elipsoidal, or lobulated, approximately 150 to 250 mm long or wide, 30 mm thick and weighing approximately 400–600 g. The weight of the placenta and the fetus are related (Graphs 2 and 3).

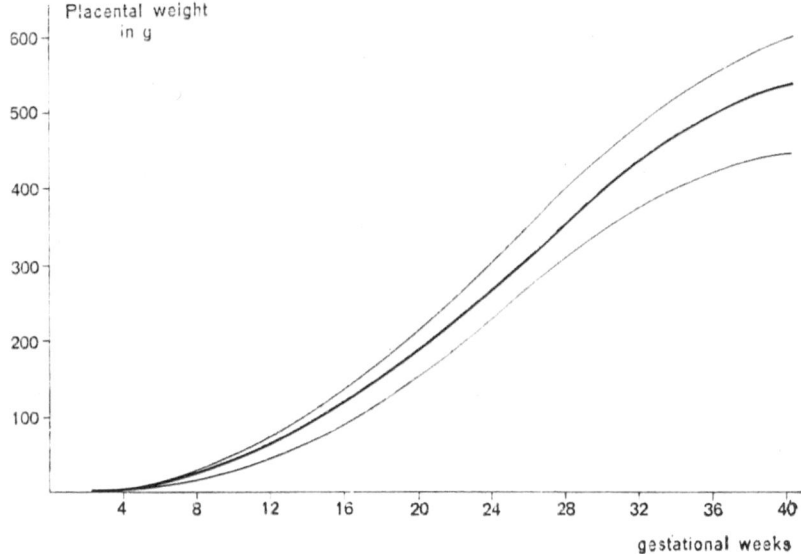

Graph 2. Placental weight during gestation.

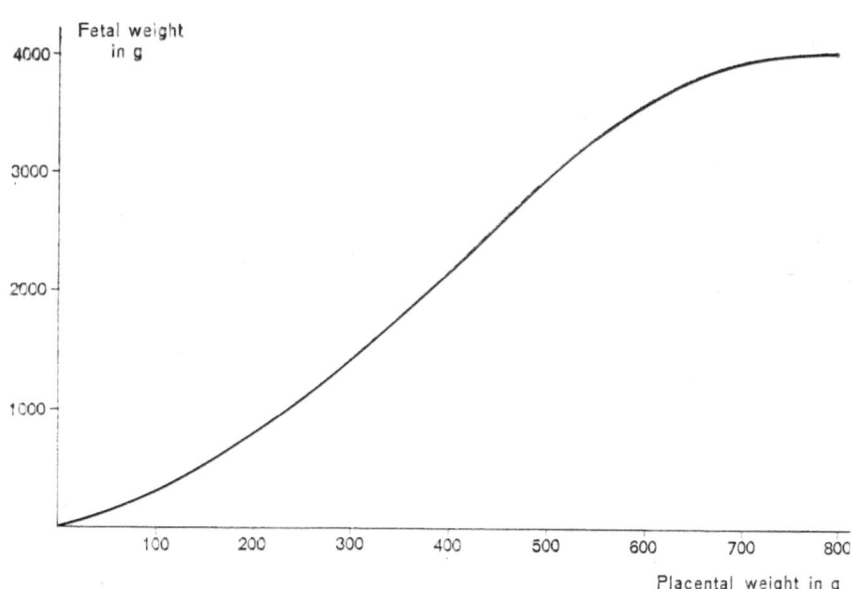

Graph 3. Relation between the weight of the fetus and of the placenta.

33

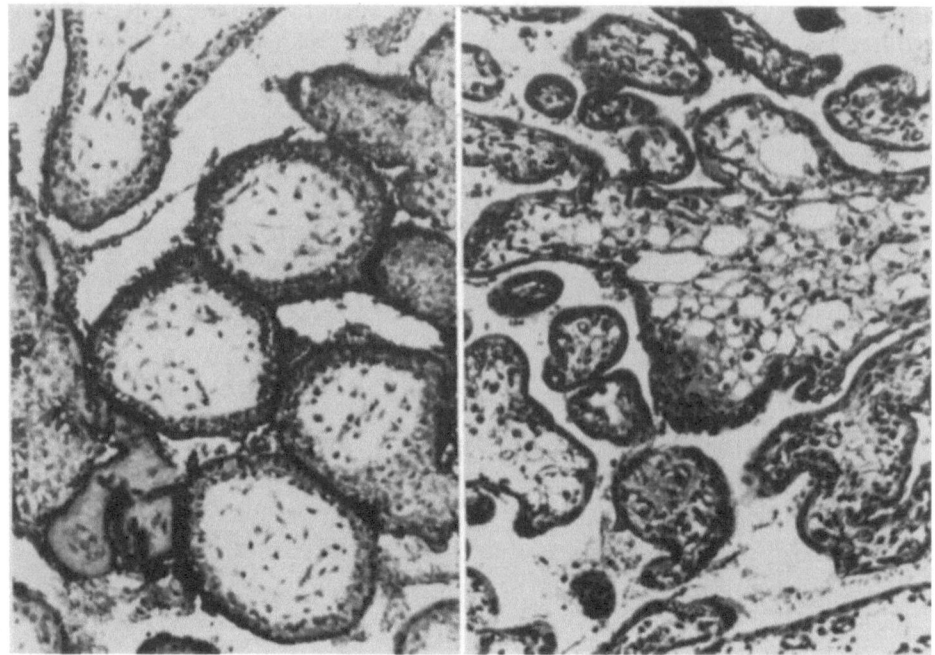

Fig. 23.—26. Section of the chorion at different age photographed at the same magnification.

Fig. 23. Chorionic villi of a 22 days old embryo. The villi are covered by a bilaminar trophoblast consisting of syncytium and a complete layer of cuboid cytotrophoblastic cells. Angioblastic cords are present in the mesenchymal connective tissue.

Fig. 24. Placental villi at 20 weeks after conception. Only scattered cytotrophoblastic cells are present undernieth the trophoblastic syncytium. Numerous Hofbauer cells are in the stroma of the villi.

Starting from the fetal side, the chorionic plate is covered by the amnion. The amnion consists of a single-layered, amnionic epithelium, which is cuboidal, becoming cylindrical at the end of gestation and a connective tissue propria, containing fibroblasts, reticular fibers and a proteoglycan-rich intercellular substance. The propria of the amnion covers the propria of the underlying chorion. The two layers are usually separated by a loose spongy layer of connective tissue originating from the reticulum of the extraembryonic coelom.

The propria of the chorionic plate extends into the chorionic stems, branches and villi contributing their "stroma". The stroma is formed by reticular connective tissue and contains paraaxial arteries and viens, and subtrophoblastic capillaries. Collagen fibers are present around vessels. Smooth muscle cells are found only in the vascular walls. As the placental villi elongate and branch, the amount of the stroma decreases (Figs. 23, 24, 25, 26). Special ovoid or spherical cells with a spherical nucleus and vacuolated cytoplasm present within the stroma of the villi are known as Hofbauer cells (*Hofbauer*, 1903). They exhibit pinocytosis and are considered to be allied to macrophages (*Horky*, 1964). They are rich in mitochondria and contain vacuoles with an electron-dense precipitate (*Panigel and Ahn*, 1964). They appear within the chorionic villi at the end of the second month. Their number reaches a maximum

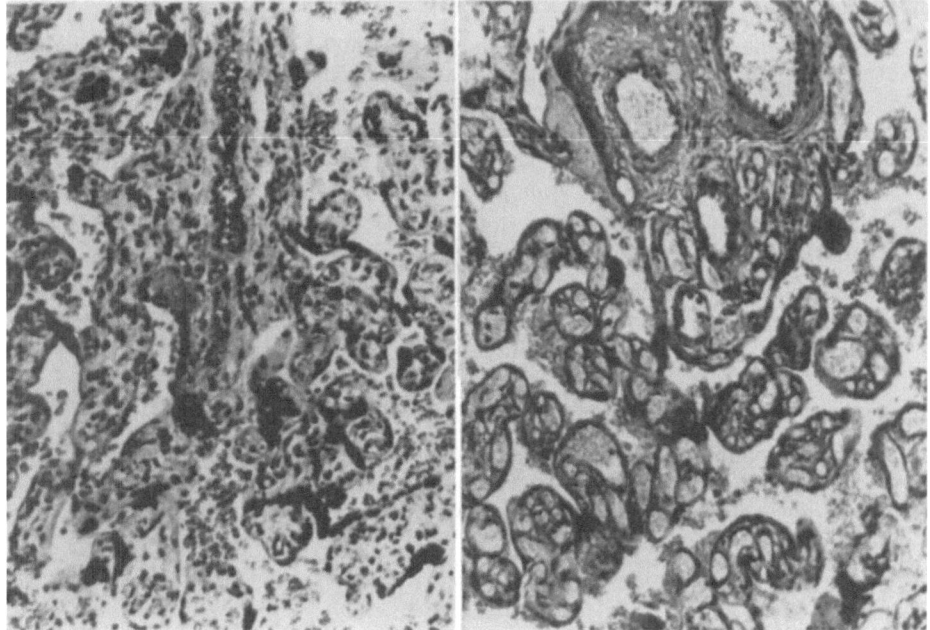

Fig. 25. Full term placenta (38 weeks after conception) showing clumping of nuclei of the trophoblastic syncytium.

Fig. 26. Full term placenta (38 weeks after conception). The fetal vessels are filled with blood. The syncytiovascular membranes are evident.

during months four and five and declines thereafter. In normal placentae, they disappear approximately a month before birth. Hofbauer cells are very numerous in villi undergoing molar degeneration (*Chaletzky*, 1891; *Neumann*, 1897).

PLACENTAL TROPHOBLAST

Topographically, the following types of trophoblast (t.) are distinguished: t. of the chorionic plate, t. of the villi, t. of the anchoring columns, t. of the islands and t. of the basal plate (including placental site cells and placental giant cells). By histologic features, the trophoblast may be classified as cytotrophoblast and syncytiotrophoblast, with some transitional subtypes. There is evidence that multinucleated syncytium originates from fusion of cytotrophoblastic cells (*Ender*, 1965).

1. CYTOTROPHOBLAST

a) Cytotrophoblast of the chorionic plate and villi

A complete layer of cytotrophoblast (Langhans layer) arranged as a single-layered, cuboidal epithelium underneath the trophoblastic syncytium is present during weeks 4—8 after conception, becoming incomplete during the third month. During the fourth month, only single cytotrophoblastic cells are present underneath the syncytium and some may remain until birth.

b) Cytotrophoblasts of the anchoring columns

Cytotrophoblastic anchoring columns are present at the tips of anchoring villi attaching to the decidua. They are separated from the mesenchymal stroma of the villus by an acid mucopolysacharide-rich, very distinct basement membrane. Cytotrophoblastic columns are formed by polyedric cytotrophoblastic cells with a strongly basophil cytoplasm. They represent a "growth center" of the villus. They disappear during the fifth month of pregnancy.

c) Cytotrophoblast of the islands

The trophoblast of the islands consists mostly of cytotrophoblastic cells. Trophoblastic islands are usually found near the basal plate, attached to the villi. Degeneration of the cells and fibrinoid depositions are common.

d) Cytotrophoblast of the basal plate

The cytotrophoblastic layer covers the decidual cells of the basal plate including placental septa. Cytotrophoblastic cells intermingle with decidual cells. In most places, however, the two components are separated by fibrinoid and other deposits, including acid mucopolysacharides.

2. SYNCYTIOTROPHOBLAST

a) Syncytiotrophoblast of the chorionic plate and villi

An epithelial type of syncytium covers the surface of the chorionic plate and villi (Fig. 27). The "free" surface oriented into the intervillous space is covered by microvilli coated with sialomucin. Beginning in the third month, as the Langhans layer of the cytotrophoblast becomes incomplete, the endothelium of the subtrophoblastic capillaries protrude into the syncytiotrophoblast, and syncytiovascular membranes are formed. They increase in number until birth (Fig. 26). The syncytiovascular membranes of the villi (especially terminal) represent the places where the most intensive materno-fetal and fetal-maternal exchange takes place. Substances are transported or passed through the thin syncytium and through the endothelium of fetal capillaries. Endocytosis and exocytosis are evident. Acid phosphatase is present in the multivesicular bodies. Lipid birefringent droplets are numerous throughout gestation and are related to the formation and metabolism of steroid hormones (Fig. 28). Rough endoplasmic reticulum is found mostly in the perinuclear localization. It has been suggested that the synthesis of placental protein hormones (hCG, hCS) takes place there. Mitochondria, some of them with an electrondense matrix, are scattered throughout the cytoplasm. At the end of pregnancy (gestional weeks 38—40) syncytial buds containing many nuclei appear on the terminal villi. Some of them are detached, pass into the maternal circulation and are deported into various maternal organs, such as lungs or kidneys, where they undergo cytolysis (*Schmorl*, 1893; *Hamilton and Boyd*, 1966; *Skle*, 1964).

b) Syncytiotrophoblast of the columns and islands

The syncytiotrophoblast of the columns and islands is mostly lamellar in type. In midtrimester placentae most of the columnar syncytiotrophoblast undergoes degeneration.

c) Syncytiotrophoblast of the basal plate

The syncytiotrophoblast of the basal plate is either epithelial or lamellar in type, providing an incomplete covering of the basal plate. Wherever the trophoblastic

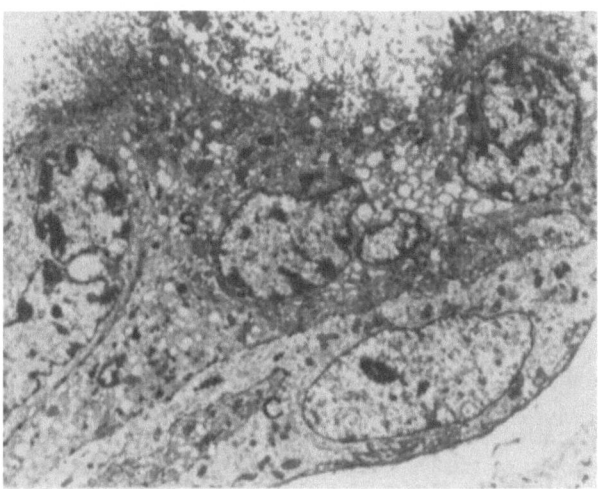

Fig. 27. Ultrastructure of the trophoblast at the beginning of 3rd month. Numerous microvilli project from the trophoblastic syncytium (S) into the intervillous space. Distended cysternae of the smooth endoplasmic reticulum are present between the nuclei. Lipid troplets are scattered in the cytoplasm. The cytotrophoblastic cell (C) is clear, the cellular organells are present in a much lesser amount than in syncytium (photographed by Dr Semecký).

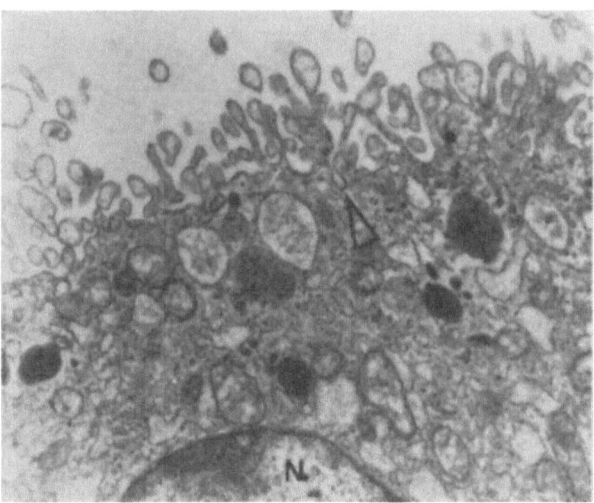

Fig. 28. Ultrastructure of the trophoblastic syncytium presenting evidence of the intense materno-fetal and feto-maternal exchange. A pinocytic vesicle is marked by arrow, N — nucleus.

surface becomes incomplete or damaged, clotting of the maternal blood occurs and fibrinoid is deposited. Cells of trophoblastic origin, some of them multinucleated, are detached throughout gestation from the syncytiotrophoblast of the basal plate. They penetrate into the decidua of the basal plate and myometrium (placental-site cells and placental-site giant cells).

FIBRINOID

Beginning with implantation, as the trophoblast comes in contact with the maternal blood and interstitial tissue fluid, maternal fibrin is deposited wherever the trophoblastic surface permits blood clotting. The term fibrinoid is applied to such a substance which originates from blood clotting. It exhibits, however, different staining properties than fibrin. Fibrinoid, in addition to fibrin, contains other blood proteins and components originating from tissue degeneration (decidua, trophoblast) which are rich in glycoprotein (*Horn and Horalek*, 1961; *Wilkin*, 1965). During chorionic and placental differentiation and growth, fibrinoid is deposited in various areas of the basal plate. The intrabasal fibrinoid lamina separates the basal trophoblast from the decidua in some places. Basal fibrinoid is known as the fibrinoid of *Nitabuch* (1887). Fibrinoid deposited on the surface of the basal plate bordering the intervillous space contributes still another portion of the basal fibrinoid. In third trimester placentae, as the oxygen supply of the chorionic plate trophoblast becomes inadequate, the chorionic plate trophoblasts degenerate and a layer of fibrinoid becomes deposited on the surface of the chorionic plate. This fibrinoid has been described as "canalized fibrin" by *Langhans* (1877), and is known also as subchorial fibrinoid (of *Langhans*). Finally, if the trophoblast of the chorionic (or placenta) villi degenerates, fibrinoid is deposited either on the surface of the syncytiotrophoblast, or between the syncytiotrophoblast and the mesenchymal stroma of the chorionic branch. This fibrinoid is known as the villous fibrinoid of *Rohr* (1899). A large amount of fibrinoid is present in white placental infarcts and in intervillous thromboses. In such lesions, fibrin is deposited on the damaged villi and subsequently becomes changed into fibrinoid. A physiologic accumulation of fibrinoid is observed at the placental margin between the placenta, the membranes and the decidua.

UTEROPLACENTAL CIRCULATION

Uteroplacental circulation begins at days 13—14 after conception (the uterochorionic circulation, see above), as the spiral arteries open into the lacunar system of the trophoblastic shell. The sinusoid veins receiving blood from the primitive intervillous space drain into the basal endometrial veins. Arteries and veins are embedded within the basal plate. As the placenta develops, the morphology of the placental vessels changes considerably with the growing and expanding uterus. In third trimester placentae, the number of maternal arteries opening into the intervillous space is estimated around 260 (*Franken*, 1954), and that of veins around 80. The counts for an individual lobe were 24 and 7 respecively. *Smart* (1962) estimates the number of arteries lower, around 100. The openings of arteries are more frequently near the center of a cotyledon; the arterial flow is considered to be responsible for the bell shape of the anchoring chorionic trunci (*Wilkin*, 1954). The blood flow coming from the uteroplacental arteries is intermittent (*Borrel and Westman*, 1958). The blood pressure in the arteries entering the intervillous space is 70—80 mm Hg (9—11 kPa) (*Alvarez and Caldeiro-Barcia*, 1950). The arterial blood washes primarily those parts of the placental villi which are near the basal plate. The blood stream under the chorionic plate is much slower. The blood pressure in the intervillous space is around 10 mm Hg (1,3 kPa), increasing during uterine contractions up to 30—50 mm Hg (4—7 kPa). The blood pressure in the uterine veins leaving the intervillous space is around 8 mm Hg (1,1 kPa). Around 600 ml of maternal blood pass every minute through the intervillous space (*Browne and Veall*, 1953). The blood pressure within the intervillous space is lower than that within the chorionic fetal vessels. The blood pressure in the umbilical arteries is approximately 48—50 mm Hg (6,4—6,7 kPa), and in the veins, 24 mm Hg (3,2 kPa), respectively (*Margolis and Orcutt*, 1960). These conditions favor the fetomaternal transport. The blood leaves the intervillous space by the way of uteroplacental veins. Their openings are more numerous at the periphery of the placenta, near the placental margin. There is not a single, unique marginal sinus around the intervillous space. Veins leaving the intervillous space penetrate through the decidua in an oblique direction. During uterine contractions, the oblique veins become compressed and the intervillous space remains filled with blood (*Caldeiro-Barcia and Posseiro*, 1960). It is also considered that during uterine contractions the terminal portions of the villi plug the venous openings.

THE PLACENTAL MEMBRANES

The placental membranes are formed by the fused (extraplacental) covered by decidua chorion laeve and extraplacental part of the amnion.

EXTRAPLACENTAL CHORION

Fetal circulation never develops in the villi of the chorion laeve. During the third month, the villi of the chorion laeve undergo an extensive degeneration. Their stroma becomes edematous, and acid mucopolysacharides accumulate between cells. The cords of the endothelial cells forming the vascular primordia disappear. The trophoblastic syncytium degenerates. This type degeneration is known as early hydatidiform swelling (*Hertig*, 1948), or micromolar degeneration (*Vojta and Jirásek*, 1965).

During the fourth month, all the villi of the chorion laeve become necrotic, and the cytotrophoblast of the chorionic plate proliferates, giving rise to a multilayered cytotrophoblast of the membranes. The cytotrophoblast is in contact with the decidua capsularis, which usually becomes necrotic before being apposed to the decidua parietalis. At birth, the extraplacental chorion consists of several layers of trophoblastic cells, with a connective tissue propria underneath. Necrotic ghost chorionic villi are present among the cells. The propria of the chorion is formed by fibroblasts, reticular fibers and an amorphous extracellular substance. Hofbauer cells are present during the 3rd—7th months.

EXTRAPLACENTAL AMNION

The extraplacental amnion, similar to the placental amnion covering the chorionic plate, consists of an epithelium and a lamina propria formed by a myxomatous connective tissue. The epithelium is single-layered cuboidal. The amnionic cells have microvilli and are attached to their basement membrane by desmosomes. Complex intercellular canals and intracellular vacuoles are present.

Fig. 29. Section of the fetal envelopes at midtrimester. A — amnion, C — chorion, K — necrotic remnant of a degenerated chorionic villus.

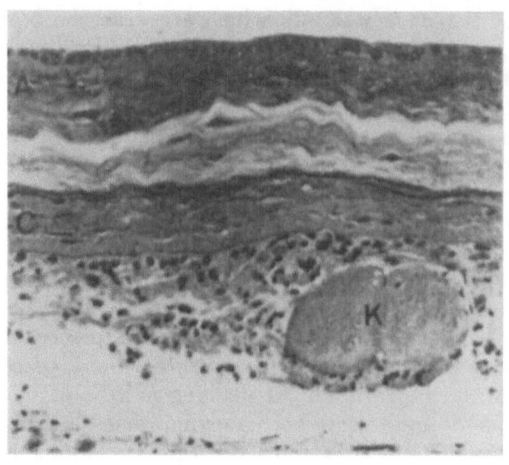

At the end of pregnancy, the amnionic epithelium become distended and some cells undergo necrosis.

The propria of the amnion is formed by a myxomatous, proteoglycan-rich, connective tissue.

A thin membrane containing fibroblasts, reticular fibers and an amorphous extra-cellular substance may sometimes be found between the amnion and chorion. This membrane, called the spongy layer by *Bourne* (1962), is derived from the reticulum of the extraembryonic coelom.

As the amnion becomes filled with an increasing amount of amnionic fluid, all layers of the placental membranes (decidua, chorion, spongy layer and amnion) are pushed together (Fig. 29).

SURVEY OF PLACENTAL FUNCTIONS

The placenta and trophoblast in particular represent a selective filter imposed be-tween the maternal and fetal circulations, not allowing the maternal and fetal blood to mix. When referring to this dividing function, the terms placental barrier, or placental membrane are used. The "membrane" is represented exclusively by fetal tissue. The placenta carries out the following:

1. all exchange occuring between the mother and fetus and vice versa
2. synthesis and secretion of hormones
3. many other anabolic and catabolic functions and conversions. The placenta is involved in the metabolism of many substances.

The transport across the placenta occurs by:

1. simple diffusion
2. facilitated diffusion
3. active transport (against gradient)
4. endocytosis
5. other mechanisms.

The simple diffusion does not require any energy. The substance passes from the area of higher concentration to lower concentration according to physical laws. Placental exchange of CO_2 and O_2 provides examples. A special kind of diffusion, which occurs faster than it would be supposed by applying physical principles, is known as facilitated diffusion. The transport of glucose across "the placental membrane" occurs by facilitated diffusion. The active transport proceeds against the concentration gradient, e. g. from the area of a lower to an area of a higher concentration. Active transport depends on energy supply. Aminoacids and some metallic ions, such as Ca^{2+}, Fe^{2+} and Mg^{2+} are transported across the placental membrane against the concentration gradient. Large molecules are taken by a selective pinocytosis (IgG, thyroid stimulating globulins). The transport of α-fetoprotein from the fetus into the maternal circulation and of some fetal leucocytes has to be elucidated. The presence of fetal erythrocytes in the maternal circulation suggests the rupture of placental villi, and bleeding into the intervillous space. The placental transfer of different substances may be substantially influenced by their binding to the maternal and fetal plasma proteins. Under normal circumstances, the placental barrier does not allow interchange of maternal and fetal somatotropin, thyreoglobulin, LH, FSH, ACTH, PRL, vasopressin, thyroxin, insulin, glucagon and calcitonin.

ENDOCRINOLOGY OF THE PLACENTA

The placenta is the most important endocrine gland during pregnancy, synthesizing proteohormones, such as human chorionic gonadotropin (hCG) and chorionic somatomammotropin (hCS), in addition to various steroids and enzymes.

HUMAN CHORIONIC GONADOTROPIN (hCG)

hCG is a specific glycoprotein produced by the trophoblasts as soon as syncytiotrophoblasts become differentiated (day 7 after fertilization). The hormone produced throughout pregnancy was discovered in 1927 by Aschheim and Zondek (originally thought to be of hypophyseal origin).

The molecule of hCG is composed of two subunits, α and β. The α subunit is identical in all gonadotropins (hCG, FSH, LH) and also in the thyroid-stimulating hormone (TSH). The β subunits of hCG, LH, FSH and TSH are dissimilar and are related to the specificity of the different glycoprotein hormones. The subunits are bound by non-covalent linkages, e. g. by hydrogen or electrostatic bonds (*Bahl et al.*, 1972; *Morgan, Kammerman and Confield*, 1972). Using immunohistochemical techniques, hCG was localized in the trophoblastic syncytium and its derivatives, like placental giant cells (*Midgley and Pierce*, 1962; *Ikonicoff and Cedard*, 1973). We observed that the immuno-competent hCG is present in the syncytiotrophoblast of an implanted 12 1/2 day-old human blastocyst. The cytotrophoblastic alone is not able to produce hCG. The hCG level reflects the cyto-syncytiotrophoblastic conversion; in other words, the amount of syncytium newly formed from the cytotrophoblast. We observed a patient with metastatic choriocarcinoma. The hCG disappeared after the treatment with cytostatics; however, the metastatic vaginal tumor was still present at this time. The tumor consisted exclusively of the cytotrophoblast. In tissue cultures, *Pattilo and Gey* (1968) grew a cytotrophoblastic cell line synthetizing hCG. It remains to be seen to what extent some of the elements of the trophoblast growing in v i t r o do correspond to the cytotrophoblast, or to the syncytiotrophoblast.

Under normal conditions, hCG and its subunit α are secreted by the syncytiotropho-blast mainly into the maternal circulation. Using specific β-subunit antisera, not cross-reacting with LH, hCG may be detected as early as days 7-8 after conception (*Braunstein et al.*, 1973; *Saxena et al.*, 1974, *Mishell et al.*, 1974). After implantation, the levels of hCG begin to rise both in the maternal serum as well as in urine. The hCG plasma and urinary levels are proportional (*Mishell, Wide and Gemzell*, 1963; *Brody and Carlstrom*, 1965). A week after implantation (approximately days 28—30 after the last menstrual period) the plasma hCG levels reach approximately 1 IU/ml. Thereafter, the concentration of hCG rises sharply reaching a maximum between days 60—75 of amenorrhea (Graph 4). The maximum level is approximately 100 IU/ml. The peak levels are maintained for some days, quickly declining thereafter. Around day 120 (G), the hCG level is approximately 20—25 IU/ml, and this con-centration does not change substantially until birth. In some cases, a small rise may be found around day 230 of amenorrhea, i. e. in the 32nd week of pregnancy. It has been reported that the hCG level in mothers bearing female infants is higher and increases between weeks 10—20, in contrast to that in women bearing male infants, and that there is a comparable increase of hCG content in the female placenta (*Broditsky et al.*, 1975).

The total daily hCG synthesis is estimated to be 50,000—1,000,000 IU a day between days 60—70, declining thereafter to a mean 100,000 IU a day (*Diczfalusy and Troen*, 1961). About 10% of the daily production is excreted by the urine. The differences in chemical properties between the serum and urinary hCG are ascribed to the hydrolysis of the carbohydrate components of the hCG molecule. In pregnancies ending in spontaneous abortions, two types of hCG curves may be observed (*Jirásek*

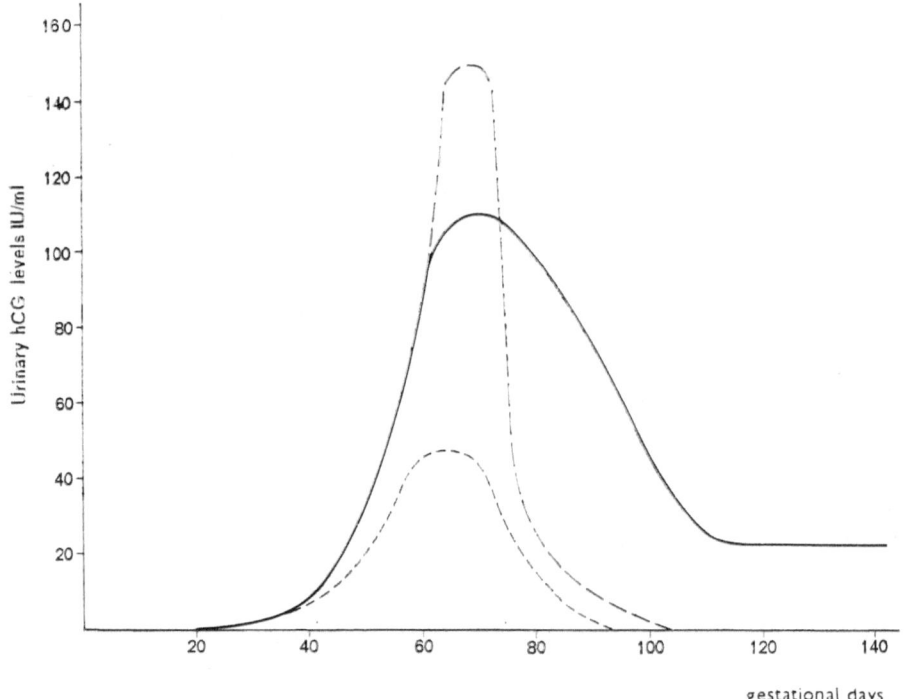

Graph 4. Maternal urinary hCG levels in early pregnancy: normal pregnancy solid line, afeta product of conception dotted line, malformed fetus unable to survive: dashed line.

and Zwinger, in press). In the first type, in which the embryo is usually malformed and chromosomal abnormalities (if found) are compatible with survival until term, the curves are characterized by an hCG peak higher than normal. The hCG levels around day 70 of amenorrhea reach 150 IU/ml, declining thereafter and falling to undetectable levels around day 100. In the second type, mostly in the conceptus showing chromosomal abnormalities incompatible with survival (resulting in blighted ova, anembryonic moles), the hCG levels do not exhibit the normal rise around day 50, the values of hCG around day 60 do not exceed 2−4 IU/ml, and decline thereafter, becoming undetectable around day 90 of amenorrhea (Graph 3). The prognostic importance of serial hCG quantitative determinations during 10−12 weeks of amenorrhea is evident. If hCG levels at this period (weeks 10−12) do not exceed 4−5 IU/ml, the prognosis for a good pregnancy outcome is poor in spite of the fact that in the same patients the hCG levels may be found normal after week 12. An abortion in such cases usually follows at the end of the second trimester (*Dykova et al.*, 1975). However, daily fluctuations in hCG levels are considerable in both normal and abnormal pregnancies. If the hCG level exceeds 200 IU/ml, the presence of a hydatidiform mole or of a choriocarcinoma has to be considered. Estimates made by *Braunstein et al.* (1973) have suggested that the hCG output per cell, however, is more rapid in the normal trophoblast than in the neoplastic. After surgical removal of trophoblastic tumors, the hCG persists for several weeks; after medical abortions of normal first trimester pregnancies, hCG is found for an additional 7−14 days; after removal of hydatidiform moles, hCG persists 2−4 weeks. In trophoblastic diseases, if hCG can be detected six weeks after the removal of the lesion, the presence of trophoblast, and the exacerbation of the disease has to be expected. After a normal delivery, the hCG disappears from maternal urine within one or two weeks, each subunit following its own excretory pattern. Fetal serum hCG levels are high at the end of the second month, declining thereafter. At conceptional days 70−90, fetal serum hCG levels are 0.8−2 IU/ml; at the end of the third month, approximately 1 IU/ml; at the end of the fourth month, 0.6; and at birth, about 0.3 IU/ml (Graph 5). During a normal pregnancy, in addition to hCG, there is a large amount of free hCG α subunit in the placental tissue as well as in the maternal serum and urine. In patients with trophoblastic neoplasia, two different groups were found. In group one, only hCG and practically no subunits were present. In group two, free hCG β was formed and was present in serum and urine. Patients belonging to group one responded to the chemotherapy. Patients of group two did not respond, and all subsequently died of a generalized choriocarcinoma (*Vaitukaitis*, 1976).

The mechanisms quantitating the hCG output are poorly understood. The hCG levels increase temporarily after the fetal circulation stops. It is supposed that fetal anoxia might be involved in the increase. In the peripheral target tissues, such as fetal testicular Leydig cells, hCG is bound to specific membrane receptors. The binding is closely related to adenylate cyclase activity and production of cAMP. Within the corpus luteum in response to hCG, there is an increase in conversion of cholesterol to pregnenolone, and androstendione to estrogens (*Channing*, 1970; *Sulijovici and Lunenfeld*, 1972). hCG has a luteotropic action in early pregnancy. hCG stimulates corpus luteum progesterone production both in vivo and in vitro (*Savard, Marsh and Rice*, 1965; *Strott et al.*, 1969). The removal of the corpus luteum during the first six weeks of pregnancy is followed by abortion, because the chorionic (placental) secretion of progesterone and estrogens is still inadequate for pregnancy mainte-nance. The function ("suf- ficiency") of the corpus luteum can be checked in early pregnancy by the deter-mination of the maternal of 17-α-hydroxyprogesterone

(*Lipsett*, 1968). During the four to five weeks following conception, both 17-hydroxy-progesterone and progesterone rise, both declining during the sixth week. During weeks seven and eight, progesterone rises again, due to its chorionic production,

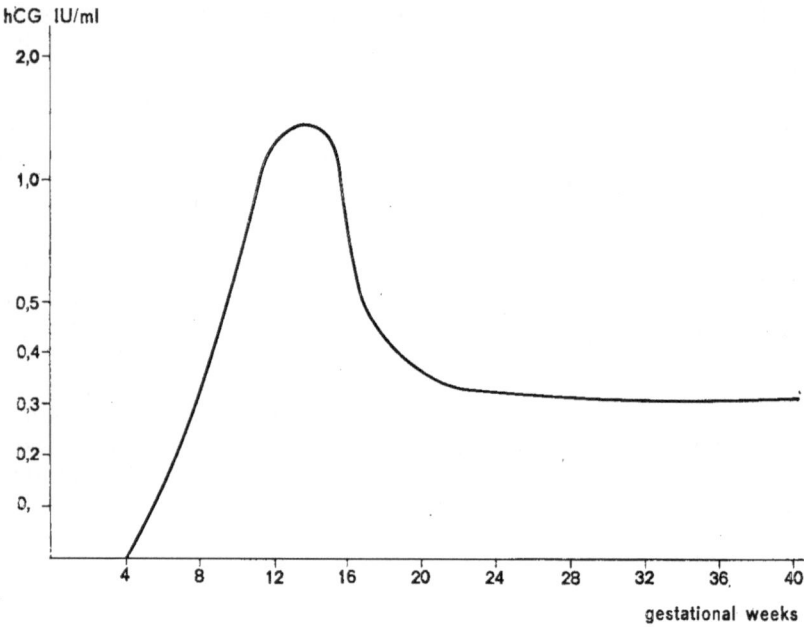

Graph 5. Fetal serum hCG levels.

whereas the 17-hydroxyprogesterone level remains low. There is no evidence of the relation between chorionic progesterone secretion and hCG. In trophoblastic disease, ovarian hyperstimulation by hCG may induce the formation of multiple large ovarian lutein cysts forming excessive steroids.

hCG, if administered to various vertebrates, promotes ovulation or sperm release. These effects are used in various biological hCG tests. In prepubertal female mice, hCG induces ovulations, and uterine weight increase. In prepubertal rats, an ovarian hyperemia is observed. In rabbits, ovulations take place. In frogs, either eggs in females (Xenopus test), or sperm in males (Bufo) are released (*Josimovich*, 1967). Immunochemical detection of hCG is used in various commercial pregnancy tests. Radioimmunoassay, using antisera against the whole molecule, or specifically against the α and β subunits, are used in highly specific assays (*Ross et al.*, 1977).

hCG THERAPY

hCG is administered to hypogonadotropic females to induce ovulation in combination with hMG (Pergonal). In the usual schema, two ampules of hMG (150 IU FSH) are administered for eight consecutive days. If there is an adequate response in urinary estrogens (total estrogens in urine more than 20 mcg/24 hours), hCG (6,000 to 10,000 IU) is administered on day 9 or on days 9 and 10 (*Thompson and Hansen*, 1970).

If the eightday hMG administration was inadequate to increase the total estrogen level substantially, 3 ampules of hMG are administered for an additional 3 days. Urinary estrogens are to be checked, and if their amount is more than 20 mcg/24 hours hCG is administered. If the estrogen level remains low, an ovarian failure is to be supposed. During hMG and hCG therapy, daily estrogen monitoring is necessary to avoid ovarian hyperstimulation.

If anovulation is treated by Clomiphene citrate (Clomid, Gravosan), hCG may be administered on the first and second day following Clomiphene application in a dose 2000—10,000 IU (*Kistner*, 1966). The complications accompanying this therapy, such as intra-abdominal bleeding from a ruptured follicle, development of lutein cysts and thromboses were reported.

In cryptorchic boys, hCG is used to achieve testicular descent. At the age of 6—8 years, 6—10 shots each containing 500—1500 IU of hCG are given during a three to five week period. If the testes do not descend, surgical intervention is inevitable. The question of testicular tubular hyalinization as a consequence of the transitory testicular hCG stimulation is to be elucidated.

HUMAN CHORIONIC SOMATOMAMMOTROPIN (hCS; HUMAN PLACENTAL LACTOGEN, hPL)

Discovery of hCS was made by *Ito and Highasi* (1961) who isolated different proteins from human placental extracts and described their properties. *Josimovich and McLaren* (1962) discovered that the placental lactogenic substance is similar to the hypophyseal growth hormone, and introduced the name, human placental lactogen (hPL). *Kaplan and Grumbach* in their studies (1964) used the term human chorionic somatoprolactin (CGP), and finally a group of authors (*Li et al.*, 1968) studying the properties of the new hormone proposed the term, human somatomammotropin (hCS).

hCS is a proteohormone with a molecular weight, in monomeric form, of approximately 21,500 (*Friesen*, 1965). The molecule is formed by 184—190 aminoacids. The C-terminal of the chain ends with phenylalanine and is very similar to the growth hormone. The N-terminal ends with valine. In diluted solutions, hCS forms dimer (*Neri et al.*, 1970). Using a histoimmunofluorescent technique, hCS was localized into the syncytiotrophoblast (*Sciarra, Kaplan and Grumbach*, 1963). hCS is also present in trophoblastic disease patients and in males with choriocarcinoma of the testis (*Samaan et al.*, 1966). Maternal hCS levels increase steadily during pregnancy (Graph 6). The serum level is proportional to the weight of the placenta (*Josimovich, Koror and Minth*, 1969). The hormone is secreted preferentially into the maternal circulation. The concentration within the fetal blood is about 1% of the maternal (*Grumbach et al.*, 1968). Only a very small amount of hCS passes into the maternal urine. hCS accumulates in the amnionic fluid (*Yen, Samaan and Pearson*, 1967). After delivery of the placenta, hCS quickly disappears, the average half-time being 12—30 minutes (*Pavlov, Chard and Letchwoth*, 1972). In trophoblastic neoplasias, the low level of hCS is in contrast to the high levels of hCG (*Yen, Pearson and Radkin*, 1968).

The determinations of the hCS levels at the end of pregnancy are of a definitive prognostic value. If the serum hCS levels after the thirteenth week of gestation are less than 0,4 g/ml, the fetus is considered at risk (*Josimovich*, 1974; *Spellacy*, 1974) of growth retardation. In abortions, the hCS disappears more rapidly after fetal death than hCG does.

The physiological importance of hCS is poorly understood. hCS may be important in the maternal regulations concerning fetal nutrition. hCS infusion to the mother increases insulin release after glucose load (*Samaan et al.*, 1966). The hormone increases fat mobilization and insulin resistance in pheriphral tissues. hCS alone is without any effect on estrogen and progesterone formation by the corpus luteum

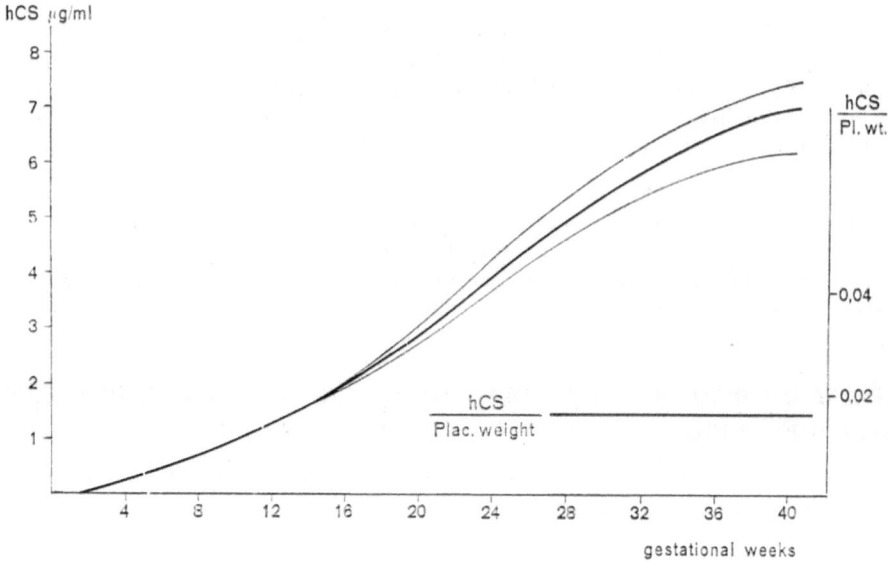

Graph 6. Concentration of hCS in maternal plasma during gestation and normal hCS, placental weight ratio.

(*Stock et al.*, 1971). The effect in preparation of the human breast for lactation is not documented (*Hwang, Guyda and Friesen*, 1971). The mechanisms of hCS secretion remain unknown.

HUMAN CHORIONIC THYROTROPIN (hCT)

Human chorionic thyrotropin still represents a controversial subject. *Hensen, Pierce and Freychet* (1969) described a protein, present in placental extracts, with similar properties as TSH. hCT reacted with the sera against bovine, or porcine TSH, but did not react with sera against human TSH. The presence of hCT was reported in patients with choriocarcinoma and hydatidiform mole (*Odell et al.*, 1964).

Recent reports fail to detect any specific placental hCT (*Harada and Hershman*, 1978). The TSH activity found in normal placental extracts, as well as in patients with hydatidiform mole is ascribed to an intrinsic, thyroid-stimulating activity of hCG (*Hershman and Higgins*, 1978).

CHORIONIC TRH

TRH is present in placental extracts. Its quantity at term is approximately 20 pg per mg protein (*Shambaugh et al.*, 1978).

46

HUMAN CHORIONIC CORTICOTROPIN (hCC)

The reports on the presence of a pituitary hCC are still inconclusive. *Genazzani et al.* (1975) and *Rees et al.* (1975) found ACTH in placental extracts as well as in the incubation media of placental cultures. It was demonstrated that in pregnant women, dexamethasone does not suppress cortisol excretion. It seems, therefore, that ACTH in the maternal circulation is both of maternal and fetal (placental) origin.

STEROID HORMONE SYNTHESIS BY THE TROPHOBLAST (PLACENTA)

There are three principal steroid-producing compartments in the trophoblast (placenta): (1) the progesterone forming, (2) the estrone-estradiol forming, and (3) the estriol forming.

TROPHOBLASTIC (PLACENTAL) PROGESTERONE-FORMING COMPARTMENT

The formation of progesterone within the trophoblast begins from cholesterol. The trophoblastic formation of "its own" cholesterol is negligible. There are two pools of cholesterol available to the trophoblast: the maternal coming with the

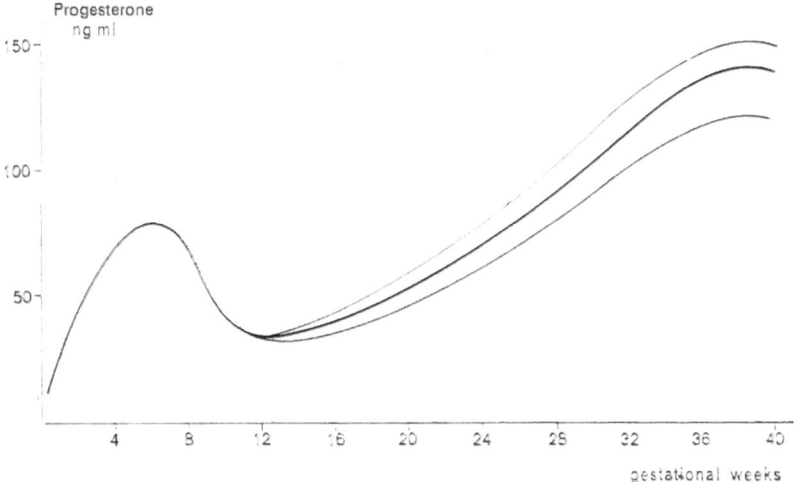

Graph 7. Maternal plasma progesterone during pregnancy.

maternal blood, and the fetal coming with the fetal blood. Fetal cholesterol is synthetized de novo from acetate, mostly in the liver and adrenals starting in the second month. Most of the trophoblastic (placental) progesterone comes from the maternal cholesterol (*Hellig et al.*, 1970). Progesterone synthesis in the trophoblast begins shortly after implantation, and its production increases with the advancing gravidity. Up to the eleventh or twelfth week of gestation, however, the main source of progesterone in pregnant women is the corpus luteum. Later on, trophoblastic (placental) progesterone takes over (*Holmdahl, Johansson and Wide*, 1971). Maternal plasma progesterone levels are depicted on Graph 7.

47

Table 5. Trophoblastic synthesis of progesterone.

Maternal blood		Trophoblast		Fetal blood
cholesterol	→	cholesterol ↓ pregnenolone ↓	←	cholesterol
progesterone	←	progesterone	→	progesterone

The pathway of trophoblastic progesterone synthesis is summarized in Table 5.

Progesterone is not used by the fetus until weeks 10—12 when the primordium of the definitive adrenal cortex develops and begins to function.

PLACENTAL 17β-ESTRADIOL-FORMING COMPARTMENT

Dehydroepiandrosterone and dehydroepiandrosterone sulphate from the maternal side and dehydroepiandrosterone sulphate from the fetal side are the main precursors of placental estrone (E_1) and estradiol (E_2). The "steroid sulphate biosynthetic pathway" seems to be advantageous. The steroid sulphates are more easily transported because of water solubility and easier transport across cellular membranes.

The pathway of chorionic E_1 and E_2 synthesis is depicted in Table 6.

Table 6. Trophoblastic synthesis of E_1 and E_2.

Maternal blood		Trophoblast		Fetal blood
DHA DHAS	→	DHA, DHAS ↓ androstenedione ↓	←	DHAS
E_1, E_2	←	E_1, E_2	→	E_1, E_2

Estrone and estradiol formed by the placenta originate from both maternal and fetal dehydroepiandrosterone sulphate or dehydroepiandresterone. Estrone and estradiol account for less than 10% of the total estrogens present in the pregnancy urine. Maternal plasma estradiol levels are seen in Graph 8.

PLACENTAL ESTRIOL-FORMING COMPARTMENT

Placental estriol, the main estrogen formed during pregnancy, accounts for more than 90 percent of total estrogen present in the pregnancy urine. The main pathway starts from 16-hydroxydehydroepiandrosterone sulphate formed by the fetal adrenals and liver. An alternative pathway covers the 16-OH pregnenolone sulphate and 16-OH androstenedione sulphate, also formed by the fetal adrenals.

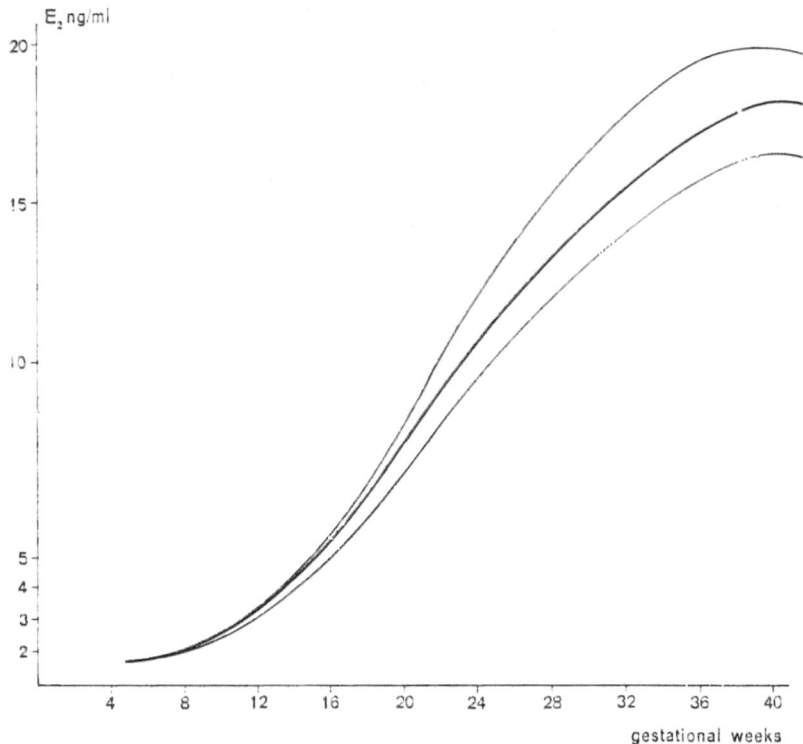

Graph 8. Maternal plasma estradiol levels during pregnancy.

Table 7. Principal pathway of E_3 formation.

Maternal blood		Trophoblast		Fetal blood
(16-OH DHA 16-OH androstenedione)	$\rightarrow$	16-OH DHAS $\downarrow$	$\leftarrow$	16-OH DHAS
E_3	$\leftarrow$	E_3	$\rightarrow$	E_3

The principal pathway of E_3 formation is summarized in Table 7.

An alternative pathway of E_3 formation (unimportant from the quantitative point) is summarized in table 8.

The alternative pathway comprises the 16-hydroxypregnenolone formed by the fetal adrenals (*Shahwan, Oakey and Stitch*, 1969); its conversion is to 16-OH progesterone by the trophoblast, conversion of 16-OH progesterone to 16-OH androstendione either

49

Table 8. Alternative pathway of E_3 formation.

Maternal blood		Trophoblast		Fetal blood
		16-OH pregnenolone sulphate	←	16-OH pregnenolone sulphate (adrenal)
		↓		
		16-OH pregnenolone		
		↓		
16-OH progesterone (corpus luteum, liver)		16-OH progesterone	→	16-OH progesterone
				↓
16-OH androstenedione (adrenal, ovary, liver)	→	16-OH androstenedione	←	16-OH androstenedione (adrenal)
		↓		
E_3	←	E_3	→	E_3

Table 9. Phenolic (negligible) pathway of E_3 formation.

Maternal liver		Maternal blood		Trophoblast
E_2	←	E_2	←	E_2
↓				
E_3	→	E_3		

by the fetal adrenals or by the maternal adrenals and the conversion of 16-OH androstendione to estriol in the trophoblast. The proposed phenolic pathway of E_3 synthesis is more of theoretical than practical importance.

The so-called "phenolic pathway" of estriol synthesis is confined predominantly to the maternal liver, and the fetus does not contribute very much to it (*Diczfalusy*, 1970).

The phenolic pathway of E_3 formation (negligible, Diczfalusy, 1970) is summarized in Table 9.

Maternal urinary estriol values are given in Graph 9.

Regulatory mechanisms controlling trophoblastic (placental) steroidogenesis are poorly understood. The dependence of the trophoblast on the precursors provided by the fetus is most evident regarding the estriol production.

The trophoblastic production of progesterone and hydrolysis of dehydroepiandrosterone sulphate seems to be inhibited by a feed-back mechanism involving circulating fetal steroids (*Townsley et al.*, 1973).

Steroids produced and secreted by the trophoblast into the maternal circulation are candidates for the monitoring of placental functions and fetal well-being. The progesterone, and its urinary metabolite pregnanediol, do not tell much about the fetus or its viability.

Maternal plasma 17—hydroxyprogesterone is used at the early stages of pregnancy as an indicator of the corpus luteum activity. Maternal estriol levels, however, reflect the steroid production of the fetal adrenal, the capacity of 16-hydroxylation occuring within fetal adrenals and liver, and dependence on fetoplacental circulation. Their determination is simple and of a practical value. Because of the complexity involved in the estriol production, it would be misleading to believe that a single determination is good enough to conclude the status of the fetus. Several daily serial estriol assays are needed especially in "high risk" patients, such as toxaemic, diabetic, or Rh-sensi-

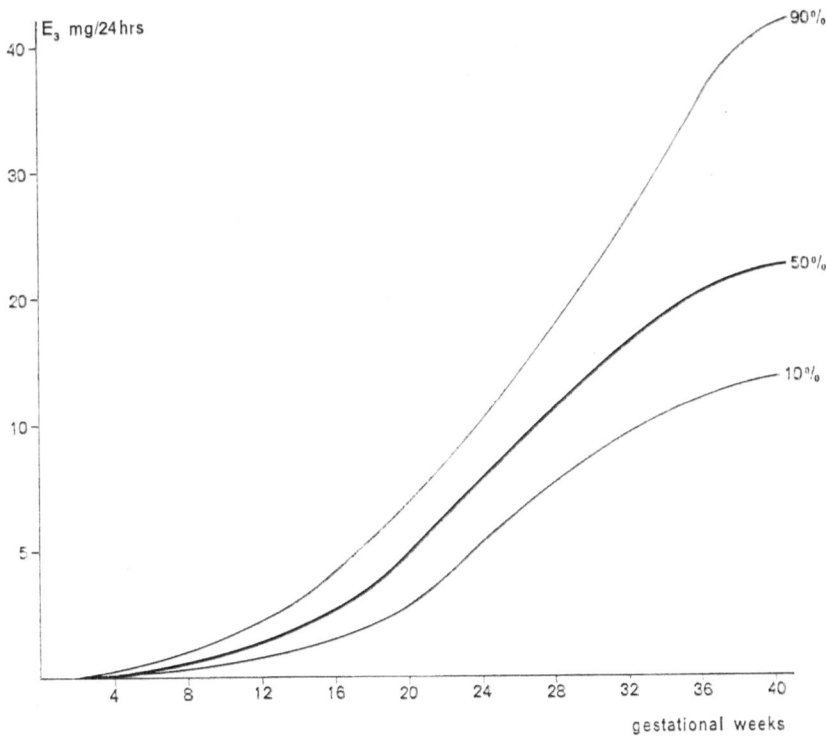

Graph 9. Maternal urinary estriol values during pregnancy.

tive women (*Gobelsmann et al.*, 1973; *Diczfalusy*, 1969). Low levels of estriol, despite fetal well-being, were reported in cases with placental sulphatase deficiency (*Cedard et al.*, 1970; *France and Liggins*, 1969).

Good reviews on the estriol value of monitoring the intrauterine fetus were presented by *Beling* (1967), *Bjoro* (1972) and *Beischer and Brown* (1972).

Estetrol, 15-hydroxyestriol, found in the maternal circulation, is considered to be exclusively of fetal origin. Its assays are of a definitive value regarding the fetal monitoring, especially in toxaemic patients (*Heikkela and Lukkainen*, 1971; *Gurpide et al.*, 1966, *Kaplan and Hershehyshyn*, 1973).

It is impossible to review the vast literature related to estriol and fetal monitoring. If exogenous DHAS is administered to the mother in a dose of 50 mg or less, only E_2 rises. If the DHAS load is more than 100 mg, and the pregnancy is normal, rise in both E_2 and E_3 occurs. Maximal E_2 and E_3 elevation takes place two to three hours after injection (DHAS test).

COMPARTMENTALIZATION OF STEROID PRODUCTION WITHIN
THE FETOPLACENTAL UNIT

During the prenatal period, steroids are produced by the trophoblast of the placenta by interstitial cells of the fetal testis, by ovarian stromal cells, by thecal cells of growing follicles of perinatal ovaries and by adrenal cortical cells. In the adrenals, the hormones produced are different according to the cortical to the cortical zone. Each cell type in a steroid-producing organ probably has its own characteristic enzyme pattern. There are, however, some general rules.

Cholesterol, regarded as a principal precursor of steroid hormones, may be derived from acetate by de novo synthesis within the steroid-producing cell. Some cholesterol originates from perfusing blood being produced by some other cells mostly from cholesterol fatty-acid esters or ingested with the food. During pregnancy, maternal and fetal cholesterol is to be distinguished. Fetal cholesterol is synthetized in large quantities within the liver. The metabolism of cholesterol within the steroid-producing cell may differ if the cholesterol available is free or sulphated. The differences in their metabolism may result in differences of transport across the cellular membranes. Cholesterol side-chain cleavage and steroid C-18 and C-11 hydroxylations were localized to the inner membrane of mitochondria. The microsomes of the rough endoplasmic reticulum are considered with steroid oxidations. The aromatization of steroids occurs both in mitochondria and in microsomes.

Recently a hypothesis has been proposed that there are not true isolatable intermediates in the synthesis of various steroids, each steroid secreted being produced by its own specific subcellular superstructure called biosynthetic particles (*Lieberman, Gurpide, Lipsett and Salhanick,* 1977). The biosynthetic particles may contain closely related, substrate-specific oxygen and electron-transporting systems involving flavoprotein, NADP reductase, iron sulphur protein and cytochrome-P-450.

The combination of oxygen, electrons and enzymes systems leads to a chain of immediately proceeding reactions such as: oxydation, hydroxylation, carbon-carbon cleavage and aromatization.

With the exception of hCG, each steroid-producing cell has a specific trophic hormone. hCG, during the first trimester of pregnancy, is closely related to the trophoblastic steroidogenesis as originating within the same cellular environment, to the maternal corpus luteum, to the steroidogenesis of the fetal testis and to the fetal adrenals. Later, in the second half of pregnancy, the gonadal steroidogenesis becomes controlled by LH and the primordium of the definitive adrenal cortex by ACTH and the renin--angiotensin system.

THE FETOPLACENTAL UNIT

"Would not the human placenta have developed, there would not be the human brain."   Dr. Jan Florian, 1936

The concept of the fetoplacental unit was introduced by *Diczfalusy* (1964). *Diczfalusy* studying placental and fetal steroid metabolism recognized that in regard to some steroids, both the placenta and fetus represent incomplete systems which alone are unable to produce the final steroid hormone. The role of the placenta and the fetus in the steroid synthesis is related to the compartmentalization of the steroid metabolism. The placenta is the primary site of cholesterol to C-21 steroid conversion

Table 10. Main steroidogenic compartments of the placenta in context of steroidogenic pathways:
progesterone forming (materno-trophoblastic
estrone-estradiol forming (materno-feto-trophoblastic)
estriolforming (feto-trophoblastic)

Main characteristics of trophoblast: a highly active 3βOH steroid dehydrogenase
a highly active ring A aromatase
absent 16 hydroxylase
absent 21 hydroxylase

Main steroids produced:
progesterone
estron, estradiol
estriol (from 16-hydroxylated fetal precursors)

MATERNO TROPHOBLASTIC COMPARTMENT	MATERNO-FETO-TROPHOBLASTIC COMPARTMENT	FETO-TROPHOBLASTIC COMPARTMENT
ACETATE		
↓		
CHOLESTEROL		
↓		
PREGNENOLONE(S) → 17-OH PREGNENOLONE (S) → DHA (S) → ANDROSTENEDIONE → TESTOSTERONE		16-OH DHA(S)
↓	↓ ↑	→
PROGESTERONE → 17-OH PROGESTERONE	ESTRONE ⇌ ESTRADIOL	ESTRIOL
↓	↓	
11 DEOXYCORTICOSTERONE 11 DEOXYCORTISOL		
↓	↓	
CORTICOSTERONE CORTISOL		
↓		
ALDOSTERONE		

(20-22-hydroxylase and desmolase), Δ^5 keto to Δ^4 hydroxy conversion (Δ^4-Δ^5 isomerase, 3β-hydroxydehydrogenase) and aromatization. Steroid sulphates are converted in the placenta into free steroids by a highly active sulphatase.

The fetus provides acetate to cholesterol synthesis (liver, adrenal) sulphurylates steroids (sulphokinases; fetal adrenal, fetal liver), and hydroxylates them at various positions. The 16α-hydroxylation, which is necessary for placental estriol formation occurs in fetal adrenals and liver. A limited C-21 to C-19 steroid conversion occurs in the fetal adrenals. In general, within the fetus there is no 3β-hydroxydehydrogenation, and a very limited C-21 to C-19 steroid conversion.

In terms of steroid metabolism compartmentalization, the placenta comprises: cholesterol, progesterone-forming compartment; DHA, DHAS-estrone, estradiol-forming compartment; and 16-OH DHAS (16-OH-C-19 steroid) estriol-forming compartment. The fetal adrenal comprises (1) acetate to cholesterol compartment, (2) progesterone to corticosterone and cortisol compartment, (3) progesterone to aldosterone compartment; (4) pregnenolone, dehydroepiandrosterone-sulphate and 16-OH dehydroepiandrosterone sulphate forming compartment (fetal zone of cortex; fetal liver are involved regarding the 16-hydroxylation). From the quantitiative point, the DHAS-forming compartment seems to be the most important. The androstendione, testosterone-forming compartment is present in the Leydig cells of fetal testes. The steroidogenic compartments of the placenta (trophoblast) in context of steroidogenic pathways is presented in Table 10.

It is evident that fetoplacental (embryochorial) circulation is of a primary importance for the proper function of the fetoplacental unit. During the early embryonal period beginning in the stage of blastocystic implantation, two quite independent biological systems are present: the chorion and the proper embryo. The early chorion is nourished by the maternal blood from the intervillous space, the embryo by a simple diffusion. The early chorion survives for a considerable period even in the absence of the fetus. The embryochorionic circulation becomes established during the fifth week. As the growth of the chorion becomes dependent on the embryochorionic circulation, the fetoplacental (embryochorionic) unit becomes established. If the embryochorionic circulation stops, the trophoblast remains viable, because of the nourishment from the intervillous space, but the mesenchymal stroma of the chorionic villi undergoes necrosis.

From the anatomical and physiological point, the fetoplacental unit becomes operational beginning at week five after conception. Regarding the steroid fetoplacental metabolism, there is evidence that fetal adrenals and liver participate in the steroid metabolism beginning at the seventh week.

PHYLOGENESIS OF THE PLACENTA

Placental diversity in different species of animals makes it extremely difficult to contribute a comprehensive survey of placental phylogenesis. Reviews on comparative placentation have been published by *Grosser* (1927); and *Amoroso* (1952). During vertebrate phylogenesis, many problems have been solved, such as nutrition of the developing organism, protection of the embryo, gas exchange, removing of the metabolic wastage, etc. From the phylogenic points, the nutrition of the embryo is primarily related to the accumulation of yolk within the oocyte. There is a general rule in vertebrates (with the exception of mammals) that the more complicated embryonal development and the bigger the animal is, the more yolk there is present in the oocyte. Considerable amounts of yolk accumulate within the oocytes of amphibia, fish, reptiles and birds. The amount of yolk determines the cleavage pattern of the oocyte as well as mechanisms by which the germ layers develop. The increased amount of the yolk increases the size of the oocyte. The oocyte becomes more vulnerable.

To protect the embryo against the environment and drying, various envelopes were formed. These are commonly known as the egg white and shell. However, at the same time as the envelopes develop, they make the oxygen supply and CO_2 removal from the developing embryo more difficult. Both gases are exchanged by a simple diffusion. It is supposed that the primitive vertebrates were living in pools containing warm water which frequently dried out. The conditions for an adequate oxygen supply varied greatly. One of the ways of overcoming environmental instability was the retention of the developing embryo within the genital ducts of the female. The fertilization outside the maternal body was changed to an internal one. The embryos developed inside the body of the mother and came out "alive". The viviparity developed independently in several species of fish, frogs, lizards and snakes. There is paleotologic evidence that the Ichthyosaurs were viviparous. The retention of the embryo within the body of the mother facilitates the metabolic exchange between the mother and her progeny. Oxygen was probably the first substance exchanged between the embryo and the mother. In viviparous sharks, oxygen is transported from the mother into the vessels of the yolk sac. The protection against drying out became "a question of survival" in mesozoic reptiles.

The hypothesis is poorly documented suggesting that the embryonal defense against drying consisted of the formation of ectodermal folds over the embryo and conserving water inside. However, that is the mechanism by which the amniochorionic folds do develop in recent terrestrial reptiles and birds. The inner sheet of the ectodermal amniochorionic fold gives rise to the amnion, the outer to the chorion.

The metabolic waste in vertebrate embryos with a terrestrial development is primarily saved in a sac evaginating from the hind gut, and known as the allantois. The opening of the allantois into the gut is located caudal to the opening of the yolk sac. The accumulation of metabolic waste expands the allantois. During embryonal development in reptiles and birds, the size of the yolk sac decreases while that of the allantois increases. The allantois evaginates under the shell of the eggs. The wall of allantois becomes highly vascular and attached to chorion. Both structures fuse to the allantochorion. The allantochorion becomes the main organ responsible for the gas exchange in sauropsid embryos. Phylogenetically, all this development occured before the mammals developed.

As all the nutrition of the mammalian embryo was provided by the mother, the amount of yolk in the mammalian oocytes decreased. Contrarily, the tissues involved in the maternofetal exchange become specialized, and at the beginning of ontogenetic development, their differentiation precedes that of the embryo itself. This is reflected in the mammalian blastocyst. The surface layer of the blastocyst is formed by the trophoblast (trophoectoderm) responsible for all the maternofetal exchange and not contributing to the embryo proper. The mammalian (ectodermal) amnion develops either from the amniogenic folds, or directly from the ectoderm of the inner cell mass (human). The extent of the amnionic development is variable. In most mammals exhibiting a rudimentary allantois, the amnion does not fuse with the chorion into an amniochorion. The mammalian yolk sac originates as an envelope of the virtual yolk sphere (mass) located inside the blastocyst. The "inversion" of germ layers observed in some species (rabbits, bats, insectivores) represents a virtual invagination of the embryo into the yolk sac.

The choriovitelline placenta found in marsupials originates from fusion of the vascularized mesenchyme of the yolk sac with the mesenchyme of the chorion. In some mammalian species, the choriovitelline placenta preceeds the formation of a proper allantochorionic placenta. In the allantochorionic placenta, the vessels accompanying allantois are brought to the chorion. The vascularization of chorion is dependent on allantoic vessels.

Allantochorionic placentae are classified from different points of view. Decidual (guinea pig, human), and adecidual placentae (ungulates, carnivores) are distinguished according to the presence of decidua. According to the distribution of chorionic villi, diffuse and cotyledonic placentae are distinguished. In the diffuse placentae, chorionic villi are all over the surface of the chorion (pig horse). In cotyledonic placentae, chorionic villi form aggregates (cotyledons). The cotyledons may be present sparsely all over the chorion (disseminate placenta in ruminants), or in a strip formed perpendicular to the equator of the chorion (zonary placenta in carnivores), or the cotyledons form a disc, single (human), or doubled (some simians). According to the endometrium-trophoblastic relation, epitheliochorial, syndesmochorial, endotheliochorial and haemochorial placentae (*Grosser*, 1927) are distinguished. In the epitheliochorial placentae, the trophoblast is apposed to an intact endometrial epithelium (occurs in horse, pig and whale). In the syndesmochorial placentae, the trophoblast penetrates into the connective tissue of the endometrial propria (in ungulates). Most of the placentae formerly considered as syndesmochorial, are reclassified as epitheliochorial (cow, sheep; *Bjorkamn and Bloom*, 1957; *Ludwig*, 1962; *Hamilton*, 1960). In the endotheliochorial placentae, the trophoblast contacts the endothelium of maternal endometrial vessels (cat, dog, carnivores). In the haemochorial placentae, the trophoblast comes in direct contact with maternal blood. Maternal blood circulates within the intervillous space covered by the trophoblast (rabbit, guinea pig, rat, primates, including human).

The placental morphology is extremely variable, and can hardly be used for phylogenic contemplations.

PATHOLOGY OF THE CHORION AND PLACENTA

AVASCULAR CHORIONIC VILLI (HYDROPIC VILLI, EARLY HYDATIDIFORM SWELLING, MICROMOLAR DEGENERATION)

An avascular chorion with degenerating chorionic villi (Fig. 30) is normally present in the area of chorion laeve during the third and fourth month of gestation. The stroma of the villi is edematous, hydropic and no vessels are present. Sometimes disintegrating remnants of vascular endothelial cords may be recognized. Thin trophoblastic syncytium with pycnotic nuclei covers the degenerating villi. Some cytotrophoblastic cells may be found underneath the syncytium (*Vojta and Jirásek*, 1965). The fluid accumulation within the stroma does not proceed to the formation of a central cavity, which is characteristic for the "true" hydatidiform degeneration. The differentiation of chorion laeve represents a partial chorionic micromolar degeneration. A complete micromolar degeneration of the chorion is found in most spon-

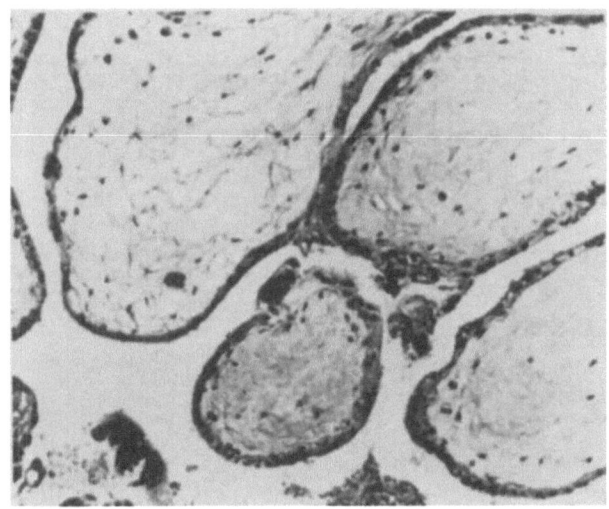

Fig. 30. Avascular chorionic villi with a edematous stroma (micromolar degeneration) in a chorion from a first trimester spontaneous abortion.

taneous first trimester abortions and occurs especially in abortions with such chromosomal aberrations, which are incompatible with embryonal survival.

As evident from the normal development, the uterochorionic (uteroplacental) circulation begins at the end of the second week. The embryochorionic circulation becomes established during the fifth week. The vascular chorionic primordia represented by endothelial cords, are present in the early chorionic villi prior to the beginning of the embryonal heart beat. However, during the fifth week of development, the further development of the vessels and the stroma of the chorionic villi depends upon the embryochorional circulation. (The trophoblast is nourished by maternal blood from the intervillous space.)

If the embryochorional circulation does not develop, embryonal chorionic vessels disintegrate and disappear. Consequently, the chorionic villi undergo micromolar degeneration. The complete micromolar degeneration of the chorion occurs in every conceptus where the embryo fails to develop or does not develop a functional heart. If the embryochorional circulation is stopped after being established (such as in incomplete artificial abortions week 6—8), the chorion, if retained within the uterus, may undergo micromolar changes if the uterochorionic circulation (uteroplacental circulation) remains preserved. In such cases, remnants of vessels still filled with blood may be distinguished within the stroma of the hydropic chorionic villi.

Usually, chorionic remnants retained within the uterus after abortion, or chorion from extrauterine pregnancies, undergo a different kind of degeneration because the uterochorionic circulation stops usually as a consequence of intervillous thrombosis at the same time as the embryochorionic circulation. If the uterochorionic (tubochorionic) circulation is disrupted, fibrin is deposited on the trophoblast and blood clotting occurs in the intervillous space. The stroma of the chorionic villi degenerates, but hydropic degeneration (edema) is not seen. A secondary inflammatory infiltrate

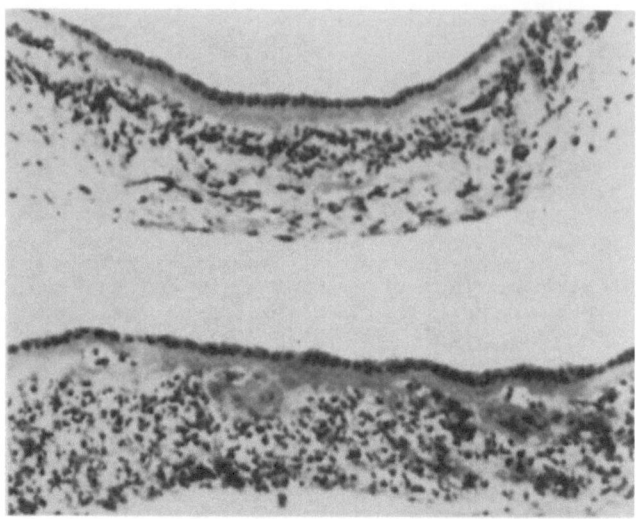

Fig. 31. Amnionitis. Inflammatory infiltrate in the amnionic stroma.

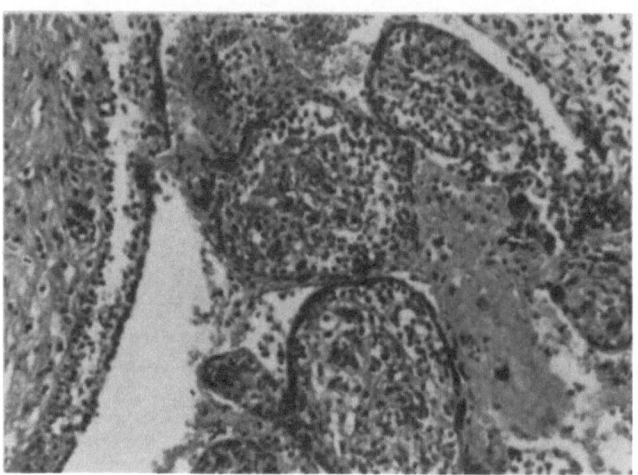

Fig. 32. Acute purulent placentitis. The stroma of the placental villi shows a massive polymor-phonuclear infiltration.

may be present. Extensive maternal blood clotting affecting the chorion and under-going organization, is known as the mola cruenta of *Breus* (1892). The degenerated product of conception, mostly only chorion, relates to the clinical syndrome of missed abortion, or to an extinct extrauterine gravidity.

CHORIODECIDUITIS AND CHORIOAMNITIS

Choriodeciduitis and chorioamnitis (Figs. 31, 32) occurring in the first trimester of gravidity is characterized by the presence of vascularized chorionic villi, fibrin deposition and extensive inflammatory infiltration, consisting mostly of neutrophil

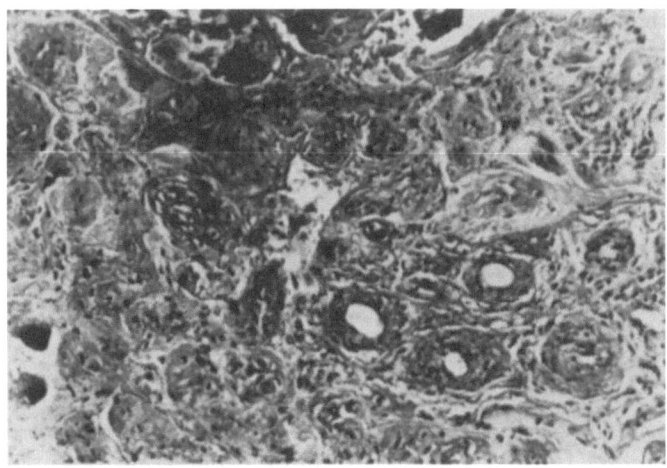

Fig. 33. Primary intervillous thrombosis. The connective tissue of the placental villi is viable. The fœtal blood vessels are patent. The intervillous space is obliterated, filled with fibrinoid.

leucocytes. Thrombi occur in the intervillous space. The decidua is infiltrated by both leucocytes and lymphocytes. Most such chorionic specimens come from septic abortions. In the midtrimester, choriodeciduitis usually develops after the membranes rupture; as usually seen in untreated women with an incompetent cervix.

PRIMARY INTERVILLOUS THROMBOSIS (PIT, WHITE PLACENTAL INFARCT)

PIT is characterized by an extensive obliteration of the chorionic, or placental, intervillous space (Fig. 33). The space between the chorionic villi is filled with thrombi, fibrinoid and fibrin (*Fox*, 1963). The connective tissue of the stroma of the chorionic branches and villi remains preserved for considerable time after trophoblast undergoes necrosis. The chorionic vessels are luminized but empty in most of the areas. Hofbauer cells may be recognized if the chorion is older than two months and less than nine months. The PIT is considered as a consequence of damage to the intervillous space, such as that occurring in soap-induced criminal abortions, or abortions done by intra-amniotic hypertonic saline.

CHORIONIC STROMAL FIBROSIS

Increase in collagen is observed within the placentae of fetuses showing growth retardation. Collagenic fibers are deposited along the paraaxial vessels. In some cases, sclerotic changes and obliteration of the chorionic vessels occurs. Obliteration of placental chorionic vessels must always be regarded as pathological. Deposition of collagen in the stroma of villi leading to the diagnosis of placental stromal fibrosis is sometimes subjective, depending on the pathologist's experience.

PLACENTAL INFARCTS (RED PLACENTAL INFARCTS)

Placental infarcts are composed of degenerating and partially necrotic chorionic branches and villi (placental villi) embedded within clots of maternal blood filling the intervillous space (*Bartholomew*, 1938; *Little*, 1960; *Sidall and Hartmann*, 1926). Most of the placental infarcts originate in consequence to obliteration of a para-axial artery in a chorionic branch. Some may be related to a primary intervillous infarction if the maternal veins draining the cotyledon obliterate. Obliteration of decidual arteries and veins frequently occurs in maternal diabetes and hypertension related to a kidney disease or in toxemia. Placental infarcts are never in consequence to the fetal intrauterine death.

Necrobiosis within the infarcts and some inflammatory infiltration around the infarcts are frequent. The most usual localization of placental infarcts is in the marginal zone.

PLACENTITIS SECONDARY TO INFECTIONS

Bacteria such as *Enterococci, Aerobacter, Proteus, Streptococcus faecalis,* or *Escheria coli* are frequently found in full-term placentae (*Morison*, 1963). The infection is usually preceded by a rupture of the membranes more than 24 hours before delivery. Bacteria proceed per continuitatem from the vagina in most of the cases. A typical accompanying histological picture is chorionitis and amnionitis. Inflammatory cells of maternal origin penetrate into the membranes and are stopped to a certain degree, by the thick basement membrane complex underneath the amnionic epithelium.

Hematogenic placental infections are more frequent during the second than during the third trimester of gestation. They are related to a severe maternal septicopyemia, such as that occurring in typhoid fever, etc.

LISTERIAL PLACENTITIS

The infectious agent is *Listeria monocytogenes*. In this infection, numerous miliary abscesses are present throughout the placenta resembling miliary tuberculoses. The miliary necrosis shows an excenssive inflammatory polymorphonuclear infiltration. Gram-negative bacteria are present within the lesions (*Potal*, 1958; *Dungal*, 1961).

TUBERCULOUS PLACENTITIS

Specific tuberculomas are more distinct within the decidua than in the chorionic or placental villi (*Warthin*, 1907). After the treatment by Streptomycin, INH and PAS was introduced, I did not see any tuberculous placentitis which could be diagnosed using morphological criteria.

SYPHILITIC PLACENTITIS

A syphilitic placentitis may occur if spirochetemia is present after weeks 16—20 of gestation. The early chorion seems to be resistant to the infection.

The histology of the syphilitic placentitis is rather unspecific, consisting mostly of perivascular chorionic infiltrates, endovasculitis and plasmocellular and lymphocytic infiltration. Pathognomonic is the demonstration of *Spirochaetae* by means of specific staining (*Dorman and Sahyun*, 1937). In recent years, I was unable to detect any placental *Spirochaetae* in patients treated with antibiotics.

60

TOXOPLASMIC PLACENTITIS

Toxoplasmic placentitis was documented only in cases of an acute maternal disease. The placental infection with *Toxoplasma gondii* is characterized by inflammatory infiltrates consisting of lymphocytes and monocytes. Characteristic toxoplasmic cysts are present in the connective tissue of the amnion and chorion (*Beckett and Flynn*, 1953). If the fetus is affected by hydrops, an extramedullary haematopoesis occurs. Erythroblasts may be present in chorionic vessels, similar to Rh incompatibility (*Bain et al.*, 1956). Two successive cases of toxoplasmosis affecting siblings of one mother were never documented (*Feldman*, 1963).

PLACENTAL PATHOLOGY IN METABOLIC DISEASES

Unspecific pathologic placental lesions, consisting mostly in the presence of "imma- ture" villi and vascular alterations are found in Rh incompatibility (erythroblasts may be seen in chorionic vessels), maternal diabetes and toxaemia.
"Immature placental villi" of a full term placenta exhibit Hofbauer cells and rem- nants of the cytotrophoblast.

Characteristic placental changes were observed recently (*Jirásek and Zwinger;* unpublished) in a case of familial mucopolysacharidosis 1 (Hurler's disease). In the placenta of a five month-old fetus diagnosed by amniocenthesis and biochemistry, numerous Hofbauer cells with an accumulated acid mucopolysacharide (stained by alcian blue at pH 2−3, after fixation in alcoholic picric acid and formol) were found.

PLACENTAL TUMORS

PLACENTAL CHORIOANGIOMA

Placental chorioangioma represents a vascular neoplasia consisting of endothelial cords and capillaries similar to those found in haemangiomas (Fig. 34). If the chorio- angioma is present within the chorionic plate, the tumor is not covered by the tropho-

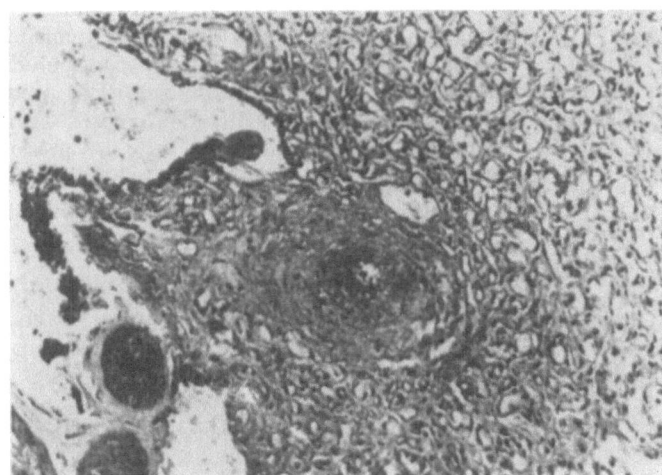

Fig. 34. Chorioangioma in a full term placenta.

blast. If the chorioangioma originates from chorionic branches (villi), the tumor is covered by the trophoblast. The frequency of chorioangioma is considered to be 1 : 245—250 term placentae. Some chorionagiomas were reported in cases associated with hydramnion, cardiovascular fetal abnormalities, and chronic fetal distress. Fetal mortality in pregnancies complicated by placental chorionangiomas is high (approximately 35%, *Decosta et al.*, 1956, *Strakosch*, 1956) due to the fetal bleeding into the intervillous space.

TROPHOBLASTIC DISEASE

Mola hydatidosa

Complete and incomplete hydatidiform moles are to be distinguished. In incomplete moles, the molar degeneration does not affect the entire chorion, and there may be some fetal survival ("moles with a living fetus"; *Uher, Jirásek and Šima*, 1963). In complete moles, the fetus is absent in most of the cases. Excessive hCG, produced by the trophoblast, is found in all patients with a trophoblastic disease. If β-hCG subunit is present in addition to hCG, the prognosis seems to be poor. In hydatidiform molar degeneration, the villi are avascular, edematous and contain fluid accumulated within a central pseudocystic cavity (*Hertig and Mansell*, 1956; *Hertig*, 1968; *Vojta and Jirásek*, 1965; *Hertig and Sheldon*, 1947). The frequency of hydatidiform mole is estimated in the U.S.A. and Europe as 1 : 2000 pregnancies. According to tropho-blastic proliferation and differentiation, hydatidiform moles were distinguished (1) without trophoblastic proliferation, (2) with proliferating differentiated trophoblast, and (3) with proliferating anaplastic trophoblast. If the invasion of the trophoblast into the myometrium is evident, a destruent mole (chorioadenoma) may be diagnosed (*Hertig*, 1968; *Novak*, 1950).

(1) *Hydatidiform moles without trophoblastic proliferation (with a degenerating trophoblast).*

Chorionic villi are transformed into multiple, grapelike-arranged pseudocysts of different diameters, ranging from 3—25 mm. The stroma of the degenerated villus, mesenchymatous connective tissue, lines the central cavity. The tropho-blast is thin, rarely bilaminar, usually formed only by trophoblastic syncytium (Fig. 35). Budding of the trophoblastic syncytium is frequently present. Small groups of cytotrophoblastic cells with pycnotic nuclei are observed. Big empty vacuoles found within the syncytium are considered to be related to a de-generative dysplasia rather than neoplasia. The presence of decidua around the hydatidiform villi suggests a good prognosis. Trophoblastic invaginations into the stroma of degenerating villi may be present. These invaginations are frequently observed in the triploid conceptus in which a hydatidiform molar degeneration of the chorion, sometimes incomplete, is a common fin-ding.

(2) *Proliferating hydatidiform moles with well-differentiated trophoblast.*

The stroma of the hydatidiform villi is similar in character to that in moles without trophoblastic proliferation. The proliferating trophoblast forms well differentiated syncytial lamellae, cytotrophoblastic columns and aggregates (Fig. 36). Anaplastic trophoblastic syncytium is not present. The prognosis for this lesion is favorable, but the patient is to be followed by regular hCG checks for at least half a year.

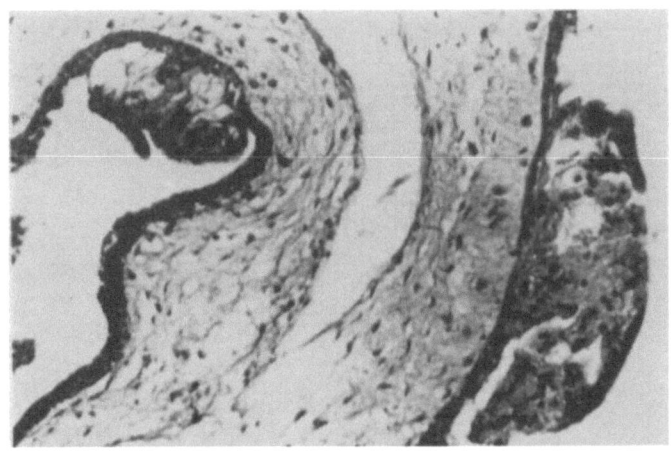

Fig. 35. Hydatidiform molar degeneration of a chorionic villus. A characteristic pseudocystic cavity is present within the stroma of the villus. Degenerative dysplasia of the trophoblast is evident.

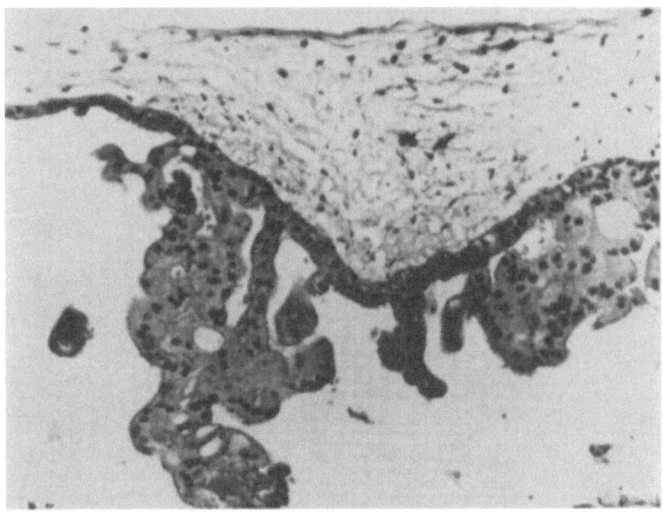

Fig. 36. Proliferation of a well differentiated lamellar syncytium (considered benign) on the surface of a villus showing molar degeneration.

(3) *Proliferating (invasive) hydatidiform mole with the anaplastic trophoblast and mola destruens (chorioadenoma destruens).*

Anaplastic syncytiotrophoblastic elements are considered to be characteristic of a malignant trophoblast. The anaplastic syncytium is "something between" the cytotrophoblast and lamellar syncytium (Fig. 37, 38). The anaplastic syncytium is represented by long thin elements formed around the cytotrophoblastic islets, or by irregular multinucleated flocks of syncytium with hyperchromatic anaplastic nuclei. The cytotrophoblast is multilayered with nuclei of different sizes (dysplasia of cytotrophoblast). The stroma of the villi exhibi-

63

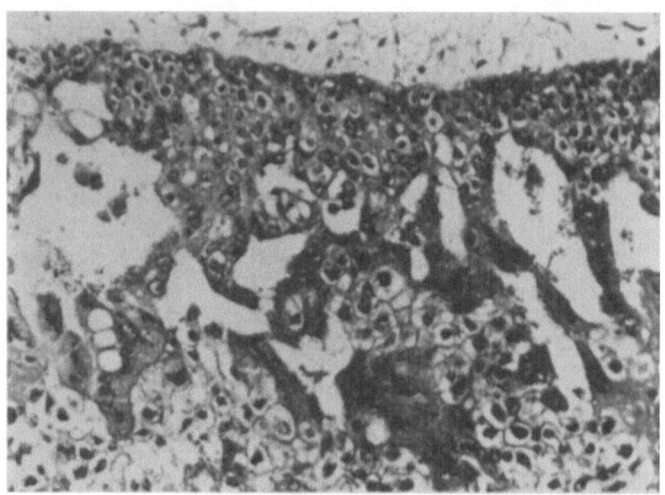

Fig. 37. Anaplastic proliferating trophoblast (considered malignant) in a proliferating mole. Anaplastic elongated syncytial trophoblastic elements with a basophil cytoplasm (arrow) are considered a characteristic of malignant trophoblast.

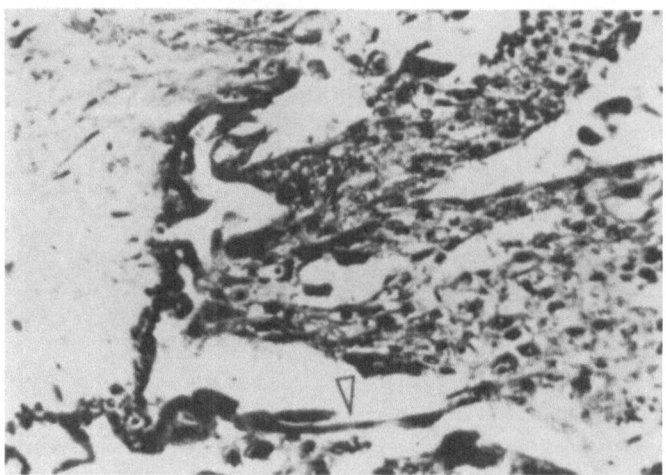

Fig. 38. Dysplastic trophoblast of a proliferating mole. The collumns of dysplastic cytotropho blast and irregular syncytial elements (con sidered as malignant) are present.

ting an extensive trophoblastic proliferation is usually degenerating, sometimes fibrotic but extensive edema and pseudocystic degeneration is rare. Decidua- lization of the endometrium, if present, is considered prognostically favorable. The final prognosis of a proliferating mole remains doubtful. The treated patient, after becoming hCG negative, has to be followed by hCG checks at six-week intervals for half a year and at two-month intervals for an additional half year. In frankly malignant moles, the trophoblast is morphologically very similar to that of choriocarcinomas, and the only difference between a malignant mole and choriocarcinoma is the presence of connective tissue stroma of the chorionic villi in moles. The prognosis for the patient is usually more dependent on how much of the trophoblast was left within the uterus after removal of the mole than on the histological character of the lesion.

Choriocarcinoma

Choriocarcinoma is formed exclusively by the malignant trophoblast. The tumor either follows a pregnancy, or may be teratogenic in origin. Teratogenic choriocarcinoma are found in ovaries (in children), in testes, or very rarely in some extra gonadal localization such as liver or epiphysis. The frequency of postgestational choriocarcinomas is regarded as 1 : 40,000 gravidities, or 1 : 17,000—20,000 deliveries. The incidence of the trophoblastic disease varies according to the geographical location. In Europe and in North America, choriocarcinomas are rare. In Southeast Asia, choriocarcinomas are among the most frequent malignancies. The frequency in Southeast Asia is considered to be 1 : 1,382 gravidities, in Hong Kong 1 : 3,708, in Taiwan 1 : 496 deliveries. In the yellow population coming from Southeast Asia to the U. S., the frequency of choriocarcinomas is low (*Iverson, 1959*).

It is supposed that most choriocarcinomas originate from the trophoblast of anchoring villi surviving after delivery or abortion. The malignant trophoblast of choriocarcinomas is formed by a solid cytotrophoblastic mass usually dysplastic, and by highly anaplastic syncytial elements. The malignant trophoblast, composed of cytotrophoblastic aggregates and present within a net of anaplastic elongated syncytial elements (Fig. 39), is known as the (malignant) reticular trophoblast (*Vojta and Jirásek*, 1965). Anisocytosis and anisonucleosis are very pronounced in the malignant trophoblast. Hemorrhages are frequent due to the characteristic trophoblastic vascular invasiveness. Necroses are regularly present because choriocarcinomas are avascular.

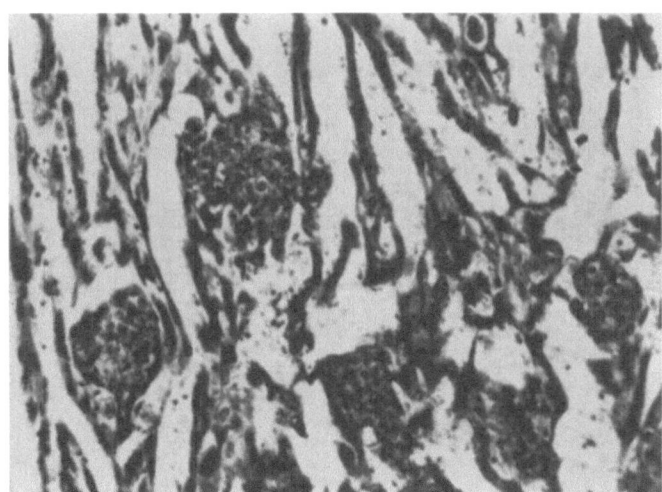

Fig. 39. Malignant reticular trophoblast of a choriocarcinoma. Islets of cytotrophoblasts are intermingled with elongated anaplastic elements of trophoblastic syncytium.

The metastases are frequent and early (*Hertig and Mansell*, 1956). Lungs are involved in 60%, vagina in 40%, brain in 17%, liver in 16%, kidneys in 13%, spleen in 9%, intestines in 9%, ovaries in 6% and lymph nodes in 6% of cases. Pancreatic, heart, skin and adrenal metastases occur in a frequency of approximately 1% of cases. Transplacental intrafetal metastases were reported (*Niercer et al.*, 1958).

Remission and even a spontaneous healing of choriocarcinomas were observed. The immunologic rejection of the trophoblastic tumor, because of the maternal tropho- blastic tissue incompatibility, was proposed in such cases. Most of the choriocarci- nomas do respond to cytostatic therapy (*Holland and Hreshchryshyn*, 1967). The syncytiotrophoblast is much more sensitive to cytostatics than the cytotrophoblast. The hCG becomes undetectable before all trophoblast is gone. In insufficiently treated patients, the "quiet" cytotrophoblast gives rise to a new malignant syn- cytium. In all treated choriocarcinoma patients, after they become hCG negative, an additional hCG regular checkup is necessary for at least a year. The prognostic value of the free β-hCG subunit determination was mentioned (p. 43).

Choriocarcinoma in situ

Driscoll (1963) found a small area of malignant trophoblast in a delivered fullterm placenta. The lesion was incidental, no metastases developed and the patient re- mained healthy. We observed a primary choriocarcinoma in a full-term placenta. The lesion was 1×1 cm, remarkably reddish. Detection by the obstetrician was the reason for the placental histological examination. The baby delivered was anemic. The lesion showed a malignant trophoblastic proliferation on the surface of fully vascularized villi (Fig. 40). The post-partum checkup of the patient was unremarkable with no clinical evidence of any tumor being present. Immunological determination of hCG was not available (1960). The patient came back six months after delivery, and subsequently died of a generalized choriocarcinoma.

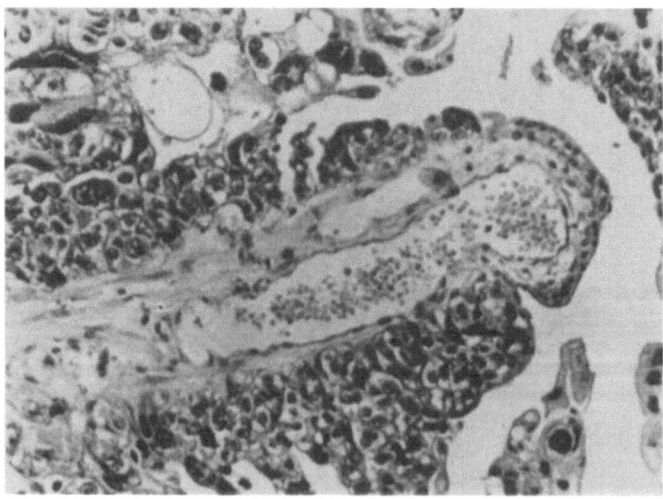

Fig. 40. Choriocarcinoma in situ. Proliferating malignant trophoblast on the surface of a nor- mally vascularized villus of a spontaneously delivered placenta.

Trophoblastic infiltration of the decidua and myometrium occurs physiologically in every pregnancy, and is known as the endometritis syncytialis or endometritis decidualis. Isolated trophoblastic giant cells and placental site cells are scattered in the myometrium, or decidua. There is always some inflammatory infiltrate around (*Hertig and Mansell*, 1956). Syncytial endometritis is not to be mistaken for a malignancy.

Trophoblastic deportation into various organs occurs in every pregnancy. Trophoblastic emboli into small lung arteries were found in 43% of women accidentally dying during pregnancy, in partum or puerperium (*Atwood and Park*, 1961). Trophoblastic deportation to the lungs, vagina or urethra commonly occurs. The deported trophoblast undergoes a spontaneous regression (*Schmorl*, 1905; *Hsu, Huang and Chen*, 1962) after delivery or after the removal of the mole. To distinguish a malignant trophoblastic metastasis from a benign trophoblastic deportation or infiltration, the scattered isolated trophoblastic elements in the absence of hemorrhages and necrosis, are regarded as benign, regardless of anaplasia sometimes observed.

PLACENTAL STEROID SULPHATASE DEFICIENCY

Placental steroid sulphatase deficiency is characterized by low maternal estrogen levels in spite of a normal fetus and fetoplacental circulation. Progesterone synthesis is unaffected, suggesting that cholesterol-3β-yl-sulphate and pregnenolone sulphate are not important for progesterone synthesis. The maternal serum and urinary estron and estradiol levels are approximately 15% of a normal level and estriol levels 5% of a normal level (at the end of pregnancy E_1 around 0.25 mg/24 hrs; E_2 0.1 mg/24 hrs; E_3 0.1 mg/24 hrs. (*France, Seddon and Liggins*, 1973). Urinary pregnandiol is normal. Fetal cord serum levels of 16-OH DHAS and pregnenolone sulphate are normal. DHA may be slightly subnormal. DHAS is not converted to estrogens by the placenta. In spite of abnormally low estrogen production, pregnancy proceeds normally and fetal growth and development are normal. In all (nine) reported cases of placental sulphatase deficiency, the sex of the baby was male.

Complication at delivery, due to the uterine cervix which remains "unripe" if the estrogen levels are low, may occur. Lactation is normal.

PLACENTAL INSUFFICIENCY

Placental insufficiency is a frequently misused term which should be used only in cases specifying the parameters of insufficiency. The low birth weight of a newborn is not adequate for the diagnosis of "placental insufficiency".

THE FETUS, FETAL MEMBRANES AND PARTURITION

The expulsion of the fetus during delivery is related to the uterine contractions. *McDonald et al.* (1974) observed that the contractions are consistently triggered by intra-amnionic administration of arachidonate, a precursor of prostaglandin F_2. It was also found that prostaglandins are accumulated within the amnionic fluid (*Hillier et al.*, 1974), in the fetal membranes (*Keirse et al.*, 1975) and within decidua (*Gustavii*, 1972).

During pregnancy, progesterone stablizes lysosomal phospholipase A_2 which is located in the fetal membranes and decidua. As progesterone production decreases before the onset of labor, free arachidonate is released from the phospholipids by phospholipase A_2. Arachidonic acid is a precursor of prostaglandins synthesized in the placental membranes and decidua.

We observed, after examining fetal membranes, that there is a constant degeneration of the amnionic epithelium (*Jirásek and Zwinger*, 1977) at the end of pregnancy. We stressed the hypothesis that degeneration of the amnionic epithelium is related to the distension of the amnion by accumulating amnionic fluid, and to the hypotonicity of the fluid. The hypotonicity of the amnionic fluid increases at the end of pregnancy because of the increasing amount of hypotonic urine contributed by the fetus. The hypotonicity of the fetal urine is related to the endocrine regulations of the fetal kidneys. According to our hypothesis, the low fetal secretion of AVP and increasing cortisol secretion by the fetal adrenal induce a "physiological fetal diabetes insipidus". The increased amount of fetal hypotonic urine makes the amnionic fluid hypotonic, damaging the amnionic cells and increasing the permeability of the membranes. The hypotonic amnionic fluid liberates the prostaglandins formed in the membranes and the decidua and uterine contractions appear. In this way, the fetus urinates through its way out of the uterus.

In anencephaly, where a low cortisol level results from the hypoplasia of the adrenal cortex (and ACTH deficiency), pregnancy is prolonged if hydramnion does not develop.

The "maternal way" of triggering parturition is mediated principally by oxytocin.

CHAPTER 4

FETAL ADRENAL

The adrenal gland is composed of two components of different origin and significance: a mesodermal cortex and a neuroectodermal medulla. The cortex of the adrenal, the gonadal interstitium and the trophoblast of the chorion are implicated in fetal steroid production. The medulla is part of the sympathetic nervous system and produce norepinephrine and epinephrine. Important contributions on the development of human adrenals were published by *Felix* (1912), *Uotilla* (1940) and *Crowder* (1957).

THE ADRENAL CORTEX

Development: The anlage of the adrenal cortex is formed by small primitive cells of coelomic origin. In embryos 35—39 days old (6—8 mm, S. H. XIV) some coelomic cells migrate from the primitive coelomic epithelium medially and cranially from the future genital ridge between the root of the mesentery and the mesonephric ridge. They penetrate into the underlying mesenchyme. In embryos 35—38 days old (7—9 mm, S. H. XV) they concentrate within the retroperitoneal mesenchyme ventrally and laterally to the aorta and medially to the upper portion of the mesonephric ridge. The blastematous condensation formed by small glycogen-rich cells is known as the adrenal blastema (Fig. 41). Although the adrenal blastema is in

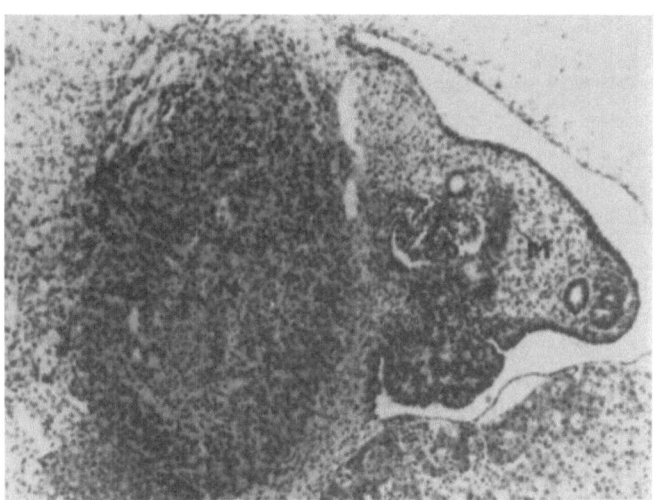

Fig. 41. Adrenal cortical blastema in a 15 mm embryo (S. h. XVII) and its relationship to the genital and mesonephric ridges. N — adrenocortical blastema, G — genital ridge, M — mesonephric ridge.

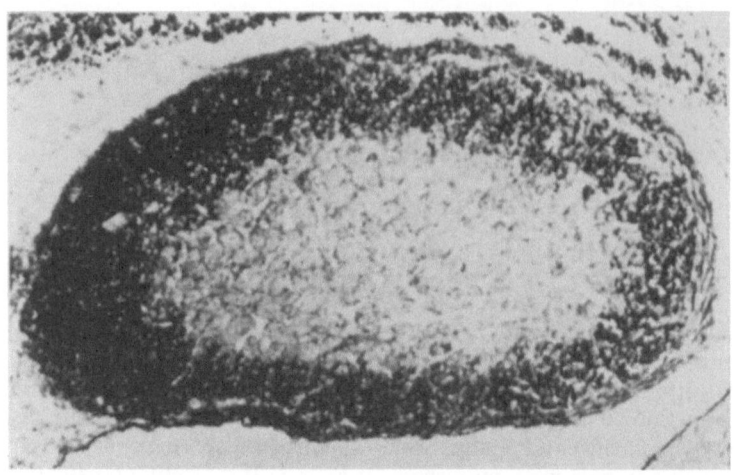

Fig. 42. Distributing of the glycogen in the adrenal of a 25 mm embryo (S. h. XXI, ca 53 days old). Large amount of glycogen is present in the blastematous subcapsular zone.

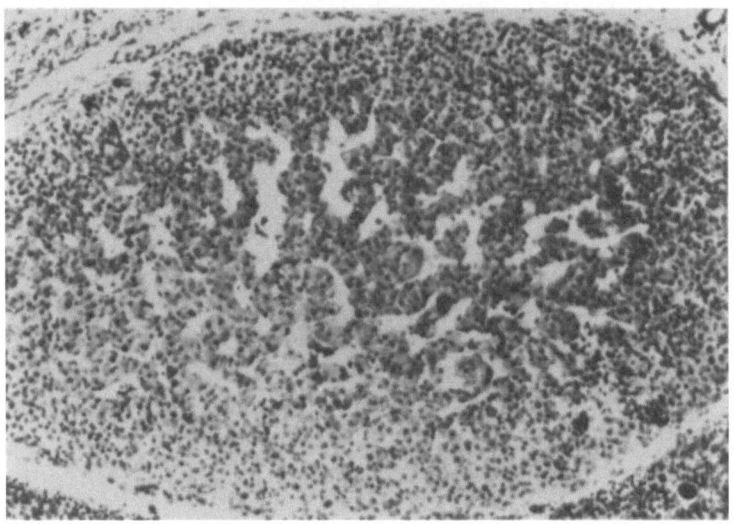

Fig. 43. Adrenal of a 25 mm embryo. The central zone of the adrenal consists of anastomosing interposed epithelial cords with capillaries. The peripheral (subcapsular) zone is blastematous composed of small poorly differenciated cells.

contact with the developing mesonephric nephrons, there is no mesonephric contribution to the adrenal (*Jirásek*, 1969). Some primordial germ cells are adjacent to the blastema. In 43—50 day-old embryos (15—20 mm, S. H. XVIII) the size of cells located in the central part of the blastema increases, and the cells differentiate into anastomosing epithelial cords. During migration from the primitive coelomic epithelium the cells contributing to the adrenal blastema contain alkaline phosphatase which disappears at the blastematous stage. The cells of the adrenal blastema are

Fig. 44. Adrenal cortex in a four month old fetus. The fetal cortex consists of a central (C) and intermediate (I) zone. The differentiated subcapsular zone (S) represents primordium of the definitive cortex.

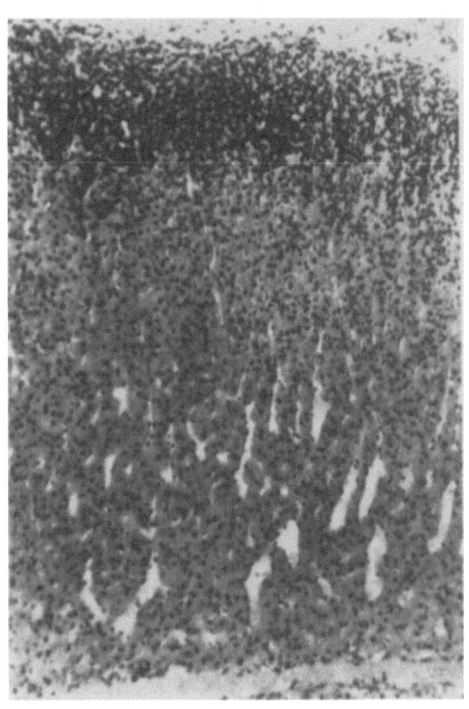

small and rich in glycogen. As they differentiate into epithelial cells of the fetal adrenal cortex, they become acidophilic. Acid phosphatase appears within the Golgi complex and the 3β-hydroxysteroid dehydrogenase can be visualized histochemically. They exhibit high activities of G-6-PD and NADP reductase. PAS-positive granules are located in the Golgi complex and a diffuse staining of cytoplasm lipids (as seen in an optic microscope) takes place (*Jirásek and Lojda*, 1960, 1964; *Vacek*, 1960; *Jirásek*, 1969).

In 50—54 day-old embryos (18—22 mm, S. H. XX), sinusoidal capillaries appear between the epithelial cords of the central zone and a connective tissue capsule differentiates around small glycogen-rich blastematous cells of the peripheral zone (Figs. 42 and 43). The blastematous peripheral cells proliferate and contribute to the epithelial cells. A zone of parallel cords is formed during the third month between the peripheral and central zone of the fetal cortex. During the third month the fetal adrenal cortex consists of three zones: a blastematous peripheral, an intermediate (fetal fasciculata) and a central (fetal reticularis). During the fourth month (Fig. 44), the subcapsular layer of blastematous cells differentiates into arcuate trabeculae of clear cells, which represent the primordium of the definitive adrenal cortex (See table 11).

Follicular-like structures containing PAS-positive homogeneous fluid are present within the definitive cortex primordium. Hypothetically, the differentiation of the fetal adrenal cortex from the indifferent subcapsular blastema might be placenta--(progesterone, hCG, PRL) dependent, whereas the hypophyseal ACTH secretion might turn the undifferentiated subcapsular blastema into the primordium of the definitive cortex. The fetal cortex represents the C-19 steroid metabolizing com-

Table 11. Development of the human adrenal cortex.

Stage	Blastematous	Early embryonal	Late embryonal	Fetal
zones	blastema (undifferentiated) →	blastematous (subcapsular) → ↓ central →	blastematous ↓ intermediate ↓ central →	arcuate - definitive cortex → intermediate ↓ central }fetal cortex
in	35—43 day embryos	43—54 day embryos	55—90 day fetuses	fetus four months and older
CR length	7—15 mm	15—30 mm	30—90 mm	90—360 mm

partment and the definitive cortex the C-21 steroid metabolizing compartment. The subcapsular cells of the definitive cortex are glycogen poor, exhibiting activities of NADP reductase, glucose-6-phosphate dehydrogenase and LDH. Histochemically, the 3β-hydroxysteroid dehydrogenase activity can be detected. The presence of the histochemically detected 3β-hydroxysteroid dehydrogenase is puzzling because little, if any, 3β-hydroxysteroids were detected in fetal adrenals using perfusion. In vivo, there is an inhibition of the 3β-hydroxysteroid activity in the fetal adrenal cortex.

Using EM, the cells of the adrenal blastema and of the blastematous peripheral zone have a poorly differentiated endoplasmic reticulum, numerous free ribosomes and glycogen particles. The cells of the fetal central and intermediate zone have a well-developed granular as well as agranular endoplasmic reticulum, a well-developed Golgi zone, and characteristic mitochondria with tubular cristae and an electrondense matrix. Lipoid droplets are present (Figs. 45, 46). The cells of the primordium of the definitive cortex in midpregnancy do not have the appearance of intensive metabolically-active, steroid-producing cells. They increase their mitotic

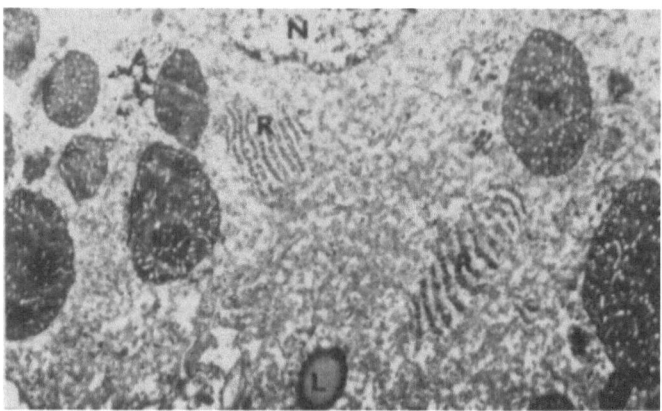

Fig. 45. Ultrastructure of a adrenocortical cell from the fetal zone. An abundant smooth endoplasmic reticulum is present. The mitochondria are charakterized by an electrondense matrix. N — nucleus, M — mitochondria, R — rough endoplasmic reticulum, L — lipid droplets.

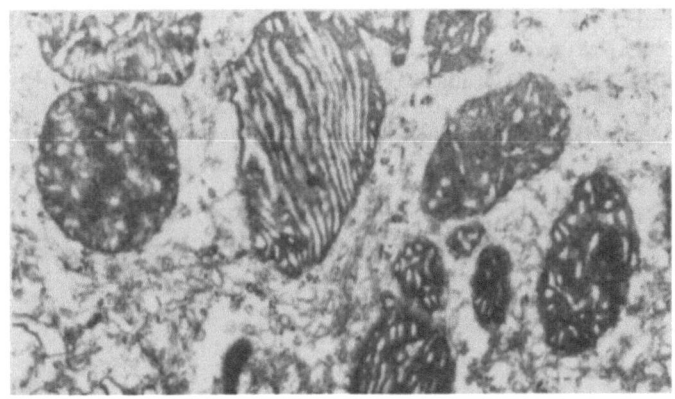

Fig. 46. Mitochondria of a fetal adrenocortical cell. Well developed tubular cristae and elec trondense matrix are evident.

activity after birth as the fetal cortex degenerates. Only the reticularis of the postnatal adrenals represents a derivative of the fetal zone. The entire reticularis disappears in early childhood and reappears before puberty.

THE ADRENAL MEDULLA

The adrenal medulla is principally a sympathetic ganglion. The evidence comes from the innervation by preganglionic nerve fibers. Chromaffin cells forming the medulla of the adrenal are sympaticoblasts which emigrated either from the neural crest, or directly from the neural tube (*Keen and Hewer*, 1927; *Ivanov*, 1927). Sympaticoblasts are first identified in paravertebral and paraaortal localization in the thoracic and lumbal segments of 8 mm embryos (35 days, S. H. XV). In 10 mm embryos (37—40 days, S. H. XVI), they concentrate near the blastema of the adrenal cortex. In 15—20 mm embryos (45—52 days, S. H. XIX—XX), they penetrate into the adrenal cortex, forming scattered islets of medullary tissue throughout the cortex. The fusion of the medullary islets into a single, centrally located mass occurs postnatally, after involution of the fetal cortex. Migrating sympaticoblasts of the adrenal medulla (Figs. 47, 48) differentiate into pheochromoblasts, and pheochromoblasts into phaeochromocytes. First, chromaffin granules, which are associated with the synthesis of norepinephrine, are present in pheochromoblasts of the medullary islets in 30—50 mm fetuse (week 9). Sympaticoblasts of the sympathetic ganglia develop earlier than those of the adrenal medulla. The differentiation of the extra-

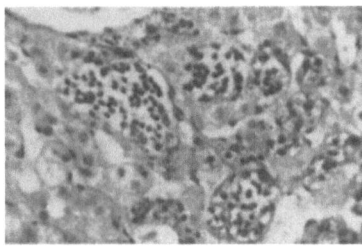

Fig. 47. Islets of phaeochromocytoblasts, representing primordium of the adrenal medulla, within the adrenal gland of a four month old fetus.

medullary sympathetic chromaffin tissue is complete in six month old fetuses (270 to 300 mm long). The extramedullary nodules of chromaffin cells in a para- and preaortic localization are known as the organ of Zuckerkandel. Other chromaffin ganglia are located adjacent to the large arteries of the neck and mediastinum and in the vicinity of gonads. The development of the chromaffin tissue of the adrenal medulla extends through the perinatal period.

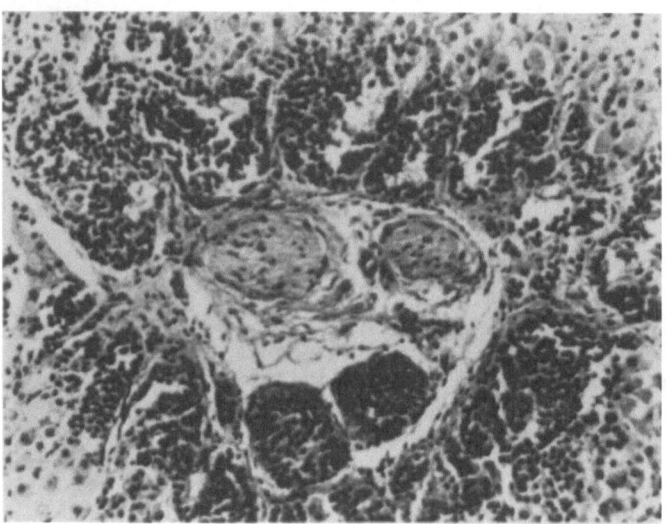

Fig. 48. Aglomerate of sympaticoblasts in the vicinity of unmyelinized nerves. Primordium of the adrenal medulla in a five months old fetus.

PRENATAL GROWTH OF THE ADRENAL

It is generally regarded that the fetal adrenals are unusually large. That is true only in relation to comparing the size of fetal kidneys. Until the end of the fourth month the adrenal is larger than the kidney, but later on the growth of kidneys is more extensive than is the growth of adrenals. At birth, the size of the adrenal is approximately one third of the kidney. Graph 10 shows the absolute and relative weights of the adrenal during prenatal development. It is remarkable that the relative weight of the adrenals during weeks 8—23 is stable, contributing approximately 0.4% of total body weight. In fullterm newborns at birth, the weight of both adrenals is 9 g and declines sharply thereafter. The average weight of adrenals in two or three month-old babies is 3.9 g. During the second year after birth the weight of the adrenals is 3.5 g (Lanman, 1962).

ACTH alone seems not to be responsible for maintaining the weight of the adrenals during the second half of pregnancy. In fetuses with hypophyseal aplasia, at six months the weight of the adrenals is about 50% of normal and at birth less than one tenth of normal. In anencephalics, the weight of adrenals is normal during the first trimester but declines thereafter (Benirschke, 1956). The adrenal hypoplasia in anencephalics at birth may be corrected by exogenous administration of ACTH (Lanman, 1961).

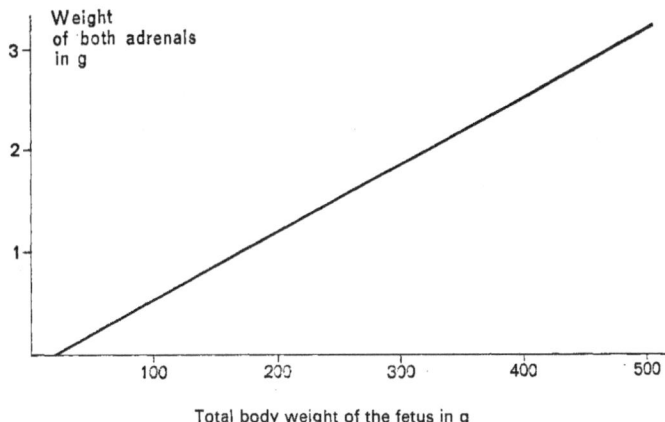

Graph 10. Relation between the weight of the fetal adrenals and total body weight

Weight of both adrenals in g

Total body weight of the fetus in g

ACCESSORY ADRENALS

Accessory adrenals commonly are found in human fetuses. They are present usually near the main adrenals in the vicinity of the plexus coeliacus. Their sites of localization include the kidneys (especially near the cranial pole under the capsule), the gonads (near the hilus), mesovarium or plica lata in females and the epididymis and the plexus pampiniformis in males (*Willis*, 1958). Accessory adrenals, if sought, are found in about $10-30\%$ of adults. In about 50% of accessory adrenals, only the cortical tissue is present. In 50%, both cortical as well as medullary tissues are found. In patients affected by adrenal hyperplasia, the accessory adrenals are always hyperplastic. Accessory adrenals develop from coelomic epithelium derivatives which do not reach the main adrenal cortex (*Jirásek*, 1969).

PHYLOGENESIS

The interrenal tissue, considered to be a homologue of the adrenal cortex, and the adrenal tissue homologue of the medulla, are first found in fish. In sharks, separate nodules of interrenal and adrenal tissue are present near the postcardial veins or at the segmental branches of the dorsal aorta, supplying the pronephros and mesonephros.

In Teleosts the interrenal and adrenal tissue are mixed, forming ovoid bodies adjacent to the cranial pole of the mesonephros. In lizards and in some reptiles, the chromaffin (adrenal) tissue concentrates at the dorsal site of the interrenal tissue. In crocodiles, interrenal tissue is embedded within the adrenal tissue. In mammals, as the metanephros becomes the definitive kidney, and as the mesonephros degenerates, adrenal tissue is embedded within the interrenal tissue forming the adrenal gland located above the definitive kidney. Nevertheless, remnants of adrenal (chromaffin) and interrenal tissue related to the development of the mesonephros are common in all mammals.

STEROIDOGENESIS IN THE FETAL ADRENAL

Cholesterol is found in large amounts in the fetal adrenal, and the fetal adrenal is able to synthesize cholesterol from acetate (*Bloch and Benirschke*, 1959). The amount of cholesterol reaches maximum at about twenty weeks, declining thereafter, especially at the end of gestation. The human fetal adrenal is able to convert cholesterol into pregnenolone, dyhydroepiandrosterone and other steroids (*Bloch and Benirschke*, 1960; *Telegdy et al.*, 1969). It is certain, however, that synthesized cholesterol is not the main precursor of the fetal adrenal steroids because of limited activities of the C-20, C-22 desmolase and 3β-hydroxysteroid dehydrogenase. Precursors of placental origin such as pregnenolone and progesterone are the main source of corticoids formed by the adrenal. As far as pregnenolone is concerned, it was demonstrated that in the fetal adrenal of 35 mm-long fetuses, 5% of pregnenolone 7-³H was converted into 17-hydroxyprogesterone and 55% into 17-hydroxypregnenolone. Androstenedione and 11-hydroxyandrostenedione were also formed (*Villee*, 1966). The steroid 17-hydroxylation is, in the fetal adrenal, very active and is immediately followed by the splitting of the side chain of the C-21 steroid, changing them into C-19 steroids. In other words, 17-OH-pregnenolone is rapidly metabolized to dehydroepiandrosterone. The conversion of Δ^5 3-hydroxysteroids into Δ^4 3-ketosteroids is very limited, suggesting a very limited activity of the steroid 3-hydroxysteroid dehydrogenase. Dehydroepiandrosterone is secreted by the fetal adrenal after conversion to dehydroepiandrosterone sulphate. The adrenal steroid sulfurylase is very active and pregnenolone and 17-hydroxypregnenolone may be sulfurized even before their conversion to dehydroepiandrosterone (*Villee and Loring*, 1969). In tissue culture, if pregnenolone is added to the medium, the activity of Δ^4-3β--hydroxysteroid dehydrogenase declines and the activity of hydroxylases increases, suggesting the dependence, repression and induction of the steroid enzymatic activities on the concentration of the substrate. These results suggest that the main steroid-forming compartment in the fetal zone of the adrenal cortex involves the formation of DHAS (and 16-OH-DHAS) from pregnenolone.

21-C glucocorticoids

Progesterone is mostly of trophoblastic origin because the fetal adrenal is unable to make progesterone since it lacks the active 3β-hydroxysteroid dehydrogenase. Within the adrenal, progesterone is subjected to hydroxylations. From eight weeks on, activities of C-16 and C-17 hydroxylases were documented; (*Villee*, 1961), C-21 and C-11 hydroxylases appear at the end of week ten and increase thereafter (*Wilson et al.*, 1966; *Bird et al.*, 1966). The significance of these hydroxylases is difficult to quantitate. Within the midtrimester fetal adrenal, when progesterone —4 ¹⁴C was administered, 39% of this substrate was converted to cortisol, 1% to corticosterone and 1.9% to 16-hydroxyprogesterone (*Villee and Driscoll*, 1965). The in vitro conversion of progesterone by the adrenals of a newborn was 33% cortisol, 17% corticosterone and 12% 16-hydroxyprogesterone. In experiments with pregnenolone, the amount of corticosterone formed by the adrenal of a newborn was 9.8% and cortisol 6.6%. It seems to be a shift to a lower cortisol — corticosterone ratio with the increasing fetal age. In the newborn, in the umbilical cord blood (*Eberlein*, 1965) and urine, the amount of cortisone exceeds that of cortisol. The amnionic cortisol levels reach an equilibrium at 24—25 weeks and remain stable between weeks 26—35. Fetal serum cortisol levels are 7.0 ± 1.2 ng/ml at 12—18 weeks, 24.0—4.5 ng before labor at weeks 38—40, and rise sharply during spontaneous labor reaching ca. 80 ng/ml (*Murphy*, 1973). Although cortisone and cortisol are formed by the fetal adrenal beginning at week 10, the synthesis of cortisol and cortisone de novo from acetate begins after birth after the involution of the fetal adrenal cortex. In pathological conditions such as in C-21 hydroxylase-deficient fetuses, progesterone is the main precursor of androgens. Androstenedione is formed by the adrenal of C-21 steroid hydroxylase-deficient fetuses starting in weeks 9—10.

The C-16 hydroxylation of steroids within the fetal adrenal is extensive affecting dehydroepiandrosterone, dehydroepiandrosterone sulphate and progesterone. Large amount of Δ^5-16 hydrolated steroids are present in the newborn urine, 16-hydroxy-dehydroepiandrosterone, Δ^5-androstenetriol and 16-hydroxyΔ^5steroids in the urine. Postnatally, in six month old babies, the C-16-hydroxyΔ^5steroids disappear.

The fetal central zone of the adrenal cortex produces mainly dehydroepiandrosterone sulphate beginning in the sixth week of gestation. 16-hydroxyepiandrosterone sulphate appears at 9—10 weeks, the fetal intermediate zone being the probable source. The primordium of the definitive cortex forms most of the C-21 steroids. There is no C-11, C-16 and C-21 steroid hydroxylation in the absence of adrenals (*Wilson et al.*, 1966). Most of the steroids leaving the fetal adrenal are water soluble sulphates. The inactive 3β-hydroxysteroid dehydrogenase represent a limiting factor for the conversion of pregnenolone, 17-hydroxypregnenolone and dehydro-epiandrosterone to androgens. The C-21 glucocorticoids (cortisol and corticosterone) represent the main steroid-forming compartment of the definitive cortex present in the fetal adrenal gland.

21-C mineralocorticoids

Fetal development occurs in an osmotically balanced medium provided by the mother. The placenta is freely permeable to small ions. Nevertheless, all the enzyme systems related to the formation of aldosterone are present early. The conversion of progesterone to aldosterone was documented in vitro using adrenals from a nine-week old fetus (*Dufau and Villee*, 1969). In perfusion experiments aldosterone was present in fetuses from the midtrimester (*Pasqualini et al.*, 1966). Steroidogenic compartments of the fetal adrenal gland are summarized in Table 12.

There are three systems controlling aldosterone secretion in adults: the renin-angiotensin system, potassium and ACTH. The effects of aldosterone and gluco-corticoids are of basic physiological significance.

THE EFFECTS OF ALDOSTERONE

In target tissues aldosterone binds to specific receptors within the cytoplasm, is transported into the nucleus and binds to chromatin (*Swaneck, Chu and Edelman*, 1970). RNA synthesis follows. Aldosterone was shown to increase nucleolar RNA polymerase activity (r RNA synthesis) relative to nucleoplasmic polymerase activity (m RNA synthesis).

The model for the of mineralocorticoid-induced transepithelial Na^+ transport suggests that Na^+ enters the cell across the apical membrane driven by the electrochemical gradient and is pumped out of the cell across the basal and lateral membranes by a magnesium dependent, Na^+, K^+ activated adenosine triphosphatase (NaK-ATP ase, *Skou*, 1965). Aldosterone (or aldosterone-induced protein) stimulates oxidative metabolism yielding an increased supply of energy for Na^+ transport. Increased cellular Na^+ entry is secondary to its increased extrusion.

Table 12. Steroidogenic compartments of the fetal adrenal gland (marked) in context of steroidogenic pathways

Main characteristics of fetal adrenal cortex: very limited 3β-OH-dehydrogenase, very active steroid sulphatase
active 17—20 desmolase (fetal zone), active 16-hydroxylase (fetal zone)
active 21 and 11 hydroxylases (definitive zone)

Main steroids produced: dehydroepiandrosterone sulfate, 16 hydroxydehydroepiandrosterone sulfate (fetal zone)
cortisol (definitive zone)

	(central zone)	(intermediate zone)	TROPHOBLAST
FETAL CORTEX	ACETATE		
	→ (CHOLESTEROL)		
	→ PREGNENOLONE (S)		
	↑		
	→ 17-OH PREGNENOLONE (S) → |DHA(S)|	↑ → |16-OH-DHA(S)|	
	ANDROSTENEDIONE → TESTOSTERONE		
	|ESTRONE|	↓ ESTRADIOL →	|ESTRIOL|
DEFINITIVE CORTEX	PROGESTERONE	17-OH PROGESTERONE	
	↑		
	11 DEOXYCORTICOSTERONE	11 DEOXYCORTISOL	
		↓ |CORTISOL|	
	CORTICOSTERONE		
	↓		
	|ALDOSTERONE|		

Many studies have demonstrated that renin-angiotensin levels and aldosterone secretion are parallel. In adults, renin is formed in the juxtaglomerular cells near the macula densa at the beginning of the distal renal tubule. Changes in blood pressure within the renal glomerulus are the main stimuli for the secretion of renin. The macula densa or the renal afferent arterioles are the baroreceptors sensitive to the beginning of the minute blood volume changes in the kidney and the changes in Na^+ concentration. Plasma potassium affects renin release also. A rise in the plasma potassium causes a fall in renin. Renin produced by the juxtaglomerular cells induces the transformation of the decapeptide angiotensin 1 into the octapeptide angiotensin 2. Although juxtaglomerular cells are present within the human fetal kidney (metanephros) from the eleventh week, the main source of renin within the fetoplacental unit is the uterus. The cells of extraplacental cytotrophoblast contribute most of the renin which accumulates in the amnionic fluid. Some renin may be produced also by the chorionic villi, the decidua and by the myometrium (*Symonds and Skinner*, 1968). The accumulation of renin within the amnionic fluid (present at week 11) is remarkable (*Brown et al.*, 1964). The angiotensin 2 derived from angiotensin 1 by renin represents the main stimulus for the secretion of aldosterone. Corticosterone, deoxycorticosterone, cortisone and cortisol are secreted to a much lesser extent. A hypotonic urine is produced by the fetal kidney beginning weeks 14—15. The contribution of urine makes the amnionic fluid hypotonic. The osmolarity of the amnionic fluid decreases until birth.

THE EFFECT OF GLUCOCORTICOIDS

Glucocorticoids have been shown to induce the synthesis of many specific proteins in different organs. Bound to specific cytosol glucocorticoid receptors (found in the liver, thymus, lymphocytes, fibroblasts, kidney, fetal lung and mammary glands), glucocorticoids are transferred into the nucleus. Increase in nucleolus RNA polymerase activity is largely responsible for the augmentation of ribosomal RNA synthesis by glucocorticoids. In response to the administration of glucocorticoids, the activity of several hepatic enzymes of the gluconeogenetic pathway was found to increase (glucose-6-phosphatase, fructose 1,6 diphosphatase, phosphoenol pyruvate carboxykinase). The increase in activities of some other enzymes is regarded as secondary to alterations in carbohydrate metabolism. The catabolic effect of glucocortocoids on lymphoid tissue, skin and adipose tissue is mediated through the decrease of glucose uptake (*Munck*, 1971), resulting in catabolism and cytolysis in some cells. It seems that during phylogenesis, glucocorticoids, which arose late in evolution in eukaryotic systems, have taken over many transcriptional functions of cAMP in low organisms. Glucocorticoids during ontogenesis are important for the appearance of some hepatic enzymes, lung surfactant and specific proteins of the retina, pancreas and mammary glands (*Tomkins and Martin Jr.*, 1970). Release of glucocorticoids is CRF ACTH mediated.

COMPARTMENTATION OF THE STEROID SYNTHESIS
IN THE ADRENAL

Different zones of the fetal adrenal, which are distinguished anatomically, possess different properties regarding steroid synthesis (*Seron-Ferre, Lawrence, Siiteri and Jaffe*, 1978).

The main secretory product of the fetal zones — central and intermediate — is the dehydroepinadrosterone sulphate (DHAS) and the 16-OH-DHAS. hCG can increase the production of DHAS (*Seron-Ferre et al.*, 1978). The main secretory product of the definitive zone during the fetal period are corticoids — corticosterone, cortisol and aldosterone to a much lesser extent. DHAS-forming cells disappear after birth and reappear in childhood forming the zona reticularis of the definitive adrenal. Postnatally, DHA and DHAS play the key role in triggering puberty.

ADRENAL ANDROGENS AND CONGENITAL ADRENAL HYPERPLASIA

Pathology: Two anatomical forms of adrenal hyperplasia may be distinguished-focal and diffuse. In the focal lipoid adrenal hyperplasia, the surface of the adrenals is nodular, and hyperplastic nodules are present within the cortex. The cells of the nodules are hypertrophic, containing cholesterol and other lipids within the cytoplasm. Inflammatory infiltrates and foreign body giant cells are present around the crystals of cholesterol. Focal adrenal hyperplasia results from enzymatic blocks in which cholesterol accumulates, such as deficiencies of steroid 20—22 desmolase and 3β-hydroxysteroid dehydrogenase (*Siebemann*, 1957; *Bongiovanni*, 1964). In diffuse adrenal hyperplasia, cells of the adrenal cortex, especially those of the inner fasciculata are hyperplastic — neither nodules nor inflammatory infiltrates are present. The adrenal cortical cells do not contain accumulated lipids and are vacuolized. Diffuse adrenal hyperplasia occurs in individuals with defects in steroid hydroxylations (C-21, C-11, and C-18 steroid hydroxylases).

In all forms of congenital adrenal hyperplasia the enzyme defect is inherited as an autosomal recessive trait. The low levels of secreted cortisol in adrenal hyperplasias are responsible for the pituitary ACTH hypersecretion. ACTH hypersecretion is the reason for the adrenal hyperplasia.

CLINICAL FORMS OF CONGENITAL ADRENAL HYPERPLASIA

1. Forms with insufficient production of all steroids (androgens, gluco- and mineralo-corticoids) affect the adrenal cortex as well as the testes. In males, insufficient fetal masculinization results in male pseudohermaphroditism. The complete blocks affecting enzymes necessary for the formation of pregnenolone from cholesterol (such as steroid C-20, and C-22 hydroxylase, and steroid C-20, 22 desmolase), or progesterone and androstendione from pregnenolone or dehydroepiandrosterone (3-β-hydroxysteroid dehydrogenase deficiency) are practically incompatible with a long survival because of extensive salt loss. If the block is incomplete and cortisol and aldosterone are produced, the affected child might survive.

2. Forms with excess androgens: In females, masculinization of the external genitalia occurs, leading to female pseudohermaphroditism.

a) Simple virilizing form of adrenal hyperplasia (adrenogenital syndrome) represents approximately 70% of all cases. A partial deficiency of steroid C-21 hydroxylase is present. Hypersecretion of ACTH normalizes the production of cortisol. The external genitalia in female infants are ambiguous.

b) Salt-losing virilizing form of adrenal hyperplasia is related to a complete steroid C-21 hydroxylase deficiency. This defect accounts for 25% of all cases affected by virilizing adrenal hyperplasia. The ACTH hypersecretion is unable to bring the cortisol production rate back to normal. The production of androgens is excessive, starting very early in ontogenesis (around week 10). The external genitalia in females usually show a severe masculinization, sometimes being male hypospadic, or even normal male in type in which an empty scrotum is formed. In both forms of virilizing adrenal hyperplasia, the plasma concentration of androstenedione is several times higher than that of testosterone.

c) Hypertensive virilizing form of adrenal hyperplasia. This congenital enzymatic block affects the steroid 11 hydroxylase (in about 3% of cases). Large amounts of desoxycorticosterone are formed which is related to hypertension. The malformation of the female external genitalia usually is not severe. Some clitoral hyperplasia is found in most cases. The increased blood pressure becomes evident at 10 years reaching $150-200/100-150$ mm Hg $(20-27/13-20$ kPa).

CONGENITAL ADRENAL HYPOPLASIA

Congenital hypocorticalism without hypoaldosteronism has been described by *Migeon et al.* (1968). The adrenals in the affected cases were very small and were composed only of a zona glomerulosa. The zona glomerulosa secreted aldosterone but was incapable of producing cortisol in response to ACTH. Although absence of an adrenal receptor for ACTH was postulated, the cause of the disorder remains unknown.

HEREDITARY ADRENOCORTICAL ATROPHY AND DIFFUSE CEREBRAL SCLEROSIS

Adrenocortical hypoplasia occurs in association with "sudanophilic leucodystrophy" of the CNS (*Forsyth, Forbes and Cumings*, 1974). The disorder affects only males, frequently siblings, sometimes in successive generations. An X-linked recessive inheritance pattern has been proposed. A manifestation of adrenal insufficiency usually preceedes the CNS disorder. The CNS disorder is fatal within a few years.

HORMONES OF THE ADRENAL MEDULLA

Hormones of the adrenal medulla are the catecholamines, norepinephrine and epinephrine. They are formed from tyrosine. Tyrosine is hydroxylated by tyrosine hydroxylase to dihydroxyphenylalanine (DOPA) which is subjected to dopadecarboxylase changing it into dopamine. Dopamine is converted into norepinephrine by dopamine oxidase. Tyrosine hydroxylase is the limiting enzyme in the production of norepinephrine. The hydroxylation of tyrosine occurs in mitochondria (*Nagatsu, Levitt and Udenfield*, 1964). DOPA is decarboxylated within the cytoplasm and dopamine is subjected to hydroxylation within the storing granules (*Von Euler and Hillarp*, 1956). Methylation of norepinephrine occurs within the cytoplasm. The intracellular amount of norepinephrine is proportional to the activity of the phenylethanolamine-N-methyltransferase.

The granules containing norepinephrine are membrane bound with an electron-dense outer portion, 150—350 μmm in diameter. They are present in the noradrenergic nerves in the CNS and within the chromaffin cells. They are rich in ATP and specific intragranular proteins, chromogranins and contain dopamine hydroxylase (*Hillarp*, 1959). Norepinephrine, ATP and proteins form a complex which is unable to diffuse. If norepinephrine is liberated, the corresponding amount of ATP is liberated at the same time (*Kirschner et al.*, 1966). The secretion of catecholamines is triggered by neural stimuli. Each chromaffin cell is innervated by a preganglionic cholinenergic nerve. Catecholamines disappear from the circulation very quickly. They are subjected to an enzyme-o-methylation occurring mostly in the liver and kidneys. The main sources for the circulating norepinephrine are the endings of sympathetic nerves as well as the adrenal medulla. The only source of circulating epinephrine is the adrenal medulla.

Norepinephrine was first detected within the paraganglia of 70 mm long fetuses (*Coupland*, 1952 and 1953) and within the primordia of the adrenal in 95 mm fetuses. Epinephrine was found within the adrenal medulla in 130 mm fetuses (*Greenberg and Lind*, 1961).

The presence of the phenylethanolamin-N-methyltransferase in the fetal adrenal medulla is still contraversial. The phenylethanolamin-N-methyltransferase is activated by cortisol (*Wurtman and Axelrod*, 1965). It has been suggested that at birth methylation of norepinephrine occurs in the abdominal paraganglia (organ of Zuckerkandl), but does not occur in the adrenal medulla. Both norepinephrine and epinephrine are present in the urine of newborns (*Stern, Greenberg and Lind*, 1961). Vasoconstrictions, affecting both arterioles as well as veins, elevation of blood glucose and of free fatty acids are regarded as the primary effects of peripheral catecholamine action. Body temperature increases as a consequence.

The physiology of catecholamines during the prenatal period is still largely unknown. At birth catecholamines are important for the newborn to survive the changes related to the transition from intrauterine to extrauterine life. Norepinephrine is necessary for the increase of chemical thermogenesis in newborns (*Stern, Lees and Leduc*, 1965).

CONGENITAL NEUROBLASTOMA

Congenital neuroblastoma occurs frequently in newborn children (*Kissane and Smith*, 1967). About 50% of these tumors originate from the adrenal medulla. The others arise in the sympathetic ganglia, in the peripheral ganglia present in abdominal organs and around vessels. Neuroblastomas are composed of small neuroblasts arranged usually in typical rosettes. There is no sexual predisposition (M1 : F1). Neuroblastomas in situ are found sometimes accidentally within the adrenal medulla of newborns (*Beckwith and Perrin*, 1963). Neuroblastoma was reported in a 28 week old fetus. If malignant, metastases are frequent. The prognosis of neuroblastoma is always uncertain.

CHAPTER 5

TESTES, OVARIES AND THE GENITAL SYSTEM

The developmental mechanisms involved in the differentiation of the genital system provide striking examples of linkage between genetics, immunology, morphology and endocrinology, and are of a basic importance for all of those who are interested in the study of reproduction.

PRIMORDIAL GERM CELLS

Primordial germ cells appear early in ontogenesis. *Hertig et al.* (1956, 1958) claim to be able to recognize a primordial germ cell within the eight cells of the inner cell mass (embryoblast) of a $4^1/_2$ day-old human blastocyst. Primordial germ cells are larger than somatic cells; they have a large round nucleus and a clear cytoplasm. Histochemically, they have a high glycogen content and show a high activity of the alkaline phosphatase.

Several authros were able to distinguish primordial germ cells incorporated in the endoderm of the hind gut or the caudal portion of the yolk sac in presomite human embryos (*Politzer*, 1928; *Florian*, 1931). Using glycogen stain, we were unable to distinguish primordial germ cells in a 13 day-old implanted embryo showing the primary yolk sac. They were distinct, however, in another presomite embryo with a chordomesodermal process (stage VIII, S. H.). At this stage, most of them are located within the endoderm of the hind gut (Fig. 49) near the cloacal membrane, or in the caudal portion of the yolk sac, and some of them are within the endodermal epithelium of the allantois. Primordial germ cells migrate by amoeboid movement into the mesoblastic gonadal primordia.

Their migration in human embryos was first traced by *Witschi* (1948) who also described pseudopodia (Fig. 50) of germ cells. Germ cell migration was later confirmed using alkaline phosphatase and glycogen stains. In the bilaminar embryos, alkaline phosphatase and glycogen are present within the endoderm, making identification of the germ cells very hard. In the trilaminar embryos, glycogen and alkaline phosphatase decrease in the endodermal cells of the gut and allantois, but remain high in the primordial germ cells. At the period of germ cell migration, in embryos 21—44 days old (S. H. X—XVII) the primordial germ cells are very distinct. In 13—20-somite embryos, germ cells are present in the endoderm of the hind gut and in the mesoderm and mesenchyme of the mesentery; in 25—28-somite embryos (27—30 days, S. H. XII) they are present in the urogenital ridge. In 7—12 mm embryos (35—42 days, XV—XVI S. H.), germ cells are present in a retroperitoneal

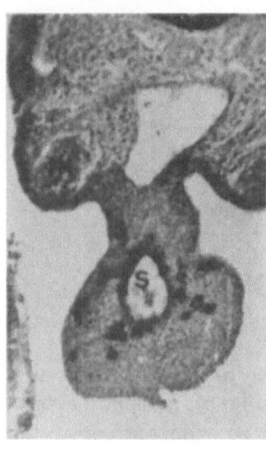

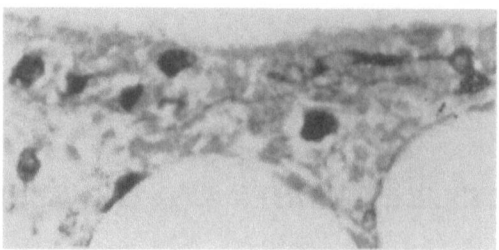

Fig. 49. Migrating primordial germ cells in a 3.5 mm human embryo (28 days, S. h. XII).

Fig. 50. Migrating primordial germ cells (dark) within and undernieth the epithelium of the urogenital ridge. Long processi (pseudopodia) of the cells are evident.

area ventral to the dorsal aorta, caudal to the primordia of the diaphragm, near or within the primordia of the adrenal glands and abdominal paraganglia and along the genital cord. Many of them are within the urogenital ridges and some are still located within the gut. After the formation of the genital ridges (stage XVI—XVII, S. H.; 40—44 days old) primordial germ cells can be classified as either genital or extragenital.Genital primordial germ cells are the only source of all spermatogonia or oogonia. Extragenital germ cells disappear after the eigth week of intrauterine development, during the early fetal period. We did not observe any differences regarding number, shape, alkaline phosphatase activity, glycogen content and migratory pattern of the primordial germ cells in 46,XY and 46,XX human embryos (*Jirásek*, 1971). Primordial germ cells were first described by *Waldeyer* (1870). Their extragenital location before the onset of gonadal differentiation was stressed by *Balfour* (1878) and *Nussbaum* (1880). In 1885, *Weismann* proposed the theory of germ plasm continuity which suggests that germ cells segregate during cleavage from the somatic cells and are passed from one generation to the other, whereas the somatic cells die. In such a way, the plasm of the germ cells was said to be "immortal" (to a certain degree). In amphibians, *Blacker* (1959) has detected areas of a special germ cytoplasm in the zygote only 40 minutes after sperm penetration.

Blandau et al. (1963) confirmed the amoeboid movement of primordial germ cells by a direct observation in vitro. In birds and in some reptiles (*Tribe and Brambell*, 1932; *Simon*, 1957), primordial germ cells migrate in vascular channels. In mammals, this vascular migration seems to be exceptional. In the cattle freemartin, where fetuses of opposite sex share a common circulation, however, *Ohno and Gropp* (1965) believe that the male germ cells may migrate from the male co-twin into the gonads of the female co-twin.

THE INDIFFERENT GONAD (GENITAL RIDGE)

Both the testes and the ovaries originate from a common primordium known as the genital ridge. The genital ridge becomes evident on the medioventral surface of the urogenital ridge (Wolffian body) in embryos 35—42 days old (7—12 mm,

Fig. 51. Indifferent gonad (G) in a 11 mm long (40 days old, S. h. XVI) embryo. The basement membrane of the surface epithelium of the mesonephric ridge ends laterally to the genital ridge. The genital ridge (G) is formed by the genital blastema containing blastematous cells of coelomic origin, primordial germ cells and some mesenchymal cells.

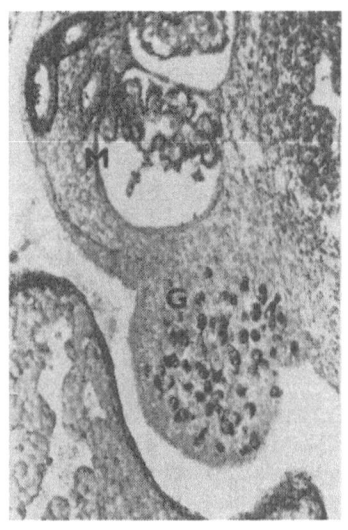

XV—XVI S. H.). The urogenital ridges (one on each side) containing mesonephric nephrons and the mesonephric duct embedded in mesenchyme, bulge from the dorsal body wall parallel to the mesentery into the peritoneal cavity. The upper end of each ridge reaches the primordium of the diaphragm and descends with the diaphragm. The caudal end becomes attached to the future inguinal area. The surface of the urogenital ridge is covered by a mesoblastic epithelium. The term "mesoblastic epithelium" is used for a primitive coelomic epithelium not separated from the underlying mesenchyme. In embryos 37—40 days old (9 to 12 mm, S. H. XVI) a distinct argyrophil basement membrane develops under the epithelium covering the lateral surface of the urogenital ridge.

The primitive coelomic (mesoblastic) epithelium on the ventromedial surface of the urogenital ridge (future genital ridge) begins to proliferate. Primitive germ cells which immigrated to the medioventral portion of the urogenital ridge become incorporated into the proliferating mesoblast. The medioventral surface of the urogenital ridge elevates, dividing the original urogenital ridge into a genital ridge medially, and a mesonephric ridge lateraly (Fig. 51). The cellular condensation representing the genital ridge is known as the gonadal blastema (*Jirásek*, 1971). The gonadal blastema is formed by (1) primitive coelomic (mesoblastic) cells, (2) primordial germ cells, and (3) mesenchymal cells located originally in the interstitium of the urogenital ridge.

The cells of the gonadal blastema originating from the coelomic epithelium or from the underlying urogenital (mesonephric) mesenchyme are undistinguishable. Some authors consider the genital blastema as an epithelium (*Nagel*, 1889; *Broman*, 1911; *Stieve*, 1930), others as a mesenchymal condensation (*Fischel*, 1930; *Pinkerton et al.*, 1961). According to the first group, all the gonadal components, except interstitial connective tissue, are epithelial in origin. According to the second group, everything within the gonads, except primordial germ cells, is mesenchymal. The genital blastema actually is a condensation of primitive cells which can differentiate either into an epithelium or into a special gonadal mesenchyme. Testicular surface epithelium, seminiferous cords and rete cords, as well as the ovarian surface epithelium, granulosa cells and the ovarian rete are epithelial derivatives. Leydig cells and the loose testicular interstitium are special mesenchymal derivatives. The ovarian stroma represents a mixture of both a special gonadal mesenchyme and an ubiquitous connective tissue mesenchyme. The tunica albuginea of testis or ovary, the testicular septa, and the connective tissue of the rete testis, are derivatives of a connective tissue mesenchyme.

DEVELOPMENT OF THE TESTIS

EMBRYONAL TESTIS

In the presence of the genetic masculinizing determinant (H-Y antigen), the indifferent gonad develops into the embryonal testis. In 43—49 day-old, 46,XY embryos (14—20 mm, S. H. XVIII) the gonadal blastema becomes divided into

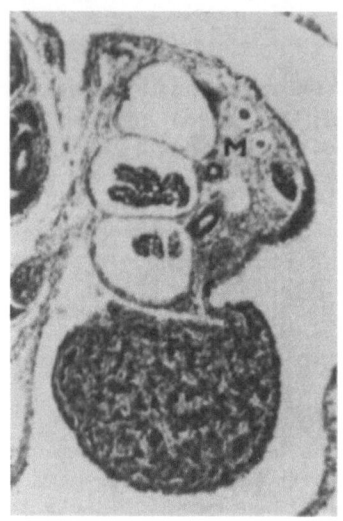

Fig. 52. Embryonal testis in a 15 mm (44 days old, S. H. XVIII) embryo. The testicular cords are evident. M — mesonephric ridge.

cords by thin basement membranes formed underneath the primitive Sertoli cells (Fig. 52). During the short period of the testicular cord formation, the primordial germ cells become irregular shaped; they temporarily lose alkaline phosphatase and glycogen and become incorporated into the testicular cords (Fig. 53). Soon after the cords make their appearence, connective tissue fibroblasts and reticular fibers become evident between the testicular cords. Differentiation of this mesenchymal tissue of the embryonal testis interstitium is closely related to the regression of the ipsilateral Mullerian duct (*Jirásek*, 1966, 1970, 1976). The deepest portions of the testicular cords communicate in an area forming the rete testis. (Fig. 54). The rete cords contact the epigenital mesonephric nephrons (urogenital junction). Fibroblasts from the mesenchyme of the mesonephric ridge contribute the connective tissue of the testicular mediastinum. As the testicular cords become separated from the surface epithelium, the primitive mesenchymal tunica albuginea becomes evident. The germ

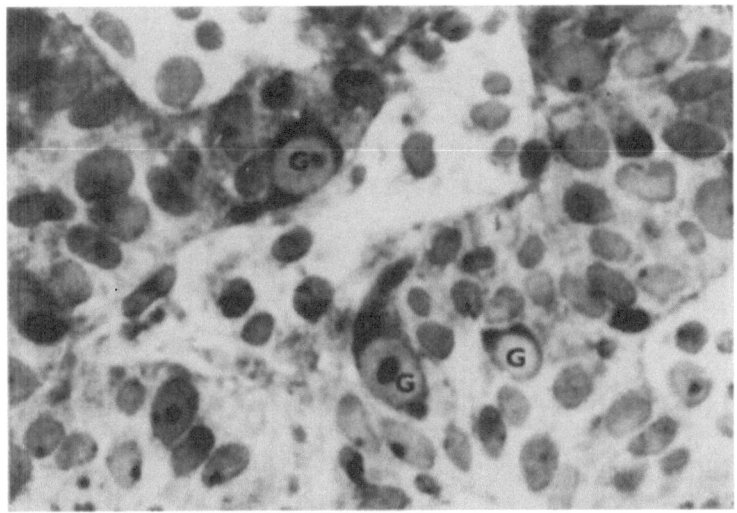

Fig. 53. Primordial germ cells incorporated within the testicular cords are known as spermato-gonia.Embryonal testis, embryo 24 mm long (52days old, S. h. XXI).

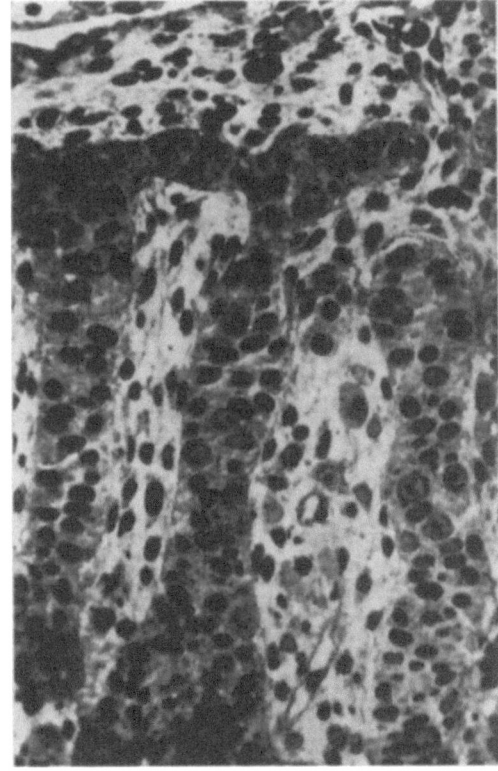

Fig. 54. Section through the embryonal testis. Primordia of the rete cords and of the seminiferous cords are evident.

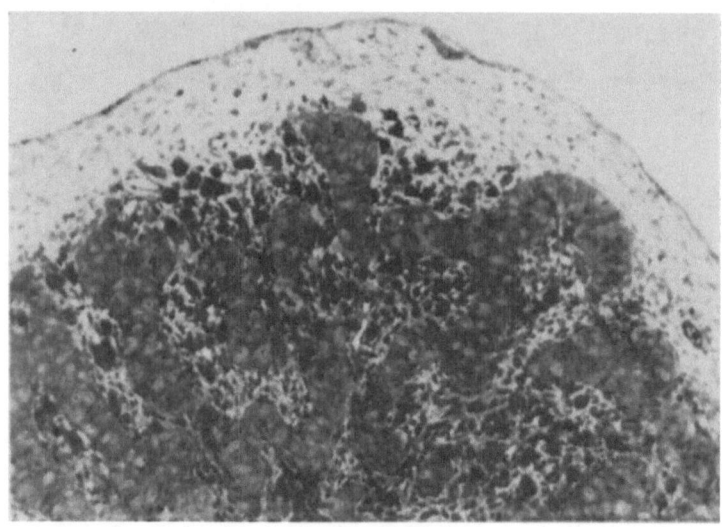

Fig. 55. Fetal testis. Epithelioid intersicial (Leydig) cells are present. (Dark cells in the intersti-cium between the cords.) 40 mm fetus, 9 weeks old.

cells located within the testicular cords are known as the spermatogonia. Germ cells incorporated within the surface epithelim are called secondary germ cells. There are no epithelioid (Leydig) cells in the embryonal testis. No 3β-hydroxysteroid dehydrogenase can be detected in any structure of the embryonal testis, suggesting that no androgens are formed at this stage.

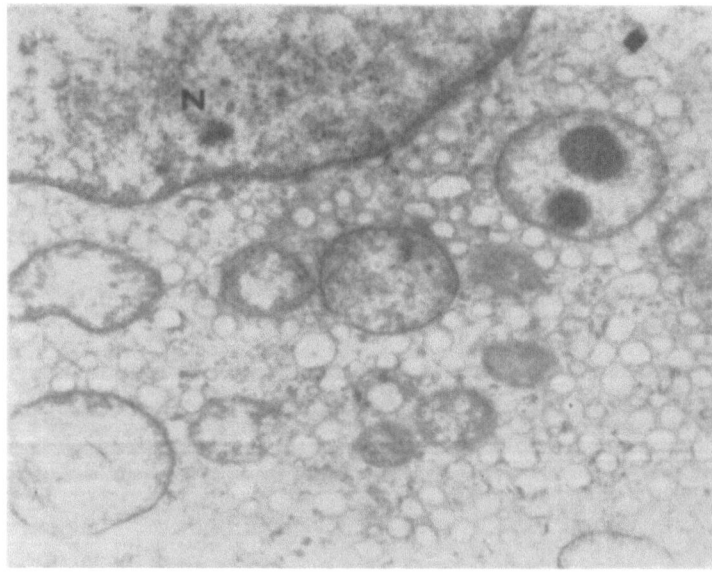

Fig. 56. Ultrastructure of the fetal epithelioid intersticial cell. Abundant smooth endoplasmic reticulum is evident in the cytoplasm. N — nucleus.

FETAL TESTIS

Embryonal testes develop into fetal testes as soon as epithelioid interstitial cells differentiate and androgen (androstenedione) production begins. Using the indirect peroxidase technique, we were able to show (*Jirásek*. 1971) that diffrentiation of

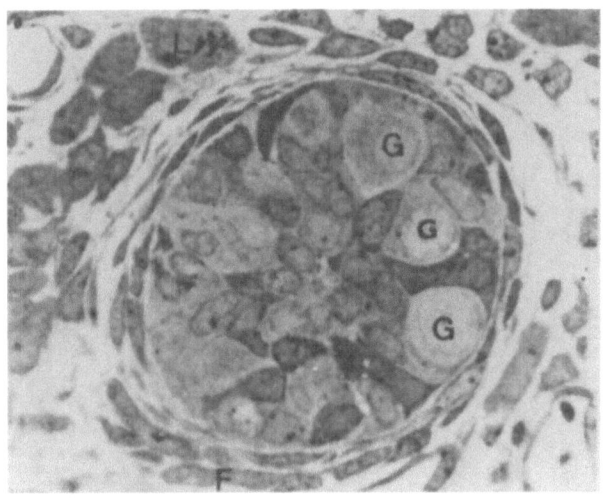

Fig. 57. Seminiferous cord containing spermatogonia (G) and im mature Sertoli-cells, fibroblasts of the lamina propria of the cord (F) and Leydig cells (L) in a fetal testis from a 12 weeks old fetus.

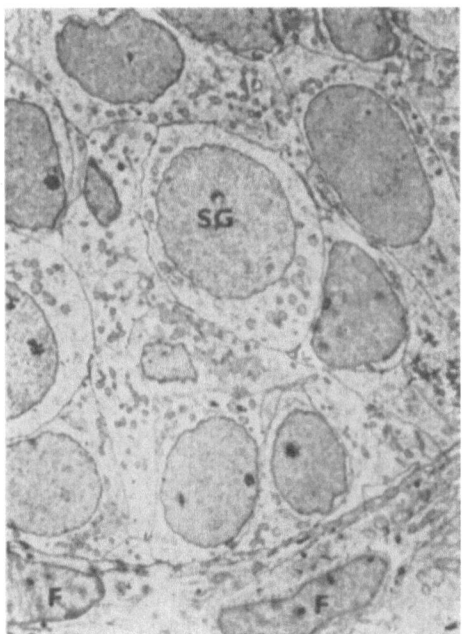

Fig. 58. Ultrastructure of the seminiferous cord. SG — spermatogonia, F — fibroblasts in the lamina propria (Photograph by Dr Semecký).

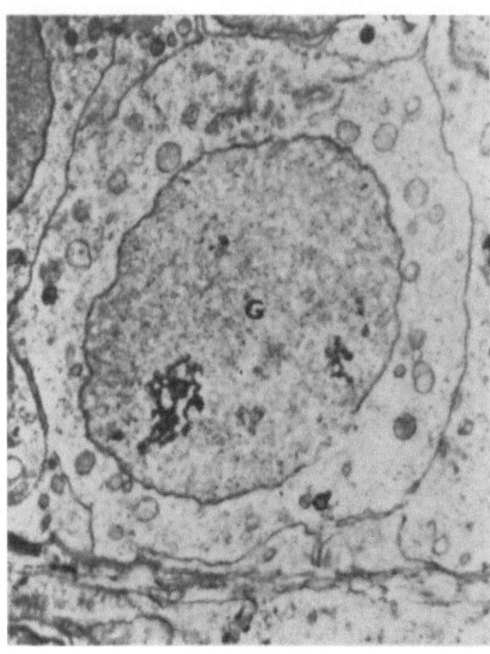

Fig. 59. The spermatogonia is adjacent to the basal membrane and is relatively poor in organells (Photograph by Dr Semecký).

the interstitial cells is accompanied by hCG binding to their cellular membranes. Fetal Leydig cells originate from the fibroblast-like cells of the testicular interstitium (Fig. 55). The first of them appear in 56—60 day-old embryos (30 mm, S.H.XXIII). Early epithelioid Leydig cells contain P. A. S.-positive granules and acid phosphatase in the Golgi complex, lipids, 3β-hydroxysteroid dehydrogenase and G-6-PD (*Jirásek*, 1967).

Abundant smooth endoplasmic reticulum (Fig. 56), a well-developed Golgi complex and tubular mitochondria are present (*Pellinimei and Niemi*, 1969). Fetal Leydig cells are able to convert dehydroepiandrosterone into androstenedione and testosterone. Androstenedione and testosterone production by the fetal testis was proven by several authors (*Acevedo et al.*, 1963; *Bloch*, 1964; *Rice et al.*, 1966; *Jirásek et al.*, 1969; *Serra et al.*, 1970). Fetal androgens are responsible for the growth of male genital ducts (epididymis, vasa deferentia), prostate and for the masculinization of external genitalia (*Jirásek, Uher, Raboch*, 1968). The number of fetal Leydig cells reaches a maximum by the end of the third month, declining threafter until birth.

From the third month until birth, the seminiferous tubules increase in length and size becoming coiled and thickened. They contain 8—10 layers of primitive Sertoli cells and spermatogonia (Figs. 57, 58, 59), dividing mitotically. Maturation of Sertoli cells, differentiation of spermatocytes and lumininzation of the seminiferous cords do not occur during the prenatal period. Cords of the rete testis and the adjacent portions of the seminiferous cords, giving rise to the straight parts of seminiferous tubules, become luminized in the last third of intrauterine life.

The connective tissue of the testes, a mesenchymal derivative, forms a dense tunica albuginea, septa of testicular lobules, connective tissue of the mediastinum testis and membranae propriae of each seminiferous cord.

After surface epithelium becomes separated from the testicular cords, some primordial germ cells are still present within the surface epithelium. These cells were called secondary germ cells (*Gruenwald*, 1934; *Jirásek*, 1960). In fetal testes, they are present until the sixth month. Transitional stages between flat surface epithelial cells and secondary germ cells were observed (*Jirásek*, 1960, 1971). They may be significant for the histogenesis of the ovotestis. Embryonal and fetal testes descend from the lumbar area as the mesonephric ridges degenerate and as the cranial mesonephric ligament disappears. The caudal mesonephric ligament representing a mesenchymal cord connecting the mesonephric ridge with the labioscrotal swelling, turns (in males) into the gubernaculum testis. As the trunk of the embryo and fetus elongates, the testes descend to the inguinal region. During the third month, a peritoneal evagination — the vaginal process — forms on each side along the gubernaculum testis. The vaginal process is accompanied by all muscular and facial layers of the ventral body wall. The inguinal canal is formed during the sixth month. Until the seventh month, the testes are located intraabdominally, near the inguinal canal. The gubernaculum shortens, pushing the testes into the scrotum. During the seventh month, testes are located within the inguinal canal reaching the scrotum approximately a month later. During the descent, the testes always remain in a retroperitonel position. The final stage of testicular descent is hormone-dependent and may be influenced by hCG, androgens and prolactin (*Rajfer and Walsh*, 1977).

After birth, Leydig cells disappear. Inactive or prepubertal testes in childhood represent a stage when neither testicular hormones nor germ cells are produced. With the onset of puberty, the interstitial epithelioid Leydig cells become differentiated (at approximately the age of 8 years) mitotic activity of the spermatogonia appears, seminiferous tubules become luminized and spermatocytes appear, starting meiotic divisions. Spermatozoa are present at the age of about 12—14 years. A normal adult testis shows luminized seminiferous tubules lined by germinal epithelium containing spermatogonia, spermatocytes, praespermatids, spermatids and spermatozoa. Leydig cells are present in the interstitium.

The prenatal development of the testis is closely related to the regression of the paramesonephric duct (embryonal testis) and masculinization of the external genitalia (fetal testis, *Jost*, 1948 — rabbit; *Jirásek*, 1966, 1968, 1978 — man).

DEVELOPMENT OF THE OVARY

In 46,XX embryos, the transformation of the undifferentiated gonad into the "embryonal" ovary occurs in 50—55 day-old embryos (S. H. XX—XXII, 18—25 mm). During ovarian development, the gonadal blastema differentiates into the interstitial connective tissue and into an epithelial component containing numerous, mitotically-active, primordial germ cells (Fig. 60). From the gonadal blastema, the so-called "ovarian rete cords" and "medullary cords" are formed (Fig. 61). The ovarian cortical cords result from the intensive proliferation of the primordial germ cells localized at the surface, mostly underneath the epithelium of the embryonal ovary (Fig. 62). The surface epithelium of the embryonal ovary is only incompletely separated by a basement membrane and by reticular fibers from the cortical cords (Fig. 63). The rete cords formed predominantly by primitive small praegranulosa cells (but also containing primordial germ cells) contact the adjacent mesonephric

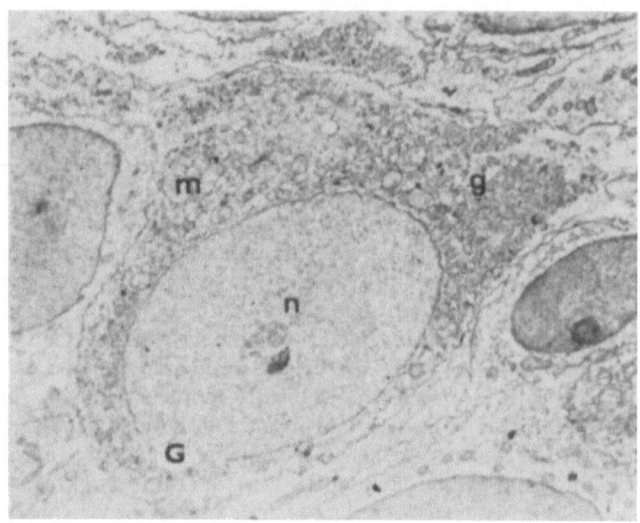

Fig. 60. Ultrastructure of a primordial germ cell (G) — oogonia — within the embryonal ovary. The cytoplasm is loaded with glycogen (g). m — mitochondria, n — nucleus (by Dr. Semecký).

nephrons. The medullary cords, irregular in shape and separated by areas of loose reticular connective tissue, contain small primitive praegranulosa cells in addition to numerous oogonia. The cortical cords are thick, irregular, roundshaped and incompletely separated from the surface epithelium by a thin primitive tunica albuginea. The cortical cords predominantly contain oogonia (Fig. 64). The term oogonia, in the embryonal ovary, refers to the primordial germ cells incorporated within the medullary and cortical cords. The cortical cords of the human ovary do not originate from an ingrowth of the surface epithelium but rather from an intensive mitotic proliferation of oogonia in situ.

The cortical area of the embryonal ovary was called the neogenic zone (*Felix*, 1912). Contrary to the testicular primordial germ cells which temporarily lose their alkaline phosphatase and glycogen during the stage when they become incorporated into the testicular cords the ovarian germ cells do not change during differentiation of the embryonal ovary (*Pinkerton et al.*, 1961). No cells containing the 3β-hydroxysteroid dehydrogenase are present in the embryonal ovary (*Jirásek et al.*, 1969; *Brandau and Lehmann*, 1970). There is no evidence of any hormonal activity of the embryonal ovary.

EARLY FETAL OVARY

In fetuses 8—9 weeks old, some medullary oocytes start the prophase of the first meiotic division (Fig. 65). The DNA is replicated in the oogonia after their last mitosis (as is normal). At the leptotene stage of the meiotic prophase, the chromosomes appear as fine individual threads; in the zygotene stage, the fine, uncoiled, homologous chromosomes pair. In the pachytene stage, the chromosomes arraned in pairs become shorter and thicker as a result of coiling, and each chromosome

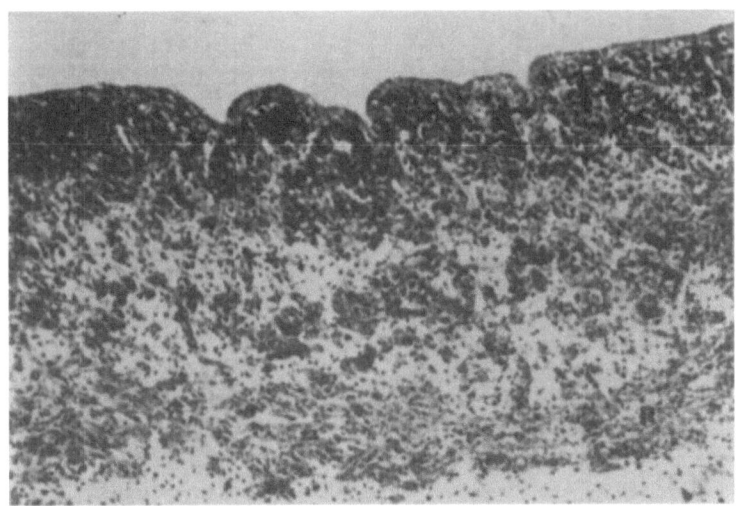

Fig. 61. Embryonal ovary of a 25 mm embryo (54 days old, S. h. XXII). The surface epithelium with the cortical zone (C), the medullary zone (M) and the rete zone (R) are evident.

splits longitudinally into two chromatids (tetrad formation). Crossing over occurs and chromatids are exchanged at this stage. At the diplotene stage, the two split-chromosomes separate except at chiasmata — that is, at places where chromatids have crossed. In the diplotene stage, the meiosis of the oocyte stops and meiosis does not proceed for about 12—50 years. The first meiotic metaphase and telophase takes place in adult women shortly before ovulation. The second meiotic division

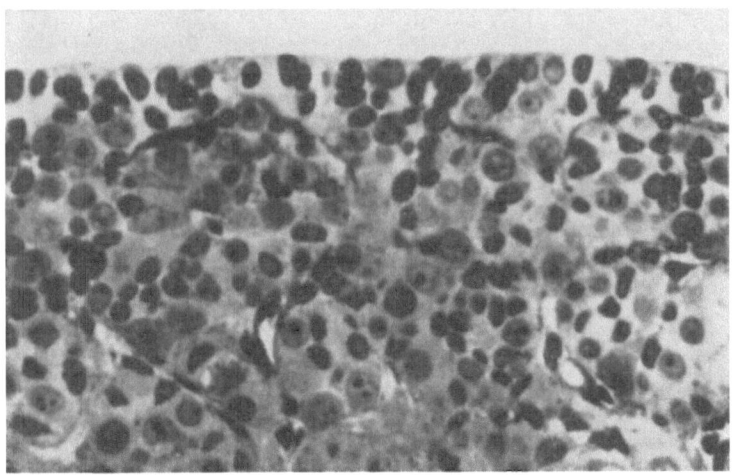

Fig. 62. Cortical cords of the embryonal ovary are incompletely separated from the surface epithelium. The ovarian cords consist of oogonia and immature granulosa cells of coelomic origin. Mesenchymal fibroblasts are scattered among the cords.

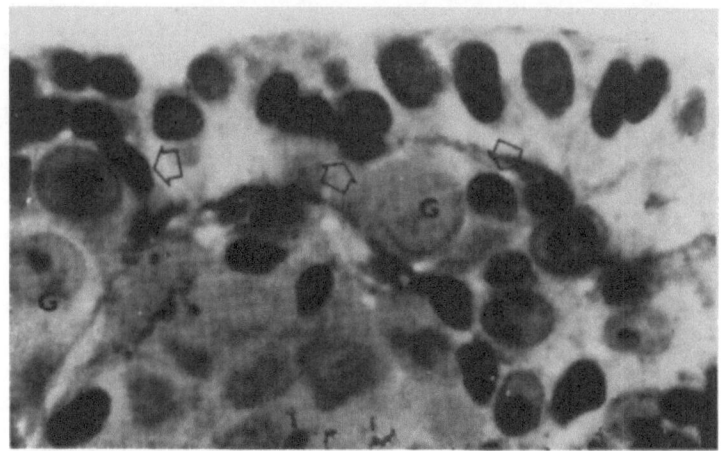

Fig. 63. Proliferation of the surface coelomic epithelium in an embryonal ovary. Immature granulosa cells are marked with arrows, G — germ cell.

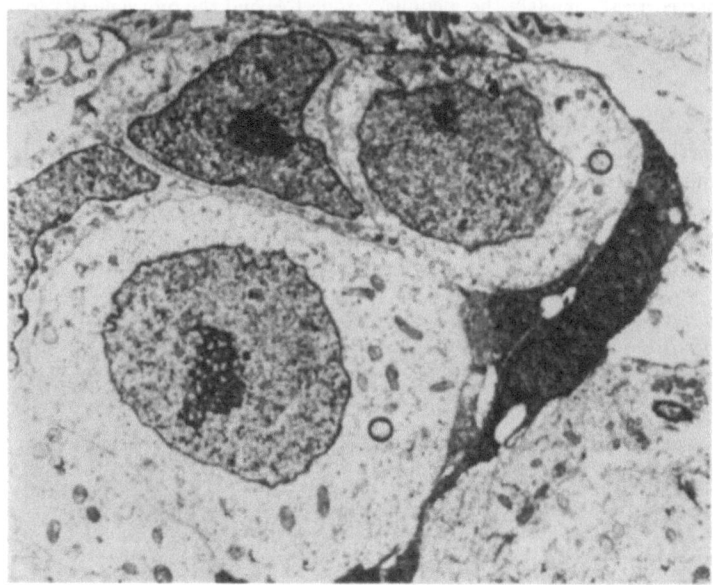

Fig. 64. Oogonia (O) poor in organells and immature granulosa cells of a cortical cord of embryonal ovary.

takes place after fertilization in an oocyte penetrated by a sperm. Oogonia are present in human fetuses from days 50—55 until birth. Meiosis first begins in the medullary oocytes and from there extends gradually to the cortex. Leptotene oocytes are present from the 9th—10th week until birth, zygotene and pachytene from 11—12 weeks and diplotene oocytes from 12—13 weeks until several months after birth. At this time, all ovarian follicles are differentiated. There is no neo-oogenesis in human ovaries after this stage. During follicular growth in the perinatal and adult ovaries, the oocytes synthesize RNA and protein and meiosis is arrested.

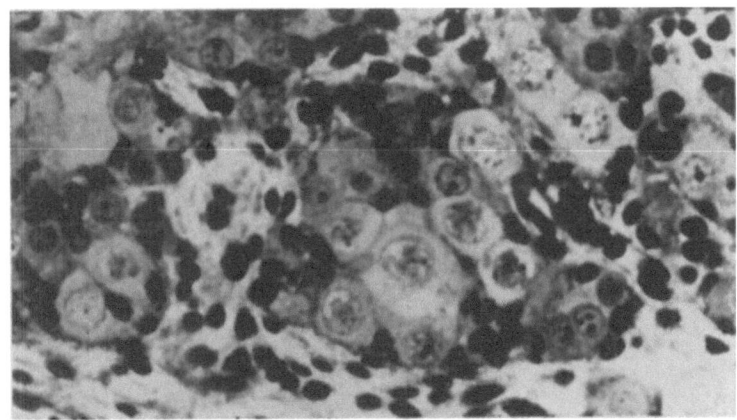

Fig. 65. Early fetal ovary. Clones of oocytes undergoing meiotic prophase in the medullary cords. No primary follicles present.

At the stage of the early fetal ovary, clones of oocytes form groups without individual oocytes being separated by granulosa cells. The granulosa cells may form a simple layer on the periphery of the oocyte clones. The term, primordial follicles, should be reserved for such groups of oocytes (*Jirásek*, 1976). The term, primary follicles, is used for follicles formed by an oocyte and a single-layered granulosa membrane which are completely separated from the others by connective tissue.

LATE FETAL OVARY

The characteristic ovarian structures at this stage are the (isolated) primary follicles (Figs. 66—69). Growing, solid follicles may also be present. The diplotene oocytes in the deep portion of the cortex and the medulla of the late fetal ovary become covered by a single layer of flattened epithelial follicular (granulosa) cells. The basement membrane of the follicular cells represents a supportive structure for the ingrowing fibroblast depositing reticular fibers. The ingrowing connective tissue separates individual primary follicles from the aggregates of pregranulosa cells present within the medullary and cortical cords. Granulosa cells not involved in the formation of primary follicles intermingle with the connective tissue contributing to the ovarian stroma. Formation of the primary follicles proceeds from the deepest part of the ovarian cortical and medullary cords reaching to the most outer parts at the perinatal stage. Numerous oocytes, which do not become completely surrounded by follicular cells, udergo degeneration (atresia).

Formation of a complete layer of follicular cells of a primary follicle is apparently controlled by genes of the two X-chromosomes. In the presence of only one X-chromosome (45,X fetuses), all oocytes of the late fetal and perinatal ovary degenerate because the follicular layer is incomplete. In the 45,X fetuses, the degeneration of all germinal cells within the late fetal and perinatal ovaries turns the ovaries into the streak gonads.

The stroma of the early fetal ovary in normal fetuses does not contain any cells containing 3β-hydroxysteroid dehydrogenase. Early fetal ovaries do not form estrogens (*Jungmann and Schweppe*, 1968.

95

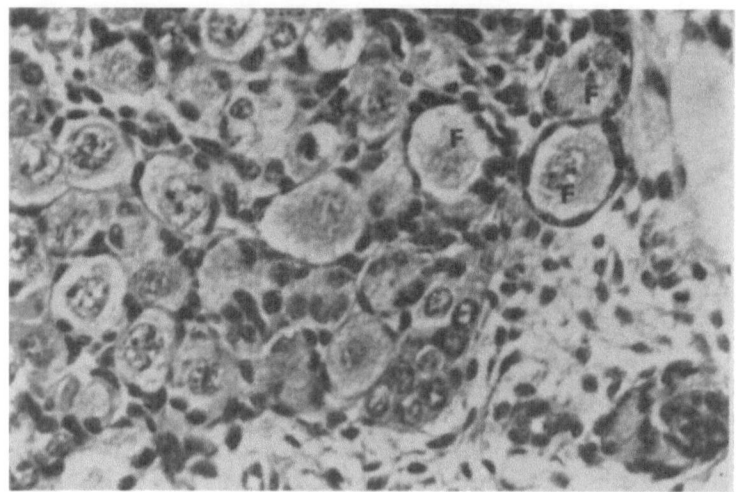

Fig. 66. Late fetal ovary. Primordial (incompletely isolated) and primary (completely isolated) ovarian follicles (F) are present.

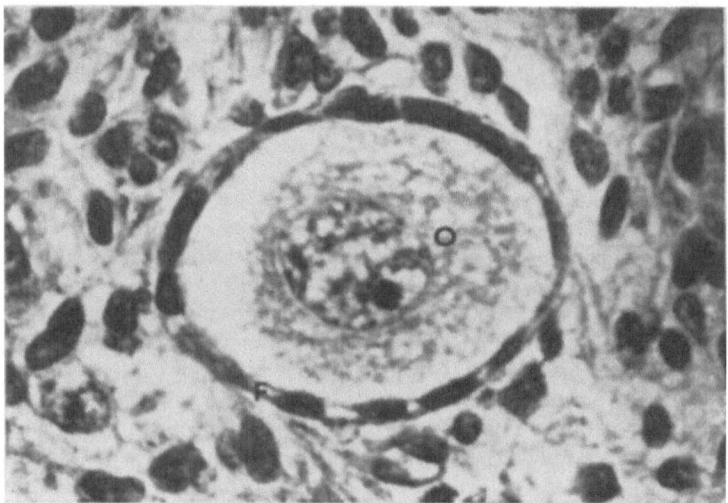

Fig. 67. Primary ovarian follicle. The oocyte (O) is completely isolated from the ovarian stroma by a singlelayered layer of flat follicular (granulosa) cells.

PERINATAL OVARY

The stage of a perinatal ovary is characterized by the presence of solid, multilayered and cavitated follicles. During the follicular growth, as the cavitation becomes evident, the ovarian stroma around the follicle differentiates into a theca folliculi interna and externa. Within the theca interna, adjacent to the future cumulus oophorus, the first epithelioid cells are formed. Thecal cells gradually increase in

96

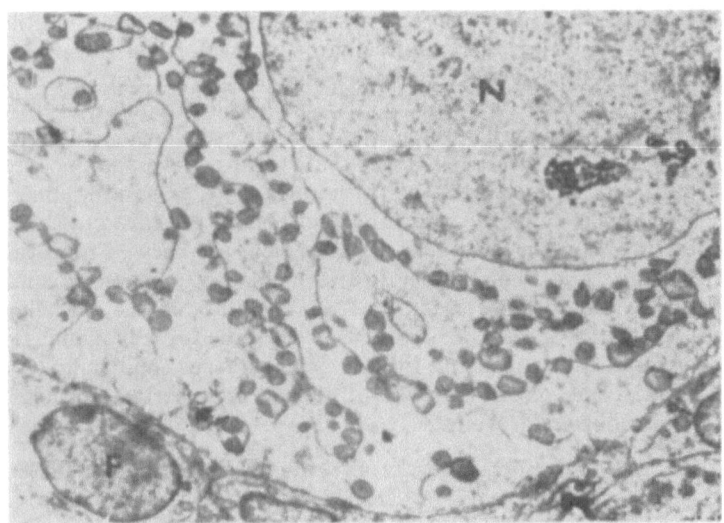

Fig. 68. The oocyte of the primary follicle. Mitochondria are interconnected by a doublemembrane originated from the rough endoplasmic reticulum. The supposed significance of this arrangement is the synchronization of the metabolism involved in the production of "yolk" granules. N-nucleus, F-follicular cell.

number and extend around the cavitated follicle. They contain the 3β-hydroxysteroid dehydrogenase, NADP-reductase, G-6-PD, non-specific esterase and lipids, suggesting their participation in the steroidogenesis. The perinatal ovary is able to transform DHA into estrogens (estradiol-17β).

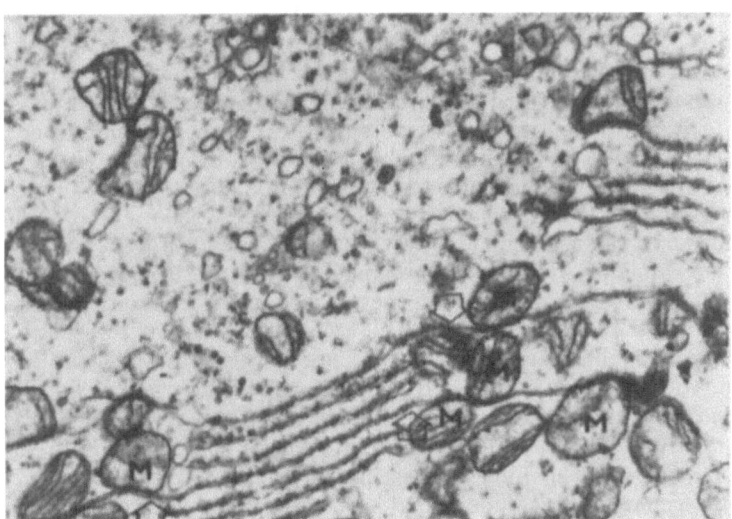

Fig. 69. Ultrastructure of the cytoplasm of the fetal oocyte from a primordial follicle. The double-membranes of the rough endoplasmic reticulum evaginate to the mitochondria (M) and connect them.

In the perinatal ovary, in addition to growing single-layered and multilayered follicles and cavitated follicles, there are remnants of the cortical and medullary cords with primordial follicles. The border between the cortex and medulla becomes indistinct. Adjacent to the medullary cords, lumenized, irregular, narrow spaces of the rete ovarii are present. The importance of the rete ovarii for triggering the formation of follicles was stressed (*Byskov*, 1973). Nevertheless, all oocytes enclosed within the rete cords degenerate in the perinatal period. There are numerous vessels and nerves in the vicinity of the rete. Some epithelioid cells are present adjacent to the nerves starting from the third month. These cells are derived from the primitive coelomic epithelium, and their affinity to the sympathetic nerves is similar to that occuring between the adrenal cortex and the medulla. If the epithelioid cells in the rete area are (more or less) dispersed, they are called extragonadal Leydig cells, or hillus or sympaticotrop cells of Berger. If they form solid nodules, they may undergo differentiation similar to that of the adrenal cortex, forming accessory adrenals. They produce androgens.

Over a period of several months postnatally, all cavitated follicles of the perinatal ovary undergo atresia and degenerate. The perinatal ovary turns into a prepubertal (inactive) ovary of a child. During puberty, first ovulations occur. Ovulatory follicles and their derivatives, corpora lutea, are characteristic for an adult ovary from the woman's fertile period (approximately 15—50 years).

Senile ovaries from menopausal women contain practically no follicles. Waved hyaline bands (corpora albicantia) are present at places where they were deposited during formation of the corpora albicantia. Many of the hillar vessels are obliterated, showing so-called "postovulatory sclerosis". There is always hyperplasia of hillus cells in senile ovaries.

PRENATAL AND PERINATAL DEGENERATION OF THE OOGONIA AND OOCYTES AND ATRESIA OF FOLLICLES

The population of the germinal cells within the ovaries reaches its maximum between weeks 18—22 prenatally. In two month-old fetuses, some 600,000 germinal cells are present in both ovaries. In 18—22 week-old fetuses, the number of oogonia and oocytes is estimated at 5—7 million (approximately two million oogonia 4.8 million oocytes) reaching the peak and declining thereafter (*Baker*, 1963). The ovaries of a newborn contain approximately two million germ cells, about half of them showing degeneration. At seven years, about 300,000 oocytes are left. All the oocytes degenerate during the woman's life except approximately 400 of them which are ovulated. The maximum number of degenerating oocytes is found in fetal and perinatal ovaries, the formation of the primary follicles with a complete layer of follicular cells being the decisive step for their further survival. The proper term for follicular degeneration prior to ovulation is atresia. During atresia of primary follicles the oocyte degenerates and follicular cells mix with the cells of the stroma. The oocytes degenerate mostly at the zygotene or pachytene stage. Chromatin cluster aggregate within the nucleus leading to pycnosis. The nuclear membrane wrinkles and fragments. In 45,X embryos, all primary follicles undergo atresia because the envelope of the follicular cells is incomplete, allowing contact between the connective tissue and the oocyte (Figs. 70, 71). The same happens in many primary follicles of normal 46,XX fetuses (Fig. 72) and is probably the main reason for their atresia. The difference between

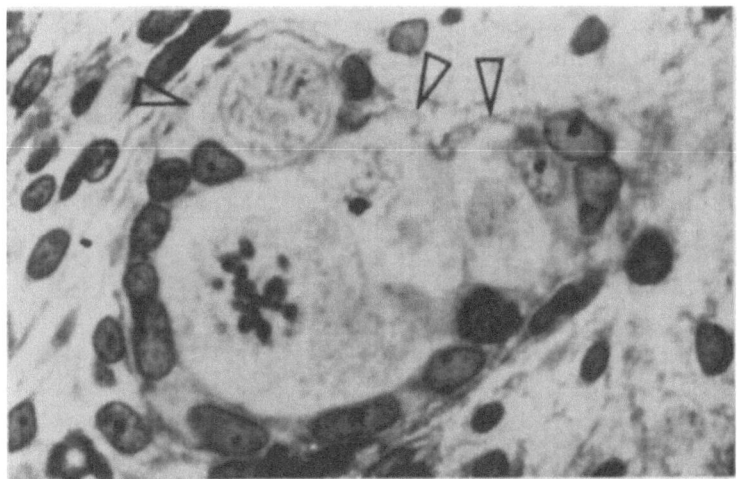

Fig. 70. Incomplete follicular layer in the ovary of a 45,X fetus. The oocytes are either in a meiotic prophase or metaphase.

the atresia of primary follicles in 45,X and sua 46,XX fetes is only a quantitative one. The meiotic prophase in 45,X embryos proceeds normally until the pachytene stage in most oocytes. In some follicles with an incomplete granulosa layer, meiotic prophase does not stop and proceeds to metaphase. Oocytes degenerate thereafter. This observation further stresses the possibility that the fetal follicular cells are responsible for the arrest of the meiotic prophase.

Shortly after the degeneration of the oocyte becomes apparent in atresic, multi-layered follicles of the perinatal ovaries, thickness of the vitreous membrane increases by collagen apposition and connective tissue penetrates between granulosa cells.

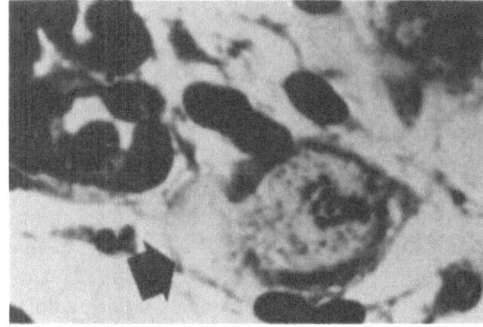

Fig. 17. Degenareting oocyte in meta- phase. The follicular layer is incomplete. Cytoplasmic herniation is marked with arrow.

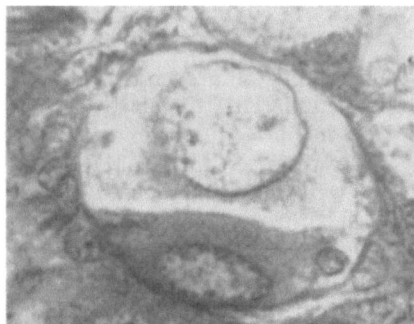

Fig. 72. Atretci follicle with two oocytes and an incomplete follicular layer in a 46,XX normal ovary. The difference in atresia between 46,XX and4 5,X fetus is only quantitative.

Granulosa cells and fibroblasts intermingle. In cavitated follicles during atresia, granulosa cells detach and degenerate leaving a cystic space lined by a thickened, hyalinized and wrinkled vitreous membrane ("cystic atresia"). The theca interna of the atresic follicles, which contains epithelioid, steroid-producing cells, undergoes hyperplasia. The steroid-producing cells derived from the theca interna of atresic follicles are the main source for the interstitial cells in the human perinatal ovary. After the atresia has been completed, only an irregular, wary hyaline band remains at the place of the former cavitated follicle.

DEVELOPMENT OF THE GENITAL DUCTS

As the gonads develop in close contact to pronephros and mesonephros, the genital ducts are closely related to the urinary primordia.

MESONEPHRIC (WOLFFIAN) DUCT

The mesonephric duct primordium is formed by a solid cellular cord appearing dorsolaterally to somites 8—13 in 25—30 day-old embryos (2—3 mm; S. H. XI, XII). Most embryologists believe that the mesonephric duct is of mesodermal origin, detached from pronephric blastema. *Jirásek* (1971) observed that the mesonephric duct primordium is glycogen rich and lacks alkaline phosphatase, whereas pronephric and mesonephric blastema do not contain glycogen and exhibit alkaline phosphatase activity. He found ectodermal buds evaginating from the surface epithelium to the pronephric blastema exhibiting the same histochemical properties as the primordia of the mesonephric ducts. Therefore, he considers mesonephric ducts to be ectodermal, a possibility already stressed by *Politzer* (1953).

This observation may suggest that the pronephric ducts of vertebrates represent a derivative of the ectodermal atrial chamber of ancient Protochordates (Amphioxus like). The mesonephric ducts grow caudally, become lumenized and reach the hind gut in 28—30 day-old embryos with 27—28 somite pairs (S. H. XII). The terminal portion of the hind gut common to both digestive and urinary tracts is known as the cloaca.

In the area of the urogenital ridge, as the mesonephric duct passes the mesonephric blastema differentiating into mesonephric nephrons, short tubules evaginate from the mesonephric duct connecting each nephron. The ureteric buds (primordia of ureters) appear in embryos 31—35 days-old (5—8 mm long, S. H. XIV) on the dorsomedial wall of the mesonephric ducts before the cloaca. They grow dorsocranially and reach the metanephric blastema located in the 4th and 5th lumbar segment. The ingrowth of the ureteric bud into the metanephric blastema is essential for the formation of metanephros. (*Grobstein*, 1957; *Winick and McCrosy*, 1968). If the ureteral buds fail to reach the metanephric blastema, the kidney does not develop, and the metanephric blastema disintegrates. After the kidney is formed, the mesonephroi (plural of mesonephros) degenerate. Approximately 20 mesonephric tubules in the epigenital and paragenital location become more or less preserved. Five to twelve epigenital, mesonephric nephrons contact the rete of the gonad. In the male, they become ductuli efferentes of the epididymis. Those remaining represent the paradidymal tubules. In the female, the epigenital and paragenital mesonephric tubules fragment and degenerate, becoming epophoron and paroophoron.

PARAMESONEPHRIC (MULLERIAN) DUCT

The epithelium of the paramesonephric ducts is derived from a primitive coelomic epithelium similar to that of the genital ridge. In 44—48 day-old embryos (15 to 18 mm, S. H. XVIII), the coelomic epithelium invaginates at the level of the third to fourth thoracic segments and grows as a solid cord to the adjacent mesonephric duct. The solid, cordlike, mesonephric duct grows on the lateral side in contact with the mesonephric duct using the mesonephric duct as a guide (*Gruenwald*, 1941; *Jirásek*, 1970). Lumenization of the paramesonephric duct begins at the invaginated abdominal opening and proceeds caudally. The paramesonephric ducts cross the mesonephric ducts ventrally, caudal to the mesonephric ridge, approach each other near the midline and run parallel between the mesonephric ducts. In 56 to 60 day-old embryos (30—35 mm long, S. H. XXIII), the tips of the paramesonephric ducts contact the endodermal epithelium of the urogenital sinus without penetrating in between the openings of the mesonephric ducts. In the area where mesonephric ducts enter and paramesonephric ducts meet, the endodermal urogenital sinus is elevated and is known as the paramesonephric eminence (Mullerian tubercle). In the area where both parallel paramesonephric ducts are in contact, their epithelium disintegrates. In fetuses 50—55 mm long (week 10), caudal portions of both paramesonephric ducts fuse into a single uterovaginal canal.

UROGENITAL SINUS

In embryos 35—39 days-old (7—9 mm, S. H. XIV), the hind gut becomes divided by a mesenchymal urorectal septum present in form of a peritoneal fold behind the allantois. The ventral part of the divided hind hut contributes to the primitive urogenital sinus (urodeum). The dorsal part is known as the anorectal canal (coprodeum). That part of the primitive urogenital sinus located above the openings of mesonephric ducts is known as the vesicourethral primordium. The portion of the urogenital sinus below the openings of the mesonephric ducts contributes to the definitive urogenital sinus. In humans, the definitive urogenital sinus is only a narrow pelvic canal. Anteriorily distended, the so-called "phalic part" of the urogenital sinus reaching the genital tubercle is provided by the anterior portion of the urogenital membrane. The vesicourethral primordium contributes to the urinary bladder, the whole female urethra, and the intramural and upper prostatic male urethra. The definitive urogenital sinus changes in accoradance with the differentiation of the external genitalia into a membranous and cavernous part of the male urethra or into a female vaginal vestibule. The cloaca is closed by a bilaminar, ectodermal and endodermal cloacal membrane. As the urorectal septum reaches the cloacal membrane (42—48 day-old embryos, 16—18 mm, S. H. XVIII) forming the primitive perineum, the ventral portion of the cloacal membrane (closing the urogenital sinus) is known as the urogenital membrane and the dorsal portion (closing the anorectal canal) as the anal membrane. Both membranes rupture and disappear in 45—55 day-old embryos (18—20 mm, S. H. XVIII—XX). The rupture of the posterior portion of the genital membrane precedes that of the anal membrane. The anterior portion of the genital membrane extends on the genital tubercle and contributes the urethral plate.

MASCULINIZATION OF THE GENITAL DUCTS

In the presence of normal developing testes, the paramesonephric ducts undergo regression. The epigenital mesonephric nephrons and the mesonephric ducts are transformed into the epididymides (plural) and ductus deferentes, and male accessory sex glands are formed around the urogenital sinus and urethra.

REGRESSION OF THE PARAMESONEPHRIC DUCT

Regression of the paramesonephric ducts begins in 60—65 day-old fetuses (30—35 mm long) in the middle of the duct in the area where the duct crosses the caudal testicular ligament. Using histochemical methods, it was possible to demonstrate at this stage that proteoglycans (first present in the testicular interstitium) reach the duct, initiating the differentiation of the connective tissue. Consequently, the activity of acid phosphatase rise within the paramesonephric epithelium of the regressing area, whereas the activities of succinate dehydrogenase and isocitrate dehydrogenase decrease. It was suggested (*Jirásek*, 1977) that changes in the lamina propria of the paramesonephric duct are induced by a water soluble mucoprotein (proteoglycan) of testicular origin. Consequently, as the activities of the oxydative enzymes within the epithelium of paramesonephric ducts decrease, acid hydrolases (acid phosphatase) stored within the lysosomes become liberated, destroying the epithelium. Once initiated, the degeneration of the paramesonephric duct extends cranially as well as caudally. The cranial end of the paramesonephric duct does not regress and becomes a cystic testicular appendix attached to the superior pole of the testes. The non-regressed caudal portion of both fused, paramesonephric ducts (uterovaginal canal) becomes incorporated within the prostate, changing into the prostatic utricle (a homologous of the vagina). This concept of the paramesonephric regression is in agreement with Josso's experiments on the so-called "antimullerian hormone". *Josso et al.* (1977) found that the substance responsible for the regression of the Mullerian duct is water soluble, having a molecular weight of approximately 180,000. In contrast to Josso, we do not classify this substance as a hormone because of its strict unilateral action (all known hormones act bilaterally), calling the substance a mullerian inhibitor.

DEVELOPMENT OF EPIDIDYMIS, VAS DEFERENS AND MALE ACCESSORY GLANDS

The epigenital, 5—12 mesonephric tubules detach from mesonephric Malpighian bodies and connect the rete testis with the mesonephric duct. As androgens are produced by the fetal testis, the epigenital tubules and the mesonephric duct extend and become coiled. The epigenital mesonephric tubules contribute the head of the epididymis. The coiled upper portion of the mesonephric duct forms the epididymal body and the cauda. The lower portion of the mesonephric duct (not included in the mesonephric ridge) runs from the epididymis to the urogenital sinus, and forms

102

the ductus deferens. The smooth musculature of the ductus deferens appears during the fourth month. A small portion of the mesonephric duct located within the cranial degenerating portion of the mesonephric ridge becomes attached to the cranial end of the epididymis and gives rise to a small vesicle known as the appendix epididymis. The paragenital mesonephric tubules, losing connection with the mesonephric duct, are known as the paradidymis. Rudimentary mesonephric tubules not connected with the rete, persisting in the epigenital area, are known as the cranial aberrant tubules.

The primordia of the seminal vesicles become distinct at the end of the third month. Each originates from an evagination of the mesonephric duct before its entrance into the urethra. The short terminal portion of the mesonephric duct between the opening of the seminal vesicle and the urethra is properly called the ejaculatory duct. The prostatic glands originate from endodermal buds evaginating from the urethral epithelium in 50—60 mm long fetuses. The prostatic stroma is a mixture of mesenchyme accompanying the urogenital sinus and mesonephric and paramesonephric ducts. Mucosal, submucosal and main prostatic glands are distinguished. The main glands contribute mainly to the lateral lobes. The submucosal glands, embedded in the stroma of paramesonephric origin, contribute the prostatic middle lobe. Mucosal glands contribute to the anterior and posterior prostatic portions (*Jirásek*, 1980). The bulbo-urethral glands originate from the endodermal buds of the pelvic part of the urogenital sinus making their appearance at the end of the third month.

Urethral glands, similar in origin, appear in the second half of pregnancy.

FEMINIZATION OF THE GENITAL DUCTS

The uterine tubes, the uterus and four fifths of the vagina are paramesonephric derivatives. Two portions can be recognized on each paramesonephric duct: a cranial portion extending from the abdomnial opening until the crossing with the mesonephric duct, and a caudal portion extending from the crossing to the paramesonephric eminence of the urogenital sinus. The caudal parts of both paramesonephric ducts fuse into a single, midline uterovaginal canal. This fusion occurs during the 9th—12th weeks. The cranial part of each paramesonephric duct becomes the uterine tube. Musculature and connective tissue of the oviducts are exclusively derived from paramesonephric mesenchyme. Both tubes are embedded within the broad ligament — a transverse peritoneal fold extending from the lateral wall of the pelvis. The uterovaginal canal represents the primordium of the uterus and most of the vagina. As tips of the paramesonephric ducts reach the endodermal epithelium of the urogenital sinus (at the paramesonephric eminence), the proliferation of the endodermal epithelium gives rise to the sinovaginal bulbs. The sinovaginal bulbs fuse with the tips of the paramesonephric ducts. Direct contact between the endodermal and mesodermal epithelium is oconstituted. Consequently, the vaginal plate develops. The vaginal plate is formed by a solid, multilayered epithelium around the lower portion of the uterovaginal canal. From this stage there is confusion about the origin of the vagina. *Koff* (1933) considers that the upper four fifths of the vagina is formed from the paramesonephric ducts; other (*Vilas*, 1932; *Bulmer*, 1957; *Matějka*, 1959) argue that the entire vaginal plate is endodermal in origin. Using alkaline phosphatase and glycogen stain, *Jirásek* (1977) was able to show that the alkaline phosphatase-rich paramesonephric epithelium si preserved as a central structure within the cranial four fifths of the vaginal plate. The point is whether the squamous epithelium of the cranial four fifths of the vaginal plate is an endodermal derivative growing along the uterovaginal canal (as stated by *Matějka*, 1959), or whether the squamous epithelium of the upper vagina differentiates from the "subcylindrical" proliferation of the mesodermal epithelium of the uterovaginal canal in situ as result of a mesoderm-endoderm induction. *Jirásek* (1977) favored the last hypothesis. The vaginal

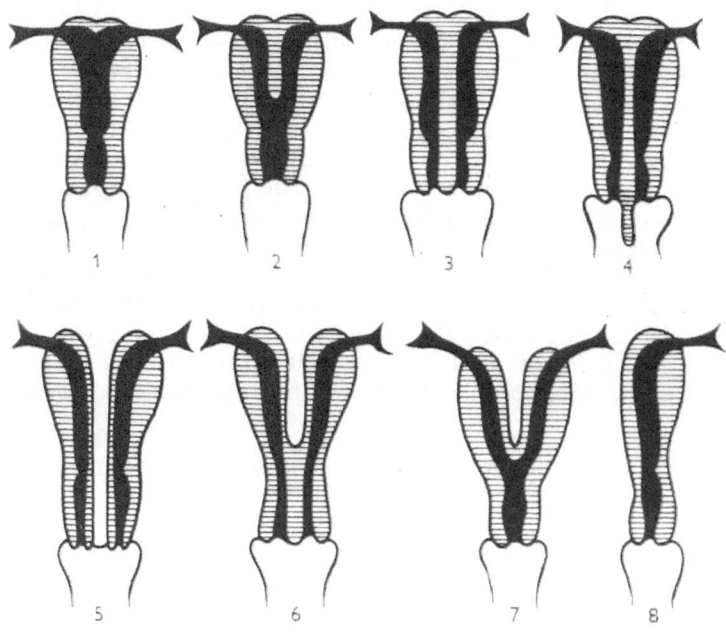

Fig. 72A. Uterine anomalies. 1 — u. arcuatus, 2 — u. subseptus, 3 — u. septuss, 4 — u. septus c. vagina septa, 5 — u. duplex, 6 — u. bicornis bicollis, 7 — u. bicornis unicollis, 8 — u. unicornis.

plate is present in 60—150 mm long fetuses. The vaginal lumen appears in 150 to 170 mm long fetuses as the cylindrical cells degenerate. The anterior and posterior vaginal fornices become evident in 130—150 mm long fetuses (*O'Rahilly*, 1973). Glycogen is present within the epithelium of the vaginal plate and its amount increases until birth. The hymen is formed as a mesenchymal septum at the level of the paramesonephric tubercle. This septum, covered by endoderm, incompletely separates the urogenital sinus and the lower vagina.

Jirásek (1971) proposed that the direct contact between the tips of the paramesonephric ducts induces endodermal proliferation of the sinovaginal bulbs. Failure of this contact results in a vaginal agenesis. The length of the vagina depends on the formation of the vaginal plate. If paramesonephric ducts regress before the vaginal plate is fully formed, the vagina is short and blind (such as in a complete testicular feminization).

The uterus develops from the upper portion of the uterovaginal canal, not involved in the formation of the vaginal plate. The mesenchyme accompanying both paramesonephric as well as mesonephric ducts, participates in the mesenchymal condensation and represents the primordium of the uterine musculature. The smooth muscle cells of the myometrium are present in 18 week-old fetuses (160—170 mm long). The definitive plexiform patterns of the myometrium are present in 260 mm long fetuses. The shape of the uterus depends on the fusion of both paramesonephric ducts. The lack of fusion results in uterine anomalies (Fig. 72A). The uterine cavity is lined by a single-layered, columnar epithelium. The buds representing the primordia of the uterine glands are found in 150 mm long fetuses. The cervical canal is lined by a single-layered, mucin-producing, columnar epithelium. The multilayered, squamous epithelium of the ectocervix originates from the vaginal plate. The primordia of the mucin-producing cervical glands appear in 100—120 mm fetuses prior to the primordia of corporal glands. The position of the uterovaginal junction is variable. In many newborns, a congenital ectropium is present. In such a case, the singlelayered, columnar, mucin-producing, endocervical epithelium extends to the ectocervix around the external uterine orificium.

REGRESSION OF THE EPIGENITAL AND PARAGENITAL PARTS OF THE MESONEPHROS

The epigenital and paragenital parts of the mesonephros, including the prostatic primordium, which is of endodermal origin, fail to grow in the absence of androgens or if the peripheral tissues are androgen resistant. When not stimulated by androgens, the epigenital and paragenital mesonephric tubules and ducts fragment. In females, epoophoron and paraoophoron, located within the broad ligament, represent remnants of the epigenital and paragenital mesonephric nephrons. The persisting mesonephric duct is known as Gartner's duct. The caudal terminal portion of this duct (if present) opens into the vaginal vestibule. The upper terminal portion turns into an appendix vesiculosa near the ovary.

DEVELOPMENT OF THE EXTERNAL GENITALIA

In 37—45 day-old embryos (S. H. XV—XVII), the cloacal membrane forms a sagittal groove with slightly elevated cloacal folds on both sides. The groove extends to the underside of the genital tubercle contributing the urethral plate (Fig. 73). As the urorectal septum divides the cloacal membrane into a genital membrane anteriorly and an anal membrane posteriorly, the cloacal folds split into the urethral folds located on both sides of the genital membrane and the anal folds on both sides of

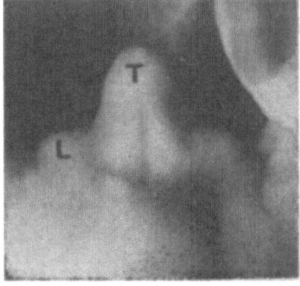

Fig. 73. Indifferent external genitalia in a 18 mm embryo (50 days old, S. h. XX). T — genital tubercle, L — labioscrotal swelling.

the anal membrane. The labioscrotal swellings appear laterally from the urethral folds in 10—14 mm-long embryos. The swellings represent areas of attachment of the caudal mesonephric ligaments (future gubernaculum testis in males, round ligament of the uterus in females). In embryos 20—35 mm long, the mesenchymal primordia of the corpora cavernosa can be recognized. One of them is formed underneath each urethral fold (corpus cavernosum penis) and one is unpaired within the genital tubercle (corpus cavernosum urethrae). As the genital tubercle elongates, the primordium of the glans becomes evident, and by now the penile primordium is known as a phallus. The urethral plate on the underside of the phallus deepens into a urethral groove. The urogenital membrane disappears (in 20—25 mm-long embryos), establishing the outside opening of the urogenital sinus. At the end of the indifferent stage of the external genitalia development, there is a phallus (with a glans and urethral groove), and paired labioscrotal swellings laterally.

MASCULINIZATION OF THE EXTERNAL GENITALIA

The transformation of the indifferent genitalia into male genitalia is androgen dependent. The masculinization consists of fusion of the rims of the urethral folds (Figs. 74 and 75). The fusion proceeds from the perineum to the glans of the penis. The rhaphe scroti and rhaphe penis are formed. On the underside of the glans,

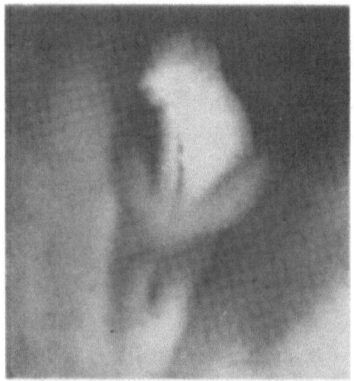

Fig. 74. Beginning of masculinization of the external genitalia in a 40 mm male fetus. The anogenital distance lengthens and labioscrotal swelling are pushed toward the midline. The urethral groove is open.

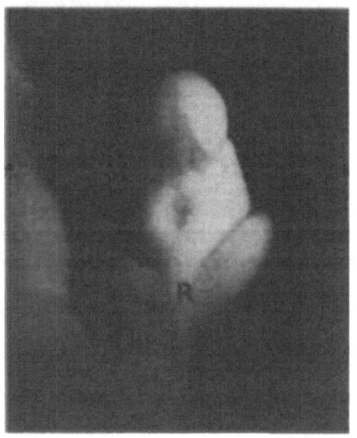

Fig. 75. Masculine external genitalia with a physiologic hypospadia in a 52 mm long (11 weeks old) fetus. The rhaphe of scrotum is formed. The penile urethra closes. The triangular epithelial plate on the ventral part of glans is derived from the most anterioe portion of the urogenital membrane.

there is an epithelial remnant of the most cranial part of the genital membrane at the place of the future preputial frenulum. The terminal portion of the male urethra is formed during the fourth month from an ectodermal plate growing from the tip of the epithelial genital membrane toward the urethra. This terminal ectodermal plate becomes luminized and becomes the fossa navicularis at the definitive external urethral meatus. During formation of the rhaphe scroti, the anogenital distance increases and the labioscrotal swellings approach the midline, each of them providing half of the scrotum.

The formation of the rhaphe scroti takes place between days 65—70 and the formation of the rhaphe penis between days 68—75. A so-called "physiological penile hypospadia" is present for approximately a week until the beginning of the fourth month. Corpus spongiosum urethrae closes around the cavernous urethra in 10—14 week-old fetuses. The penile skin becomes separated from the glans by an ectodermal glandopreputial lamella in 5—6 month-old fetuses. At the time of birth, this lamella splits, liberating the foreskin.

FEMINIZATION OF THE EXTERNAL GENITALIA

In 9 week-old female fetuses (40 mm long), the anogenital distance does not increase, and no rhape is formed. The labioscrotal swellings remain separated and the urethral groove does not close. The phallus bends caudally. The labioscrotal swellings trans-

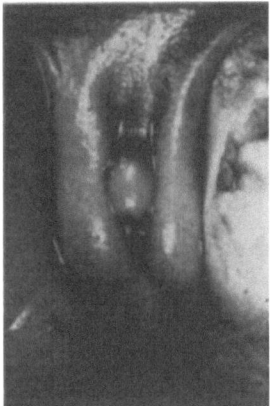

Fig. 76. Feminized external genitalia in a 120 mm long fetus.

form into the labia majora, the urethral folds develop into the labia minora and the phallus changes into the clitoris (Fig. 76). Consequently, the opening of the urogenital sinus elongates sagitally. The vaginal and urethral openings become separated, and the vestibulum of the vagina is formed. There is nothing homologous to the male cavernous urethra in females. The cavernous tissue in males contributing to the spongy body of the urethra, is, in females, involved in the formation of bulbus vestibuli. The epithelium lining — the vaginal vestibule — is ectodermal in origin. The external surface of the labia minora is lined by an ectodermal epithelium, whereas the inner surface is covered by an endodermal epithelium.

107

GENETIC CONTROL AND SEX-DIFFERENTIATION

CONTROL OF GONADAL DEVELOPMENT

The basic gene (masculinizing determinant) responsible for the differentiation of testicular cords is the H-Y antigen coding gene (*Wachtel et al.*, 1975). The gene is related to the differentiation of the embryonal Sertoli cells and to the formation of basement membranes around the testicular cords. The schema of our concept of testicular differentiation is presented in Fig. 77. The H-Y antigen coding gene is normally present on the short arm of the Y-chromosome, but may be translocated on the X-chromosome, or to another chromosome (such as in 46,XX males). The action of the H-Y antigen on the Sertoli cell differentiation is cell-to-cell mediated. The differentiation of testicular cords is defective if H-Y antigen is not present or expressed in all cells. The expression of H-Y antigen may be limited by an unknown product of an X-linked gene, which, if present in an active X-diploid state, interferes with the differentiation or growth of the testicular cords. This H-Y antigen-limiting gene, if present in a diploid active state, can prevent or suppress testicular development such as in 46,XY pure gonadal dysgenesis (*German et al.*, 1978). There is some evidence to suggest that the H-Y antigen-limiting gene normally is located in the part of X-chromosome, which is inactivated as X-chromatin. In some animals, the diploid active state of X-chromosome-located H-Y antigen-limiting gene may be responsible for "sex-reversal" (XY females).

The differentiation of the embryonal testicular cords induces the synthesis of the substance inhibiting the development of the paramesonephric ducts. The chemical

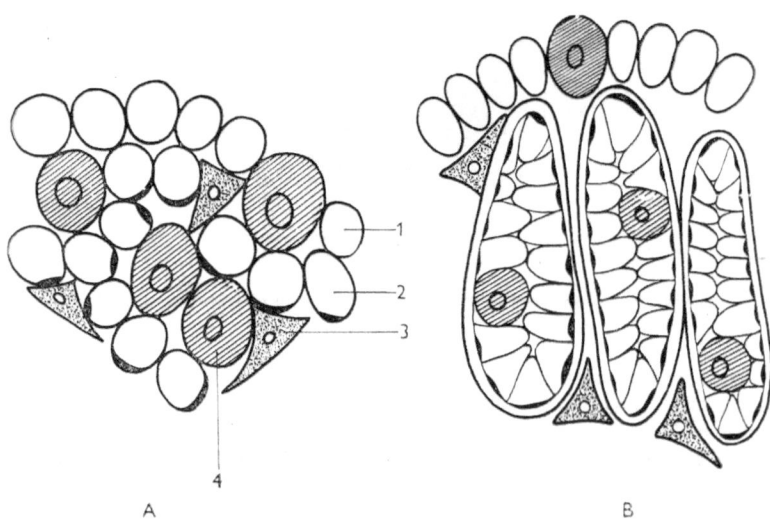

Fig. 77. Schema of testicular differentiation. A — Gonadal blastema. 1 — primitive mesoblastic cells, 2 — mesoblastic cells recognizing H—Y antigen, 3 — mesenchymal cells, 4 — primordial germ cells. B — Embryonal testis. Orientation of the Sertoli cells (recognizing H—Y antigen) and formation of the basement membranes of testicular cords.

character of this substance, as well as the gene/genes necessary for its synthesis, are unknown. The mechanisms involved will be discussed later.

The differentiation of the seminiferous cords stops proliferation of the blastema of the genital ridge. The germ cells are incorporated into the cords; they are temporarily arrested in their mitoses and are prevented from proceeding into meiosis until puberty.

The following chromosomal combinations are compatible with a normal embryonal and fetal testicular development: 46,XY; 47,XYY; 47,XXY. If the male determinant is not present in all cells (45,X/46,XY, etc), or if the X-chromosome-bound gene interferes with H-Y antigen expression, the testicular development is irregular and deficient, resulting either in a testicular dysgenesis or into a "streak gonad". The streak gonad in 46,XY individuals contains, in contrast to streak gonads in 45,X individuals, deposits of hyalin.

In 46,XX normal individuals, and similarly in 47,XXX, or 48,XXXX individuals, the genital ridge continues its proliferation in 18—25 mm-long embryos, 45—52 days old (S. H. XIX—XXI). The genital ridge extends more caudally in females, reaching into sacral segments. In the absence of H-Y antigen, primordial germ cells (later becoming oogonia) continue their mitotic divisions and after a certain number of mitoses enter meiosis according to their genetic program. The meiotic prophase in the oocytes is interrupted as the oocytes become incorporated into the primary follicles. The formation of the follicular envelope is apparently controlled by determinants on X-chromosomes. A double dose of ovarian determinants — that means two X-chromosomes (respectively one euchromatic X and "something from the other X") — are needed for the differentiation of the complete layer of the granulosa cells of a primary ovarian follicle. Granulosa cells do not only stop the meiotic prophase in oocytes, but also prevent oocytes from having direct contact with the connective tissue.

In 45,X individuals, the ovarian development proceeds normally until the formation of primary follicles in fetal ovaries. At this stage, the formation of the granulosa layer of all primary follicles becomes defective, and all oocytes come in contact with the connective tissue and degenerate. There are no differences in shape, number, migratory pattern, glycogen and alkaline phosphatase content of the primordial germ cells in human 46,XY and 46,XX embryos, suggesting that primordial germ cells do not play a decisive role in the primary sex determination.

CONTROL OF PARAMESONEPHRIC DUCT REGRESSION

The regression of the paramesonephric duct is closely related to the development of the ipsilateral testis. *Jost* (1947) showed that if the embryonal testis is removed, the ipsilateral paramesonephric duct develops into the oviduct and uterus. The chemical structure of the paramesonephric inhibitor remains unknown. *Josso* (1972 a, b) demonstrated that the substance responsible for the paramesonephric duct regression is non-steroid water soluble, has a molecular weight of approximately 18,000 and considers this substance to be produced by the Sertoli-cells. Based on histochemical evidence, *Jirásek* (1976, 1977) estimates this substance to be a water-soluble proteoglycan formed within the testicular interstitium. The substance is an inductor rather than a hormone because its effect is local and unilateral, in contrast to all hormones.

The regression of the middle and caudal portion of paramesonephric ducts in androgen insensitive individuals suggests that androgen sensitivity is note ssential for the
paramesonephric duct regression. The length of the vagina in the androgen-insensitive
patient depends on the extent of paramesonephric regression at the time of the
formation of the vaginal plate.

ANDROGENS OF THE FETAL TESTES: TESTOSTERONE SYNTHESIS

The necessity of morphological differentiation of the fetal epithelioid interstitial
(Leydig) cells for the androgen secretion is usually overlooked. The differentiation
of Leydig cells is gonadotropin dependent, and primarily hCG rather than fetal LH
stimulation is to be considered. Binding of hCG to the human Leydig cells was
demonstrated using the peroxidase method (*Jirásek*, 1971). Synthesis of the hCG-LH
receptor protein within the Leydig cells represents a prerequisite for androgen
synthesis. The formation of androgens in the embryonal testis does not occur until
Leydig cells are present (*Jirásek*, 1966). The formation of androstenedione begins
in the testes of the 30—35 mm-long fetus (56—60 days) and the presence of testosterone was demonstrated about 5—7 days later (*Jirásek et al.*, 1969; *Šulcová,
Jirásek and Stárka*, 1973). There is this question: what is the main pathway for the
formation of the fetal testosterone? *Serra et al.* (1970) demonstrated in vitro the
possibility of a "de novo" synthesis from acetate. *Siiteri and Wilson* (1974) considered
that the main testicular testosterone synthesis starts from pregnenolone and progesterone which are converted to their 17-hydroxy derivatives. The 17α-hydroxypreg-
nenolone and the 17α-hydroxyprogesterone are converted by the 17—20 desmolase
into corresponding C-19 androgens, dehydroepiandrosterone and androstenedione.
Dehydroepiandrosterone is converted to androstenedione by the 3β-hydroxysteroid
dehydrogenase. Androstenedione is converted to testosterone by the 17β-hydroxy-
steroid dehydrogenase. *Huhtaniemi et al.* (1970) isolated pregnenolone and testosterone as main steroid components present in fetal testes. The biosynthesis of
androgens in the testis is summarized in Table 13.

Table 13. Biosynthesis of testicular androgens.

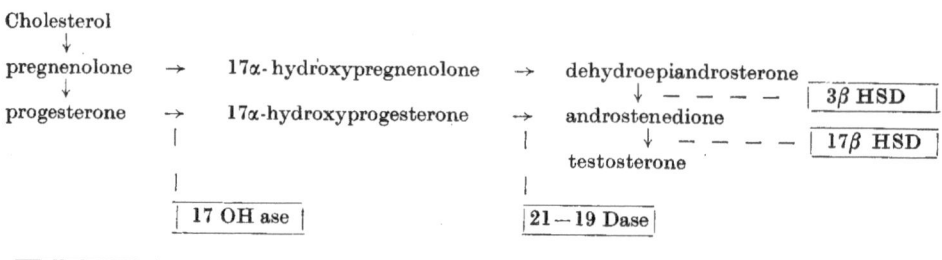

Because of the high activity of the testicular 3β-hydroxysteroid dehydrogenase
favoring dehydroepiandrosterone, and because of the activity of the steroid sulphatase
in the fetal testes (*Lamont et al.*, 1970), we consider that at least part of the testosterone synthesized early in ontogenesis by the fetal testes originates from the
circulating dehydroepiandrosterone sulphate. No estrogens were found in the fetal

testes (*Reyes et al.*, 1973). Testosterone production by the fetal testes reaches (see Graph 11) its peak in 70—100 mm long fetuses (weeks 11 and 12) and declines thereafter. The serum testosterone in male fetuses from 11—17 weeks is 300—500 ng/ml

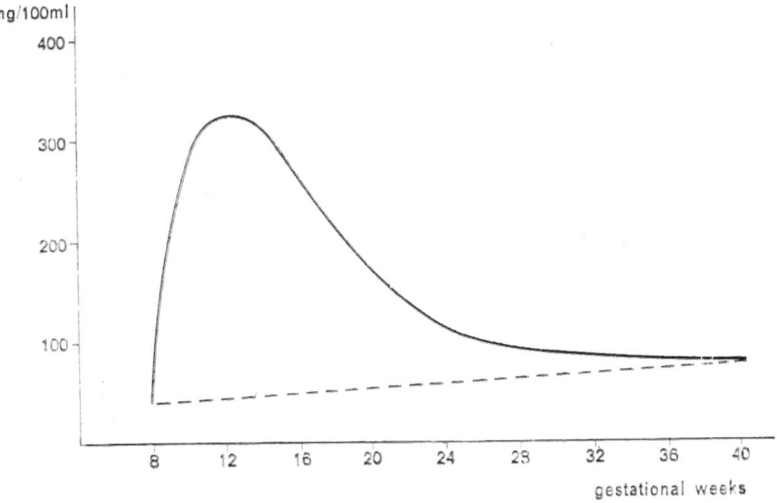

Graph 11. Fetal serum testosterone levels. Males dotted line, females full line.

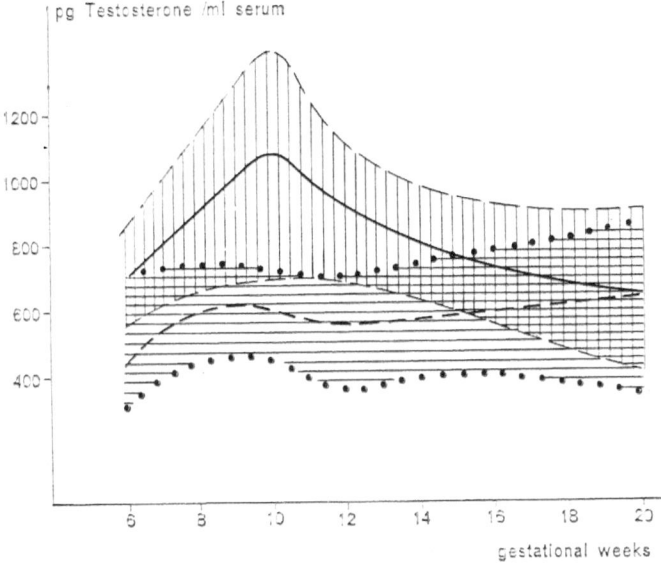

Graph 12. Maternal serum testosterone levels during weeks 7 to 20 of pregnancy (according to Klinga, Bek and Runnebaum, 1978)

Values in pregnancies with male fetuses represented by horizontal lines, with female fetuses by vertical lines.

and is significantly high^r r than in female fetuses of similar age (20—130 ng/100 ml) (*Reyes et al.*, 1974).

In the amniotic fluid, the determination of the testosterone level is a useful tool for the prenatal sex determination. Amniotic fluid testosterone in male fetuses between 12—25 weeks gestation is 223 ± 10 pg/ml, and female fetuses 40 ± 2 pg/ml. The highest mean level in males was found during week 17 (*Judd et al.*, 1976). If the amniotic testosterone around week 17 of gestation exceeds 100 pg/ml there is more than 95% probability of a male fetus.

Differences in maternal peripheral testosterone levels during the first half of pregnancy were also noticed (*Klinga, Bek and Runnebaum*, 1978) (see Graph 12). The mean serum testosterone level in ca. 12 week-pregnant women with male fetuses is 828 ± 298 pg/ml and 597 ± 167 pg/ml with female fetuses. The peripheral testosterone concentration in women with male fetuses showed an increase beginning in week 7, reached a maximum during weeks 9—11 and was followed by a decrease. Although there is some over lapping, if the maternal peripheral testosterone level during gestational weeks 9—13 is more than 800 pg/ml, there is more than a 95% probability that the fetus will be male. If the levels are below 500 pg/ml, the fetus will be female.

FETAL TESTOSTERONE EFFECTS

In fetal testes, there is no evidence of any testosterone-dependent differentiation. Sertoli cells of the fetal testes remain immature even in the presence of testosterone produced by the Leydig cells. Androgens are necessary for the growth of male genital ducts and for the masculinization of the external genitalia. Testosterone in blood is partially bound to a testosterone binding globulin (Te BG). The midtrimester fetal plasma capacity to bind testosterone is low, $1.5—12.8$ mol/l — about one tenth of the maternal (*Hampl et al.*, 1973). In the peripheral tissues, either testosterone or its reduced metabolite 5α-dihydrotestosterone are bound to a specific cytosol receptor. The complex consisting of testosterone or dihydrotestosterone and their receptors are transported into the nucleus of the cell where they remove the specific repressor from the DNA (*Ohno et al.*, 1971), which results in a specific RNA synthesis. These mechanisms are essential for the androgen-dependent differentiation. Androgen-dependent structures are external genitalia, genital ducts, male accessory sex-glands and hypothalamic centra. Mesonephric structures (epididymis, vas deferens, seminal vesicles) seem to be testosterone dependent; external genitalia, prostate and hypothalamus depend on dihydrotestosterone. Testosterone is converted to dihydrotestosterone by the cell-membrane bound 5α-testosterone reductase. 5α-testosterone reductase is present in the indifferent embryonal external genitalia before the production of testosterone becomes evident (*Šulcová, Jirásek, Stárka*, 1973). The term peripheral testosterone sensitivity involves the reduction of testosterone to dihydrotestosterone, the binding of testosterone (or dihydrotestosterone) to a specific cytoplasm receptor, the transport of this complex into the nucleus, the intranuclear binding, the removal of the specific repressor from the DNA, the nuclear synthesis of all classes of RNA, cytoplasmic ribosomal translation of the newly-formed RNA and the formation of new proteins.

The blocks of enzymes participating in the formation of testosterone and dihydrotestosterone are present in some of the androgen-sensitive male pseudohermaphrodites without a uterus. Blocks of 20 hydroxylase, 22 hydroxylase and 20—22 cholesterol desmolase, 3β-hydroxysteroid dehydrogenase and $\Delta^4-\Delta^5$isomerase affect both testes as well as adrenals. The blocks in 17α-hydroxylase, $17-20C$ desmolase and in 17β-hydroxysteroid dehydrogenase leave the adrenal cortex unaffected. Blocks of enzymes participating in the steroid metabolism are inherited as autosomal recessive traits. The defects in the specific plasma receptors involved in the peripheral binding of testosterone and dihydrotestosterone are X-linked.

STEROID PRODUCTION BY THE FETAL AND PERINATAL OVARY

There are no reports finding steroid-production within the fetal ovaries unless growing follicles with a multilayered granulosa are present. Apparently, the granulosa cells secreting the follicular fluid are necessary to induce the differentiation of the theca interna fibroblast-like cells into the steroid-releasing thecal cells. The 3β-hydroxysteroid dehydrogenase can be first detected in the epithelioid theca interna cells of growing follicles of the perinatal ovaries at the beginning of their cavitation. Presumably, thecal cells are involved in the production of estrogens. No estrogens were detected in normal, late fetal ovaries from the second trimenster of pregnancy (*Jirásek et al.*, 1969; *Ryes, Winter and Faiman*, 1973). There may be some synthesis of dehydroepiandrosterone and androstenedione, probably within the ovarian stroma (*Jungmann and Schweppe*, 1978; *Payne and Jaffe*, 1974). The serum estradiol level in $9-25$ week-old fetuses is variable — from less than 8 to more than 800 pg/ml. Although the mean estradiol level is higher in females, the values in both sexes are overlapping. This estradiol is of placental origin. In adult ovaries, granulosa cells begin to participate in the steroid production shortly before ovulation. After ovulation, they turn into the granulosa-lutein cells of the corpus luteum, becoming the main source of progesterone (*Savard et al.*, 1965). In prenatal ovaries, no activity which could be related to the formation of any steroid was documented in the granulosa cells. Recently, the capacity to form estrogens was found at the stage of early fetal ovaries, "before histological differentiation of the tissue" (*George and Wilson*, 1978). The development of ovaries is without any influence on the formation of the genital ducts and external genitalia. The prenatal "feminization" can be explained by the absence of testes and of androgens. Ovarian prenatal androgens may be involved in the prenatal LH RH feedback. Estrogens (probably mostly of fetal placental origin) are involved shortly after birth in vaginal cornification and colostrum production observed in most female newborns. The gonadotropin stimulation of ovaries in newborns immediately after birth is related to the formation of cystic ovarian follicles (*Peters et al.*, 1976).

In premenarcheal ovaries, no preovulatory follicles are present. An age-related increase in diameter of largest atretic follicles has been observed.

PHYLOGENESIS OF SEX-DETERMINATION

Specific germ cells appear very early in phylogenesis. In colonial Protozoa, like Volvox, two types of germinal cells are present: microgametes and macrogametes. In Coelenterates (Hydra), germ cells multiply and ripen in specific organs, known as the gonads. Hydras are monochoristic, in either males or females. The transition from the vegetative type of reproduction to the sexual type can be induced in them by environmental factors, such as the lowering of temperature. In some worms which are not hermaphrodites, sexual differentiation depends on materno-larval contact (Bonellia viridis). Larvae developing in contact with the mother are masculinized and develop as males (*Baltzer*, 1935). External stimuli may be essential for sexual differentiation in many low invertebrates. In insects, special sex-chromosomes are present, stressing the importance of genetic control. In some vertebrates and in some insects, the males are heterogametic X, Y, and the females are homogametic X, X (Drosophila type). In others, the females are heterozygotic Z, W, and the males are homozygotic Z, Z, (Abraxes type). In Drosophila, the development of either testes or ovaries depends on the relation between heterochromosomes and autosomes (*Bridges*, 1939). Diploid Drosophilas with two X-chromosomes develop as females; diploid flies, with only one X-chromosome (without any Y) develop as males. Triploid flies with only two X-chromosomes (3A, XX) are intersexual. No special female determinant was found on the X-chromosome. If any part of the second X-chromosome is added to diploid X-monosomic animals, they develop into females (*Dobzhansky and Schultz*, 1934.) In vertebrates, no specific heterochromosomes were found in fish and amphibians. Heterochromosomes are present in some reptiles and in all birds and mammals. In birds, the males are homozygotic Z, Z and females heterozygotic, (Abraxes type). In mammals, the males are heterozygotic, XY and females homozygotic XX (Drosophila type). In crossing experiments, the males are heterozygotic (XY) in frogs, and homozygotic (ZZ) in turtles and newts. There is evidence that the Y-chromosome originated from the X-chromosome by a pericentric inversion (*Ohno*, 1967).

The genes of the X and Z chromosomes are homologous, contributing approximately 5 % of the genome. The male determination of the Y-chromosome in some mammals is closely related to the H-Y antigen (*Wachtel et al.*, 1975). The genetic male determinant is responsible for the differentiation of seminiferous cords within embryonal testes. Regarding gonadal differentiation, some lower vertebrates are hermaphrodites since testicular tubules and ovarian follicles are present in the same individual. In some fish, the same individual is able to produce eggs and sperm (functional hermaphroditism). In synchronous hermaphrodites, both eggs and sperm are formed at the same time. In asynchronous hermaphrodites, eggs are formed in one period of time and the sperm in another period of time. In hermaphrodites, either both testis and ovary are present, or both sperm and eggs are formed by one bisexual gonad (ovo-testis). Synchronous hermaphroditism occurs in some teleostei (*Serranidae and Perziformes; Atz*, 1964). In amphibia and reptiles, hermaphroditism is exceptional. The interference of external stimuli may be substantial for the sex determination in many species of fish, amphibia and birds. Environmental stimuli are successful in changing the genetic sex if "undifferentiated" gonadal tissue is present in the affected individual. When the testis is removed in toads where the undifferentiated gonadal tissue is present in the Bidder's organ located above the testis, an ovary develops from the Bidder's organ. If the ovary is removed in a newborn chicken, the right-sided gonad develops into a testis (*Benoit*, 1923). (In normal female chickens, the ovary is present only on the left side, while the right-sided gonad remains undifferentiated). If kept under maximum water temperature (*Witschi*, 1929), the tadpoles of a frog (Rana sylvatica) develop into males, regardless of their genetic background. Even visual stimuli may be important for sex determination in fish. In Red fish (Anthias squamipinnis), where only females are present in the tank, one fish will change to a male. If a male is kept in the same tank separated from others by glass, the sex change does not occur (*Fischelson*, 1970).

Sex hormones may be effective in changing the gonadal development during the embryonal period. In Xenopus tadpoles, if estradiol-17β is added to the water (50 g/l), they develop into ZZ-females. If fertilized by normal ZZ-males, the reversed genetic males are fertile ZZ-females producing only males.

In mammals (with the possible exception of oviparous and marsupials), the genetic control of gonadal differentiation becomes so decisive that it is impossible to change it by any of the known external stimuli.

MALFORMATIONS AFFECTING GENITAL ORGANS

SYNDROMES RELATED TO A COMPLETE BILATERAL GONADAL DEVELOPMENTAL FAILURE

(Streak gonads- eunuchoid stature syndromes; syndromes of prenatal castration)

Complete absence of gonads is rare. Genetic males with a normal 46,XY karyotype are more often affected than genetic females with a 46,XX karyotype. Absence of both gonads is related to the syndromes of pure gonadal dysgenesis, true agonadism, true anorchia or the syndrome of vanishing testes.

PURE GONADAL DYSGENESIS (INCLUDING XY-GONADAL DYSGENESIS SWYER'S SYNDROME)

Karyotype: normal 46,XY in most cases, in some others 46,XX.
Phenotype: eunuchoid stature, female external genitalia, oviducts, uterus and vagina, no female breasts. No gonads, streak gonads in some cases.

Pathogenesis: failure in gonadal development prior to the regression of paramesonephric ducts. In some XY individuals dysgenetic gonadomas (gonadoblastomas) may be present. Gonadoblastomas originate from a poorly differentiated gonadal tissue. In 46,XY cases, absence of the H-Y antigen coding gene or its suppression by the X-chromosome-located genes regulating H-Y antigen expression might be suspected.

TRUE AGONADISM (AGONADIA)

Karyotype: normal 46,XY, in most cases.
Phenotype: eunuchoid stature, female clitoris, no vagina or uterus. No female breasts. No gonads.

Pathogenesis: failure in testicular development in the period after the regression of the paramesonephric ducts started, but before the masculinization of the external genitalia began (sometime between weeks 8 and 9). Suppression of H-Y antigen by diploid amount of H-Y antigen limiting gene is suspected.

ANORCHISM (SYNDROME OF "VANISHING" TESTES)

Karyotype: normal male 46,XY.

Phenotype: normal stature becomes eunuchoid after 13—15 years of age; small, normally formed penis; normal empty scrotum. Epididymis and ductus deferens are sometimes present. Paramesonephric derivatives are absent.

Pathogenesis: anorchia is considered to be secondary due to a prenatal bilateral torsion or occlusion of the spermatic artery, or to a genetically determined testicular degeneration which occurs after masculinization of the genital ducts and external genitalia, sometimes after weeks 10—12 and is related to the H-Y antigen limiting gene.

TURNER'S SYNDROME AND ITS VARIANTS
(streak gonads - short stature syndromes)

The following conditions listed below include a short stature and either so-called "streak gonads" or "rudimentary ovaries", which show no maturation of the germinal cells.

GONADAL DYSGENESIS: COMPLETE FORM

(a) Karyotype 45,X (50—60% of affected individuals), 46,Xi(Xq), 46,XX-.
Phenotype: short stature, adults 145 cm average; female external genitalia, vagina, uterus and tubes bilaterally, no female breasts, sparse sexual hair. Primary amenorrhea. Streak gonads.

Pathogenesis: ovaries develop in 45,X individuals until the stage of late fetal ovaries. During differentiation of the primary follicles, all oocytes degenerate because of incomplete granulosa layer.

(b) Karyotypes other than 45,X, usually mosaics such as 45,X/46,XX; 45,X/XY; 45X/47,XYY; or 46,X del (Xp): 46,X del (X) (q ter q 26) or 46,X, i (Yq); 46,XX.

In summary, every chromosomal abnormality affecting gonadal determinants of chromosomes X or Y may result in streak gonads. Absence of Y or the absence of short arm of X results in a short stature.

GONADAL DYSGENESIS: INCOMPLETE FORM
(RUDIMENTARY BILATERAL OVARIES,
OR ALTERNATING STREAK-OVARY)

Karyotypes: 45,X/46,XX; 46,XX in most cases; 45,X/46,X del (Xq).

Phenotype: short stature (if some normal diploid cells are present, the average high is 152 cm), female external genitalia, vagina, and uterus, tubes bilaterally, sparse sexual hair. Some breast development may be present. Primary amenorrhea in most cases. Ovaries containing primary follicles which do not ripen are present. If only one ovary is present, a streak gonad may be found contralaterally.

Pathogenesis: The genetic background compatible with the development of ovarian follicles; short stature is related to the defective or absent "stature" determinants located normally on the short arm of X-chromosome. Reasons for the lack of ovarian follicles to grow and mature are unknown and may be different in individual cases.

PSEUDO-TURNER SYNDROME (NOONAN SYNDROME)

Karyotype: 46,XY; 46,XX.

Phenotype: short stature, webbed neck, congenital cardiac defects, mild neural retardion. *Noonan* (1972) pointed out that males and females may be affected. Cryptorchism, small testes and hypospadia are the common genital anomalies. Ovarian development including ripening of the oocytes in females.

OVARIAN DYSGENESIS AND EARLY OVARIAN FAILURE ASSOCIATED WITH X-CHROMOSOME ABNORMALITIES IN PATIENTS WITH A NORMAL STATURE

Ovarian dysgenesis or early ovarian failure may occur in patients with abnormalities of the X-chromosome. If their stature is of a normal height, a mosaicism with a normal 46,XX cellular line is present in most of the cases.

46,X, i (Xp-) FEMALES

Normal stature, breasts in some, some menstruate for a limited period, becoming amenorrheic around 30 years of age.

MALE PSEUDOHERMAPHRODITISM (M. P.)

Male pseudohermaphrodites are individuals with one or both testes present and no ovarian tissue in addition. Their external genitalia are ambiguous or female. In some, female genital ducts are present. The following classification is proposed:

Testicular dysgenesis syndromes (androgen sensitive m. p. with a uterus):
    mixed gonadal dysgenesis
    bilateral testicular dysgenesis
    unilateral testicular dysgenesis in males

Testosterone deficiencies syndromes (androgen sensitive m. p. without a uterus)
    with an enzyme deficiency: (a) adreno-testicular (b) testicular forms
    eunuchoid form related to the absence of Leydig cells
    with undetected metabolic defect and pseudovaginal hypospadia

Testosterone insensitivity syndromes (androgen insensitive m. p.)
    complete testicular feminization
    incomplete testicular feminization
    (Reifenstein's syndrome: androgen insensitive males)

Testicular dysgenesis syndromes:

The mechanisms of androgen sensitivity as well as of the paramesonephric regression were discussed. The presence of a uterus in individuals with testes is related to a severe disturbance of early testicular development (testicular dysgenesis) which may be linked either to the absence of the male determinant in some cells, or to the presence of an active X-linked gene suppressing the male determinant. By definition (*Jirásek*, 1970), the dysgenetic testis is unable to induce mullerian regression. Androgen production of a dysgenetic testis is low.

MIXED GONADAL DYSGENESIS

Karyotype: 46,XY/45,X in most cases; other karyotypes such as 47,XYY/45,X; or 46,XY/47,XYY/45,X are rare,

Phenotype: stature 155—165 cm in most cases, no female breasts, external genitalia ambiguous to different degrees, exceptionally complete female. Vagina and uterus present in all cases.

Gonads: dysgenic testis on one side, a streak gonad contralaterally. Dysgenic gonadal tumor in about 50% of cases.

Pathogenesis: dysgenic testis is characterized by a thin, poorly developed tunica albuginea and aberrant, irregular testicular tubules embedded in a cellular connective tissue stroma. Seminiferous tubules are irregular; they do contain spermatogonia. Testicular dysgenesis is regarded as a consequence of the presence of some cells bearing the male determinant (XY cells) in addition to other cells lacking the determinant. In familiar cases, the presence of an X-linked gene suppressing the masculinizing determinant is proposed (*German et al.*, 1978).

Streak gonads probably result from degeneration of the "indifferent" gonadal tissue. During degeneration, hyaline is deposited around undifferentiated supportive (primitive granulosa) and germ cells. Dysgenic gonadal tumors (gonadoblastomas) which are found in more than 50% of dysgenetic testes, originate from the "indifferent" gonadal tissue which fails to differentiate or degenerate in the perinatal period.

BILATERAL TESTICULAR DYSGENESIS

Karyotype: 46,XY in most cases; 46,XY/45,X; 45,X/46,XY/47,XYY reported exceptionally

Phenotype: normal stature with no female breast development, pubic hair present in adults, external genitalia malformed showing different degrees of masculinization ranging from a slight clitoris hypertrophy to a penis-like phallus. Vagina, uterus and both oviducts are present. Intraabdominal dysgenic testes are found bilaterally; dysgenic testicular tumors (gonadoblastomas) are common (about 50% of cases).

Pathogenesis: persistence of paramesonephric (Mullerian) derivatives and ambiguous or female external genitalia result from an improper early testicular development. Dysgenic testes are unable to induce regression of the paramesonephric ducts and do not produce enough androgens to fully masculinize external genitalia. Proposed insensitivity of paramesonephric duct to the paramesonephric inhibitor seems unjustified.

UNILATERAL TESTICULAR DYSGENESIS ("UTERUS IN MALES")

Karyotype: 46,XY

Phenotype: normal male. Hypospadia is present in some cases. Uterus and oviduct either prolapse into an inguinal hernia, or are present intraabdominally on the side of an undescended testis. The testis on the side of the developed paramesonephric derivatives is dysgenic, the contralateral may be completely normal, producing sperm. The incidence of dysgenic gonadal tumors is similar as in other dysgenic testes.

Pathogenesis: failure of dysgenic testis to produce a paramesonephric inhibitor is supposed. The hypothetical insensitivity of paramesonephric ducts to the paramesonephric inhibitors does not elucidate the unilateral involvement.

DYSGENETIC GONADAL TUMORS (GONADOBLASTOMAS)

Dysgenic gonadal tumors are common in patients with dysgenic gonads, especially in dysgenic testes. Most of such patients show chromosomal mosaicisms with two chromosomal lines, one of which (usually 45,X) interferes with a normal gonadal differentiation, such as development of primary ovarian follicles or formation of the seminiferous cords. Remnants of undifferentiated gonadal tissue in dysgenic gonads are composed of small cells and gonocytes. Round-shaped, small, multilayered cells are considered primitive granulosa cells; small single- or double-layered cylindrical cells are considered primitive Sertoli cells. Epithelioid Leydig cells may be present within the stroma. Calcifications and hyalinization are common. Dysgenic gonadal tumors rarely metastasize, but if they do, the metastases always have the character of a pure dysgerminoma. Tumors containing Leydig cells masculinize and are called gonadoblastomas. Further subclassification of dysgenic gonadal tumors is possible according to the differentiation of the germ cells, supporting cells and Leydig-like cells.

TESTOSTERONE DEFICIENCIES SYNDROMES (ERRORS IN TESTOSTERONE SYNTHESIS)

M. p. steroid deficiencies — all are inherited in an autosomal recessive fashion. The proof of a specific enzyme deficiency in infancy may be difficult, and induction of gonadalsteroidogenesis by exogenous hCG administration is necessary in most cases. Forms with adrenal insufficiency:

20,22-desmolase type — affected children have ambiguous external genitalia and severe salt-losing syndrome. Adrenal lipoid hyperplasia is characteristic.

20,22-hydroxylases deficiency was reported in an eight year-old phenotypic female with adrenal hyperplasis and without paramesonephric derivatives (*Kirkland et al.*, 1973).

119

3β-hydroxysteroid dehydrogenase deficiency — siblings of both sexes have been described. In males (46,XY), the defect is associated with a phenotype of a male pseudohermaphrodite. Because of decreased levels of androgens as well as cortisol and aldosterone, the salt-losing syndrome is extensive. Adrenal lipoid hyperplasia is always present.

17α-hydroxylase deficiency was demonstrated in some 46,XY male pseudohermaphrodites. External genitalia are ambiguous, sexual hair present in adults. Gynaecomastia appears at puberty. Testosterone and cortisol levels are decreased, corticosterone and deoxycorticosterone are increased.

The phenotype may be similar to that of an incomplete testicular feminization. In contrast to incomplete testicular feminization which is X-linked, 17α-hydroxylase deficiency is autosomal recessive. 17α-hydroxylase deficiency was found in some cases diagnosed as Reifenstein's syndrome.

Forms without adrenal insufficiency:

17,20-desmolase deficiency — two children reported by *Zachman et al.* (1972) had ambiguous external genitalia and no paramesonephric derivatives.

17β-hydroxysteroid dehydrogenase deficiency — affected individuals are unable to convert dehydroepiandrosterone to testosterone. External genitalia in males are ambiguous. At puberty, female breast development may occur.

EUNUCHOID M. P.

Karyotype: 46,XY

Phenotype: eunuchoid, no sexual hair, no uterus, vagina is shallow or absent, no pubertal changes of breasts and sexual hair. Low serum gonadotropins in some, elevated in others (*Jirásek*, 1965; *Part et al.*, 1975); extremely low levels of testosterone in adults. Leydig cells are not present in the testes.

Pathogenesis: lack of gonadotropins cannot be supposed during fetal period as Leydig cells are stimulated by hCG of placental origin. Insensitivity to LH and hCG due to the absence or binding failures of hCG-LH receptor is hypothetical. Leydig cell agenesis was proposed (*Berthezene et al.*, 1976).

M. P. WITH PSEUDOVAGINAL HYPOSPADIA

Karyotype: normal male 46,XY.

Phenotype: male, except ambiguous external genitalia, exhibiting a vaginal vestibule, scrotiform labia, a phallus of various-size. This type of genitalia was suggested to be a pseudovaginal perineoscrotal hypospadia (*Simpson and German*, 1970). Virilization occurs at puberty.

Pathogenesis: malformations of the external genitalia result from a diminished production of androgens by the fetal testes. Various enzyme defects may be present in many affected individuals, 5α-testosterone reductase deficiency was reported. In infancy the enzyme defect may be inapparent. To some degree m. p. with pseudovaginal hypospadia represents a "mixed bag" for male individuals with ambiguous external genitalia and unknown biochemical background (if any).

TESTOSTERONE INSENSITIVITY SYNDROMES

The term applies to all male individuals showing feminization at puberty because their peripheral tissues do not properly respond to androgens. Peripheral androgen insensitivity is characterized in most affected individuals by loss of a repressor binding affinity for its inducer, (either testosterone or dihydrotestosterone). This defect is X-linked (*Ohno*, 1976). In some other individuals with an incomplete testosterone insensitivity, 5α-testosterone reductase deficiency was found.

COMPLETE TESTICULAR FEMINIZATION (t. fm.)

Phenotype: female, female breast development, sparse or absent sexual hair. Normal female external genitalia. Shallow, blind vagina. No uterus. Frequent inguinal herniae. Bilateral testes with seminiferous tubules lined with immature Sertoli-cells.

Pathogenesis: embryonal testicular development adequate for paramesonephric duct regression. Female external genitalia related to the peripheral androgen insensitivity present throughout life. Postnatal feminization related to androgen resistance, whereas the sensitivity to estrogens is normal. The defect is X-linked.

INCOMPLETE TESTICULAR FEMINIZATION

Phenotype: similar to complete testicular feminization, except for external genitalia which are malformed, usually only a hypertrophied clitoris being present. In some individuals a partial labioscrotal fusion may occur.

Pathogenesis: similar to complete t. fm. The reason for the malformed external genitalia remains obscure.

Testosterone insensitivity in testicular feminization syndromes may be heterogenous. In some cases, the amount of receptor protein is low; in others, the testosterone binding to the genetic repressor is defective, in others the nuclear binding of the testosterone-receptor protein complex does not occur (*Arnheim et al.*, 1976).

5α-TESTOSTERONE REDUCTASE DEFICIENCY

The affected enzyme reduces testosterone to dihydrotestosterone in peripheral tissues, especially in the external genitalia and prostate where preferentially dihydro-testosterone is bound by the cytoplasmic receptor. The phenotype of untreated adults is similar to those with an incomple tetesticular feminization. The masculinization of the external genitalia is usually more expressed than in testicular feminization syndromes.

MALFORMATIONS OF GENITAL DUCTS

In males: persistence of paramesonephric structures leading to the development of an oviduct and uterus is always related to the dysgenesis or absence of the ipsilateral testis. A well-formed uterus is never present in androgen-insensitive male pseudo-hermaphrodites. If a uterus is present in an individual with a testis, the diagnosis of androgen sensitive male pseudohermaphroditism or true hermaphroditism is to be considered.

MESONEPHRIC DUCT APLASIA

Mesonephric duct aplasia is associated with absence of the epididymis, vas deferens and seminal vesicle. If the mesonephric duct never developed, the ipsilateral ureter and kidney are missing. Bilateral aplasia of mesonephric duct may be supposed in some cases of bilateral renal aplasia (Potter's syndrome).

In females: if a mesonephric duct never developed in females, not only the ipsilateral kidney and ureter would be missing, but the paramesonephric structures (on the affected side) would also be absent, resulting in an unicornuate uterus.

Incomplete fusion of the paramesonephric ducts is a common reason for uterine anomalies such as uterus duplex, uterus septus, uterus subseptus, uterus arcuatus and uterus bicornis. Sometimes even the vagina may be affected (vagina septa or duplex). The absence of one paramesonephric duct is related to the unicorn uterus.

ROKITANSKY-KÜSTNER SYNDROME (PARAMESONEPHRIC APLASIA)

The syndrome is characterized by a normal 46,XX karyotype; vagina is either completely absent or very short; uterus is absent. Upper portions of the oviducts may be present. Stature, breasts and sexual hair are normal, female.

Pathogenesis: the syndrome is regarded as being a consequence of a failure of the paramesonephric ducts to cross the mesonephric ducts and to fuse into the uterovaginal canal in most cases. In others failure of attachment between the uterovaginal canal and the urogenital sinus was proposed.

VAGINAL ATRESIA

Two types of vaginal atresia are to be distinguished.
Type 1 — atresia resulting from a transverse septum formed between the endodermal contribution from the urogenital sinus and the uterovaginal canal.

Type 2 — atresia resulting from a septum formed at the paramesonephric tubercle (as a consequence of developmental failure of the endodermal vaginal contribution).

In Type 1, the vagina seems to be short and blind, and in Type 2, the vagina is seemingly completely absent. A normal uterus is present in both types. Haematocolpos and haematometra usually develop at puberty and bring the patient to the medical office.

RUDIMENTARY UTERUS

The rudimentary uterus is narrow duct lined with a columnar epithelium with a muscular wall. No glands are present. Rudimentary uterus represents the persistent uterovaginal canal and usually opens into a persistent urogenital sinus. The urogenital sinus, if present, provides a common opening for both the vagina and the urethra.

MALFORMATIONS OF THE EXTERNAL GENITALIA

Androgen-dependent and androgen-independent (teratogenic) malformations are distinguished. Androgen dependent malformations result from an improper fusion of the labioscrotal swellings and rims of the urethral plate, including the formation of the cavernous (and glandular) urethra. The same malformations may occur in chromosomal males and females: in males, as a result of an androgen deficiency or insensitivity, in females as a result of androgen overstimulation. Because of much confusion in nomenclature, the following is proposed: ambiguous external genitalia (or pseudo- vaginal hypospadias) are characterized by the presence of vaginal vestibule, no fusion of the labioscrotal swellings, nor of rims of the urethral plate. The derivative of the genital tubercle is called the clitoris (normal hypertrophic, peniform), if no cavernous urethra is present and if the openings of urethra and vagina are separated (Fig. 78). If both vagina and urethra open into a persistent urogenital sinus, the derivative of the genital tubercle is called the phallus (Fig. 79, 80).

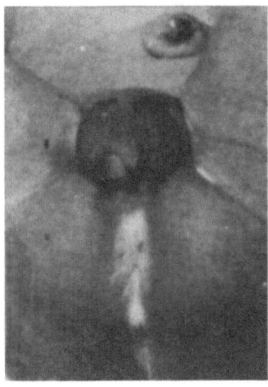

Fig. 78. Hypertrophic clitoris in a newborn.

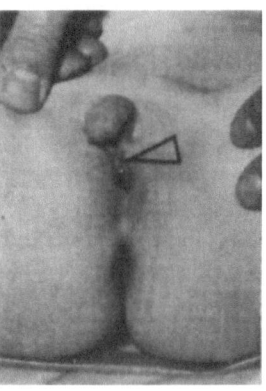

Fig. 79. Ambignous external genitalia with a peniform clitoris. The openings of the urethra and vagina are separated.

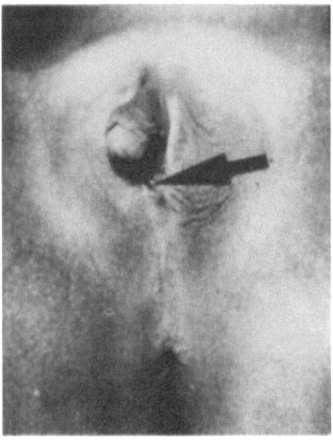

Fig. 80. Ambiguous external genitalia with a phallus. The opening of the urogenital sinus (common opening of both, the vagina and the urethra) is marked with an arrow.

Ambiguous genitalia are found in different forms of male pseudohermaphroditism, in female pseudohermaphroditism and in true hermaphrodites.

HYPOSPADIAS

Hypospadic external genitalia are characterized by an ectopic opening of the cavernous urethra. The genitalia are considered as male hypospadic if at least a part of the raphe scroti is present. Hypospadias, by definition, are defects of the cavernous urethra. Perineal, scrotal, penile and glandular hypospadias are to be distinguished. Combinations, such as peniglandular h., or peniscrotal hypospadia are common. Hypospadia may be a symptom of a syndrome or may represent an isolated malformation. Hypospadias occur as an isolated malformation in otherwise completely normal boys without any other congenital malformations (except cryptorchism in some cases). Hypospadia is present in some male and female pseudohermaphrodites, true hermaphrodites and in many multiple-anomally syndromes. A so-called "hypospadia in females" represents defects in the urethrovaginal septum, and is not comparable to the "male" hypospadia. A narrow external opening of the female urethra is usually associated with the "female" hypospadia.

ANDROGEN-INDEPENDENT (TERATOGENIC) MALFORMATIONS OF THE EXTERNAL GENITALIA

Conditions listed below are involved in this group: duplication of the phallus, penis or of the whole external genitalia; absence of penis, or clitoris, epispadia, retroscrotal penis; micropenis; absence of labia majora; bilateral or unilateral persistence of labioscrotal swellings, bifid scrotum, scrotiform malformation of the external genitalia (Fig. 81).

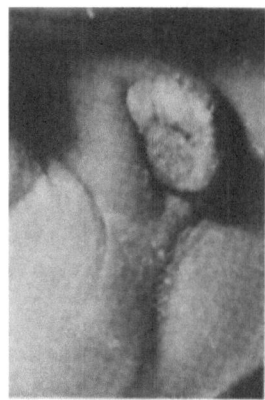

Fig. 81. Scrotiform teratogenic malformation of the external genitalia in a newborn with imperforated anus and some other congenital anomalies.

CRYPTORCHISM

Failure of testis to descend into the scrotum occurs either bilaterally, or unilaterally. The ectopic testis may be present retroperitoneally within the abdominal cavity, or within the inguinal canal. Cryptorchism is related either to the improper development of the gubernaculum testis, or to the failure of the gubernaculum to contract and bring the testis down. The testicular descent is androgen dependent, and may be influenced by the hCG administration (*Rajfer and Walsh*, 1976). Dystopic testes are found usually under the skin of perineum or within a femoral hernia. They do not have a proper gubernaculum.

The descent of ovaries is arrested by the developing uterus and by the absence of androgens. However, sometimes at birth the ovary may be present, in a shallow peritoneal pocket within the inguinal canal (diverticulum of Meckel), or even under the skin within the labia majora.

FEMALE PSEUDOHERMAPHRODITISM

All female individuals with a 46,XX karyotype whose external genitalia "do not look female" may be classified as female pseudohermaphrodites. Ovaries, oviducts, uterus and vagina (sometimes malformed) are present in all of the cases.

Virilization of the female fetus is usually related to an enzyme defect affecting adrenal steroidogenesis or to the administration of exogenous androgenic steroids to the pregnant women or to the presence of an androgen-producing lesion in pregnant women (such as carcinoma of the adrenal cortex, cortical stromal hyperplasia of the ovary, arrhenoblastoma). Various enzyme defects affecting steroidogenesis are listed below. All of them are inherited as an autosomal recessive trait. All of them are characterized by adrenal hyperplasia.

Enzymatic defects in androgen-dependent female pseudohermaphrodites:

Steroid 21-hydroxylase deficiency:

(a) without sodium loss (simple virilizing adrenal hyperplasia)

(b) with a salt-losing syndrome (salt-losing adrenal hyperplasia)

Steroid 11β-hydroxylase deficiency (hypertensive adrenal hyperplasia)

Steroid 3β-hydroxydehydrogenase deficiency and steroid 17α-hydroxylase deficiency are related to a low production of androgens and estrogens leading to male instead female pseudohermaphroditism. The sodium wasting in 3β-hydroxysteroid dehydrogenase deficient individuals is usually lethal during infancy. The males express the phenotype of the androgen sensitive male pseudohermaphroditism without uterus.

Steroid 17α-hydroxylase deficiency

Females with 17α-hydroxylase deficiency have normal external genitalia, but do not feminize at puberty. Affected males have ambiguous external genitalia compatible with diagnosis of male pseudohermaphroditism.

In teratogenic forms of female pseudohermaphroditism, the external genitalia show an androgen-independent malformation.

TRUE HERMAPHRODITISM

The true hermaphrodites are individuals with both ovarian as well as testicular structures. Histologically verified seminiferous cords or tubules and primary ovarian follicles or their unquestionable derivatives are required for the diagnosis. Presence of spermatogonia, spermatocytes, praespermatids, spermatids and sperm is not required. Ovarian-type stroma or Leydig cells are not significant for the diagnosis. The following anatomical forms are distinguished:

(1) Unilateral hermaphroditism:
   (a) with a testis (testis present on one side, ovotestis, or testis and ovary on the other); 7% of cases
   (b) with an ovary (ovary present on one side, ovotestis or testis and ovary on the other); 32% of cases
(2) Lateral hermaphroditism (h. alternans): a testis on one side an an ovary contra-laterally); 33% of cases
(3) Bilateral hermaphroditism: ovotestis (or testis and ovary) on both sides; 28% of cases

Karyotypes: 46,XX/47,XY; 46,XX (in most cases); 47,XXX/46,XX; 47,XXY; 46,XY; Phenotype: ambiguous or hypospadic external genitalia; vagina, uterus and oviducts present in 80% of cases. Abdominal ends of the tubes are often closed. Epididymis and vas deferens are present on the side of testis, and usually on the side of the ovotestis. Both spermatozoa and mature follicles were demonstrated in some cases of lateral hermaphroditism. In ovotestis, ovarian follicles do mature, but the testicular part is represented by seminiferous tubules lined with Sertoli-cells only.

Feminization, including female breast development, becomes evident at puberty.

Comment: a masculinizing determinant must be present for the testicular development. Two X-chromosomes are responsible for differentiation of the ovarian follicles. The presence of undifferentiated gonadal tissue in the fourth month, or later, is a prerequisite of ovarian development within the fetus. In true hermaphrodites, part of the genital ridge differentiates into the testis during the 7th and 8th week, leaving undifferentiated genital tissue, this tissue undergoes "ovarian" development, resulting in ovarian follicles formed during the second half of pregnancy.

Within the ovotestis, because the proliferation of the germ cells is not completely arrested during testicular differentiation, ovarian tissue is either under the surface of the gonad or at the caudal pole. In 46,XX cases the translocation of the male determinant from Y-chromosome to the heterochromatic area of the paternal X-chromosome (as stressed by *Ferguson-Smith*, 1966) is most plausible. In the 46,XY cases, the translocation of the euchromatic part of second X-chromosome to another chromosome would be the simplest explanation.

KLINEFELTER'S SYNDROME

Karyotype: 46,XY/47,XXY (incomplete form); 47,XXY (complete form) and 46,XX (complete form) are distinguished.

Phenotype: similar in all forms; eunuchoid male, normal male external genitalia and genital ducts. Testes descended in most cases, small in all of them. Gynecomastia may appear at the time of puberty. In patients affected by the incomplete form (46,XY/47,XXY) spermatozoa may be formed; 47,XXY and 46,XX patients are sterile.

Histologically, focal testicular tubular hyalinization and Leydig cell hyperplasia and hyalinization are the characteristic findings in adults.

Comment: polysomy X results either from meiotic errors, or from mitotic non-disjunction occuring in the zygote. In 46,XX cases the most probable explanation would be the translocation of the male determinant from the Y-chromosome either to the euchromatic part of the paternal X-chromosome, or to another chromosome. The reason for the testicular degeneration present in adults is unknown.

MULTI X SYNDROMES IN MALES

Karytotype: 48,XXXY; 49,XXXXY.

Phenotype: somatic anomalies and mental deficiency are present in all cases. Testes are small, affected by intensive hyalinization. Androgen deficiency becomes evident at puberty.

TRISOMY X IN FEMALES

Karyotype: 47,XXX.

Phenotype: affected females are phenotypically normal. Primary amenorrhea, menstrual disorders and premature ovarian failure was observed in some cases. Affected females have a 50% chance to produce 24,XX oocytes. The frequency of 47,XXY or 47,XXX individuals among their sibling does not exceed 15%, and is probably even lower.

Genital anomalies are frequently encountered in multiple somatic anomaly syndromes. Some of them are listed below.

TRISOMY 9 SYNDROME

Common features: lethal prenatally. Mongoloid palpebral fissures, prominent nose, low set ears, micrognathia, small penis and cryptorchism.

TRISOMY 13 SYNDROME

Common features: holoprosencephaly, mental retardation, deafness, polydactyly, heart defects. Hypoplastic ovaries and uterine anomalies in females, abnormal scrotum and cryptorchism in males.

CORNELIA DE LANGE SYNDROME

Common features: microcephaly, fused eyebrows, small nose, long hair, hirsutism. Undescended testes in most males, sometimes hypospadia. In females, uterine anomalies, small ovaries.

FETAL FACE SYNDROME (ROBINOW SYNDROME)

Common features: peculiar face with broad forehead, triangular mouth with down-turned angles, anteverted nostrils. The growth is inadequate, forearm brachymelia is remarkable. Hemivertebrae. Micropenis in boys. Hypoplastic clitors and labia in females.

HYPERTELORISM-HYPOSPADIAS SYNDROME (OPITZ)

Common features: hypertelorism, mild mental retardation, hypospadias, cryptorchism, inguinal herniae.

HYPOSPADIAS-DYSPHAGIA SYNDROME (G-SYNDROME)

Common features: hypertelorism, marked parietal and occipital eminences, mild micrognathia. Hypospadias of variable degree, scrotum bifidum in some boys. Normal genitalia in females.

LEOPARD SYNDROME

Common features: multiple lentigines, cardiac defects, minor skeletal abnormalities, hypospadias or bilateral cryptorchism. Absence or hypoplasia of an ovary. Late menarche.

MECKEL SYNDROME (DYSENCEPHALIA SPLANCHNOCYSTICA)

Common features: lethal; holoprosencephaly, encephalocele, internal hydrocephalus. Cystic liver, kidneys and pancreas. Polydactyly and syndactyly. Hypoplastic penis and cryptorchism in males, septate vagina and uterus anomalies in females.

MULTIPLE PTERYGIUM SYNDROME (BONNEVIE-ULLRYCH SYNDROME)

Common features: small stature, pterygia of neck, cubiti, poplitei and fingers. Cleft palate. Normal genitalia. Defferential diagnosis includes gonadal dysgenesis and male Turner's syndrome.

MYOTONIC DYSTROPHY (STEINERT SYNDROME)

Common features: myotonia, masklike facies, ptosis of lids, partial alopecia, mental deficiency common. Testicular atrophy in males, ovarian cysts, amenorrhea in females. Diabetes and hypothyroidism are common.

POTTER SYNDROME (OLIGOHYDRAMNION SYNDROME)

Common features: lethal, bilateral renal agenesis, peculiar face, low set ears, ectrodactyly. Gonadal hypoplasia, absent uterus, or uterine anomalies, absent vagina.

128

Masculinization of external genitalia in a 46,XX individual was observed (*Potter*, 1965).

PRADER-WILLI SYNDROME
(HYPOTONIA-HYPOMENTIA-HYPOGONADISM-OBESITY SYNDROME)

Common features: in addition to symptoms listed above, small penis and crotum, undescended testes in 90% of males.

RUSSEL-SILVER SYNDROME

Common features: birth weight around 2200 g, relatively small face, prominent forehead. Congenital asymmetry, cafe-au-lait spots, short fifth fingers, elevated STH, FSH and LH levels. Enlarged clitoris, or hypospadia may be present. Tumors of adrenal and kidney were noticed.

SMITH-LEMLI-OPITZ SYNDROME

Common features: microcephaly, epilepsy, cutaneous syndactyly of second and third toe. Small testes, ambiguous genitalia, cleft scrotum, cryptorchism in boys.

CHAPTER 6

THE HYPOPHYSIS

The hypophysis is composed of two parts of different origin. The adenohypophysis originates from the ectoderm of the primitive oral cavity and the neurohypophysis from the neuroectodermal evagination from the bottom of the diencephalic vesicle (*Altwell*, 1926; *Romeis*, 1940; *Falin*, 1961; *Levina*, 1965; *Conklin*, 1968). The area of hypophyseal development is determined very early by adhesion between the neuro-ectoderm of the brain plate and the surface ectoderm near the rostral end of the notochord (stage IX, 20—21 days). As the brain vesicles develop, and the oral pit becomes evident, the area of contact between the surface ectoderm and neuroectoderm is above the oral membrane. At this stage, (S. H. XIII, XIV), the ectodermal pocket underneath the brain primordium may be recognized as Rathke's pouch. The notochord ends at the posterior wall of Rathke's pouch and the ectoderm of the posterior wall of Rathke's pouch extends over the oral membrane. The endoderm of the oral membrane is contributed by the prochordal plate (Stage X, 20—22 days). As the mesenchyme between the brain vesicles and foregut increases in amount, Rathke's pouch deepens. There is no evagination of Rathke's pouch, or "growth from the stomodaeum".

In embryos 32—39 days old (S. H. XIII—XV) the Rathke's pouch is an anterio-posteriorly-flattened pocket lined by a single-layered, cylindrical, glycogen-rich epithelium. The anterior end of the notochord still contacts the posterior wall of Rathke's pouch (Fig. 82). In embryos 37—42 days-old, 8—12 mm (S. H. XVI), the diencephalic evagination of the neurohypophyseal primordium becomes evident (Fig. 83). The neuroectodermal evagination is formed behind the optic chiasma and is lined by a pseudostratified cylindrical neuroepithelium. The anterior portion of the diencephalic epithelium is attached to the superior part of the posterior wall of Rathke's pouch (Fig. 84). In embryos 52—60 days-old, 25—30 mm (S. H. XXII to XXIII) the primordia of the hypophyseal lobes can be seen. The posterior wall of Rathke's pouch adjacent to the neurohypophyseal evagination becomes the pri-mordium of the pars intermedia, the rest of the posterior wall of Rathke's pouch contributes the pars tuberalis. The anterior wall of Rathke's pouch transforms into the pars distalis of the anterior lobe. The formation of epithelial cords formed by endocrine cells begins in 51—53 day-old embryos, 19—24 mm (S. H. XX). The first epithelial cords grow into the mesenchyme from the anterior wall of Rathke's pouch. In 55—60 day-old embryos, 25—35 mm (S. H. XXII, XXIII) the epithelial cords are present in all parts of the anterior lobe and capillaries between the cords begin to appear (*Streeter*, 1951). The mutual growth of epithelial cords and capillaries give rise to the typical structure of the adenohypophysis (Figs. 85, 86, 87). The arteries providing blood for the capillaries come from the internal carotids into the middle of a mesenchymal center into which the epithelial cords grow. The two paired mesenchymal centers are adjacent to the anterior wall of Rathke's pouch. The

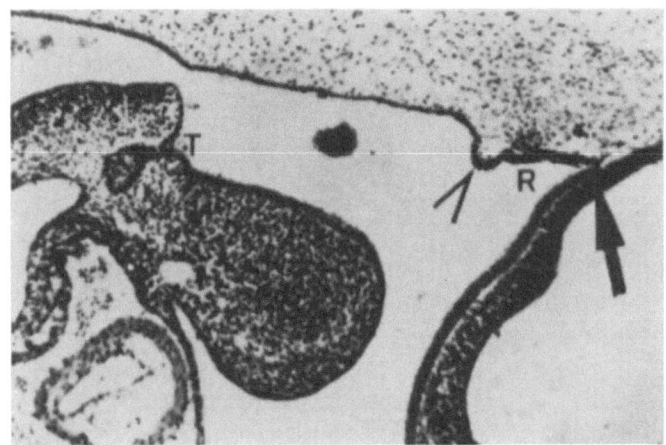

Fig. 82. Sagittal section through the oral cavity of a 5 mm embryo (34 days-old, S. h. XIII). Rathke's pouch (R) is formed between the ectoderm apposed to the proencephalic vesicle and the anterior end of notochord. The attachement of the Rathke's pouch to the brain vesicle is marked by a full arrow. The border between ectoderm of the mouth cavity and endoderm of the primitive pharynx is marked <. T — invagination of the medial thyroid primordium.

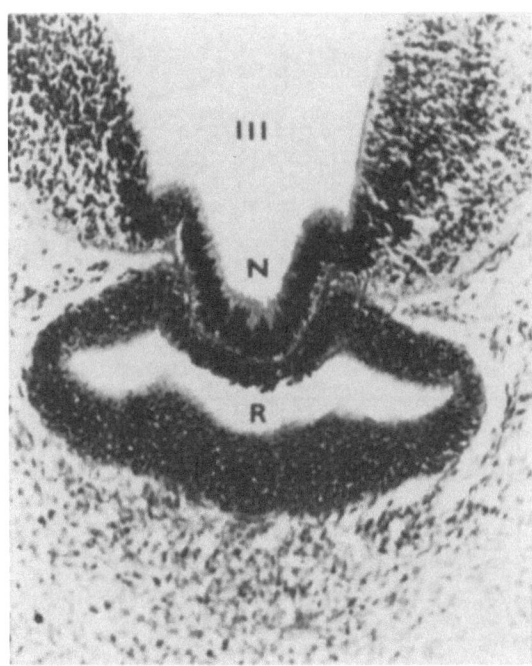

Fig. 83. Frontal section of the hypophyseal primordium in a 12 mm embryo (40 days, S. h. XVI). R — cavity of the Rathke's pouch, N — invagination of the neurophypophysis, III — 3 rd cerebral ventricle.

10

131

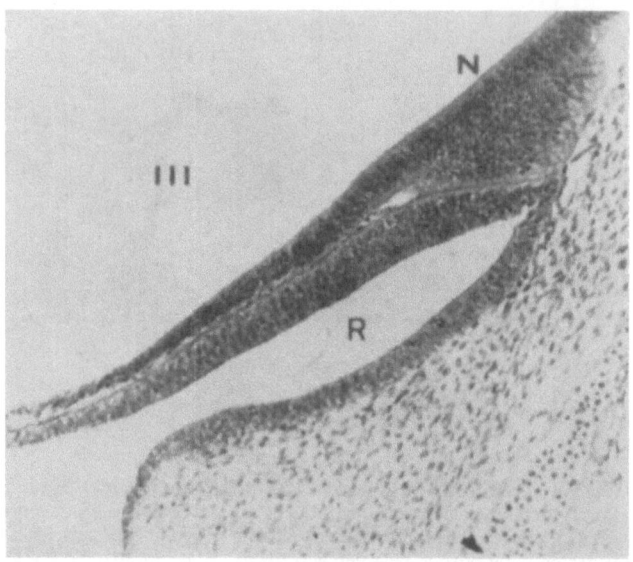

Fig. 84. Sagittal section through the hypophyseal primordium in a 14 mm embryo (42 days, S. h. XVII). R — Rathke's pouch, N — primordium of the neurohypophysis, III — third cerebral ventricle.

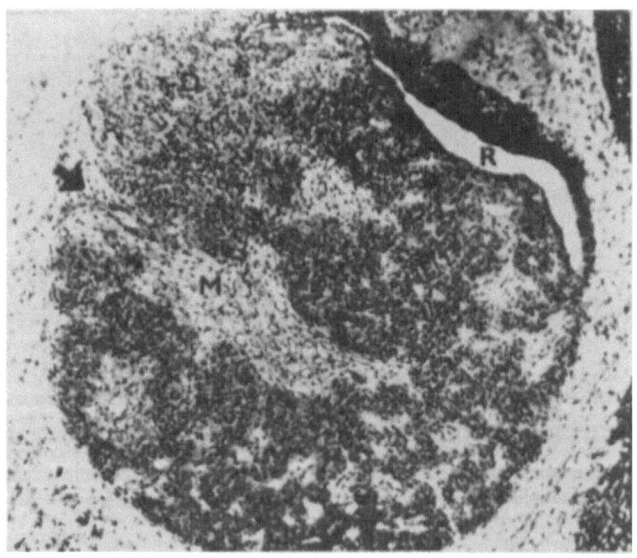

Fig. 85. Parasagittal section through the hypophysis of a 10 weeks old fetus. R — lumen of the Rathke's pouch, N — neurohypophysis, D — distal part of the adenohypophysis. The epithelial cords of the adenohypophysis are are growing into the mesenchymal centre (M) with capillaries.

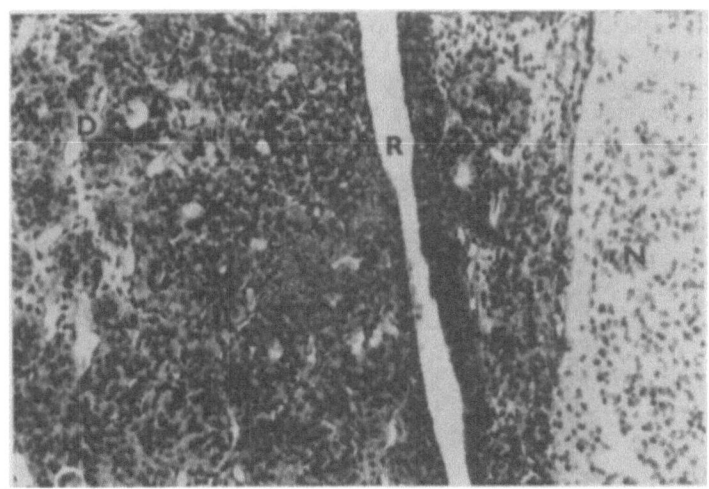

Fig. 86. Hypophysis from a 14 weeks old fetus. N — neurohypophysis, I — pars intermedia o-
the adenohypophysis, R — cavity of the Rathke's pouch, D — pars distalis of the adenohypof
physis.

original lumen of Rathke's pouch remains preserved between the pars intermedia
and the pars distalis. Rathke's pouch is connected by a stalk with the floor of the
primitive oral cavity. Later on as the oral and nasal cavities are formed, Rathke's
pouch open into the masopharynx. The epithelial stalk of Rathke's pouch fragments
in 50—55 day-old embryos, 20—25 mm (XXI S. H.) disappearing completely, except
for a small pharyngeal remnant in 55—60 day-old embryos, 25 mm (XXII, XXIII
S. H.).

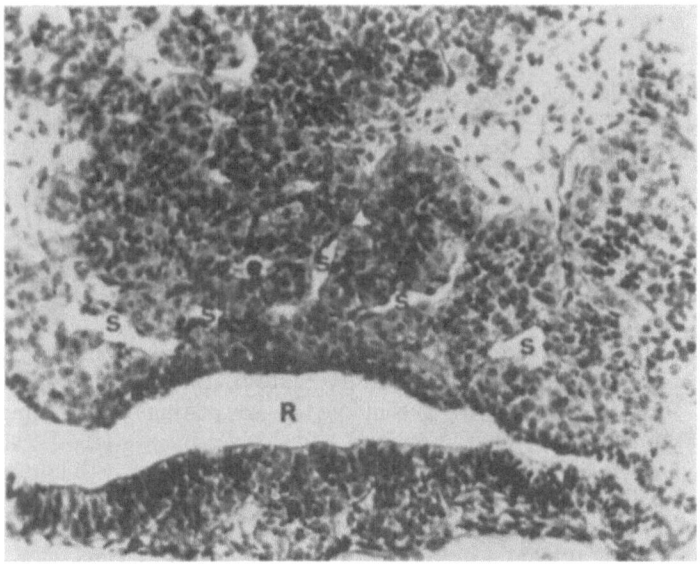

Fig. 87. Epithelial cords of the fetal hypophysis growing into the mesenchymal connective
tissue. Capillaries (S) are present. R — lumen of the Rathke's pouch.

The blood for the sinusoid capillaries of the anterior lobe is derived from direct branches of the superior hypophyseal arteries and from superior hypophyseal arteries, which first enter the capillary plexus of the tuber cinereum. The veins entering hypophysis from the tuber cinereum are known as the hypophyseal portal vessels. The blood to the neural lobe is supplied by the inferior hypophyseal arteries. Both superior and inferior hypophyseal arteries originate from the internal carotid).

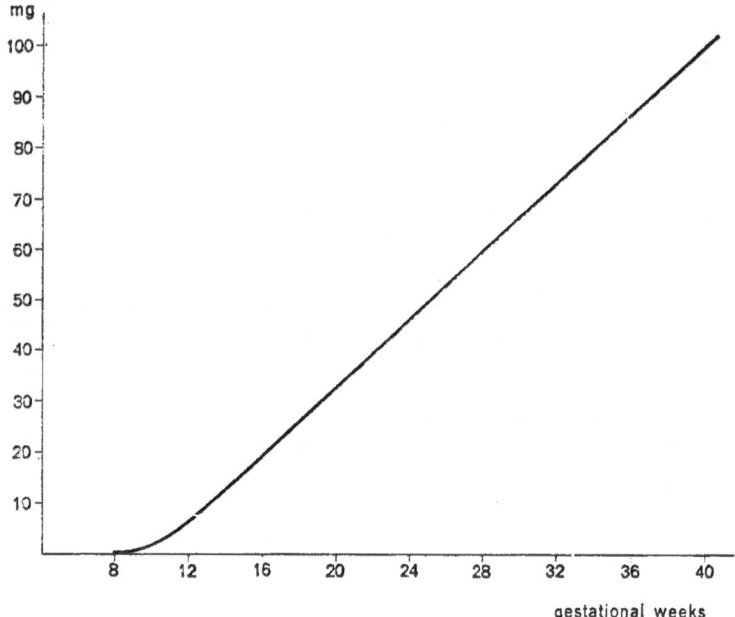

Graph 13. Weight of the fetal hypophysis.

The veins, venae laterales from the anterior lobe, veane posteriores and inferiores from the posterior lobe, enter the sinus cavernosus. The hypophyseal blood supply develops during the ninth and tenth week (*Jirásek, Rychter*; unpublished), the portal system is formed at the end of the third month. The growth of the fetal hypophysis is demonstrated on Graph 13.

CELLS OF THE ADENOHYPOPHYSIS

The classification of the endocrine cells of the adenohypophysis depends on the staining procedures. Using the classical H-E stain, the acidophilic (eosinophilic) cells, the basophilic cells and the chromophobes are distinguished. Using the azan stain (azocarmine, aniline blue, orange G and eosin), *Romeis* (1940) classified the cells, α, β, γ, δ, ε, η. The α-cells are acidophils producing the growth hormone, β-cells are basophilic cells producing the thyreotropic hormone, γ-cells are chromophobes. The δ-cells are gonadotropin-producing basophils. The η-cells are thought to be acidophils producing prolactin. According to the classical work of Romeis, β-cells are present in a 30 mm, fetus, γ-cells in a 40 mm and α-cells in an 80 mm fetus. All cellular types were found in 240—260 mm long fetuses (Figs. 88, 89). Similar findings were reported by *Daikoku* (1958). Improvement in classification of adenophyseal cells followed the introduction of histochemical stains such as aldehyde fuchsine, aldehyde thionine, P. A. S. and alcian blue, and their combinations (*Conklin*, 1968; *van Oordt*, 1965; *Rosen and Ezrin*, 1966; *Waidl*, 1960). The most important advance in the classification of adenohypophyseal cells was achieved by immunohistochemical methods, allowing an exact identification of various cells according to the hormones

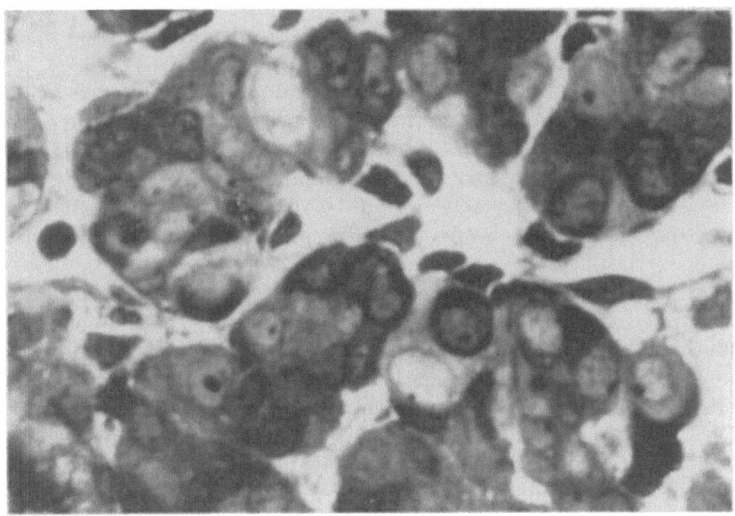

Fig. 88. Various hormone producing cells in the hypophysis of a 4 month old fetus.

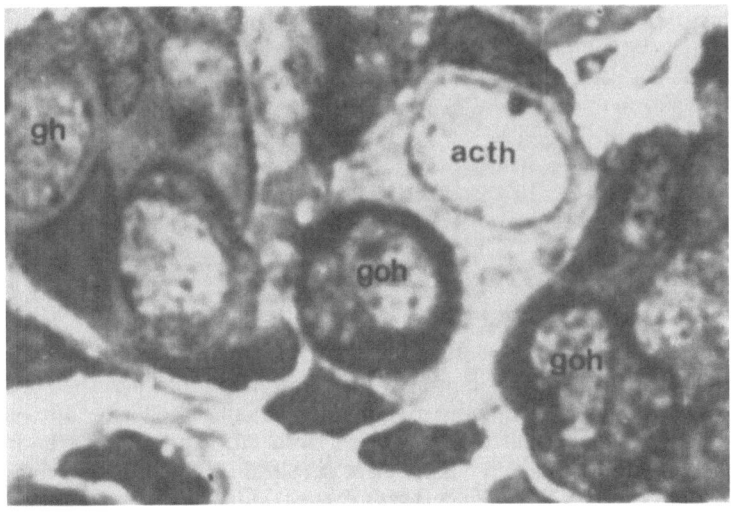

Fig. 89. Growth hormone producing cell (gh), gonadotropin producing cells (goh) and ACTH producing cell (acth) in the adenohypophysis of a 4 month old fetus.

they contain. The subcellular organization of various cells was contributed by electron microscopists.

1. GH-cells (growth hormone or somatotropin-producing cells), are acidophilic cells, or α-cells. They are recognized in the 10th week, in good agreement with the finding of the immunoreactive GH in the hypophysis of a 68 day-old fetus (*Kaplan et al.*, 1976; *Gitlin and Biasucci*, 1969). *Matsuzuki et al.* (1971) detected GH in some embryos at seven and eight weeks. The hormone-containing granules are produced at the rough endoplasmic reticulum. The granules are round and densely packed, 350—400 mm in diameter. Granules are secreted into the pericellular space unchanged.

2. PRL-cells (prolactin-producing cells, carmosinophilic cells) are acidophils, or ε-cells. Cells with the identical granules to those found in the "pregnancy cells" in adenohypophysis of pregnant women were described in the fetal hypophysis by *Pasteels* (1963). They appear at fourth month (*Levina*, 1968). They are irregularly shaped with an extremely well-developed rough endoplasmic reticulum. In the cytoplasm, sparse, large, prolactin granules, over 600 nm in diameter are found.

3. TSH-cells (thyrotropin-producing cells) are basophilic, or β-cells. Although Romeis claimed to recognize them in a 30 mm embryo (8 weeks), others did not find them until the ninth week (*Rosen and Ezrin*, 1966). Immunoreactive TSH is present by 12—14 weeks (*Fischer et al.*, 1970; *Fukuchi et al.*, 1970). TSH cells are polyedral, they have small glycoprotein granules (taking aldehydefuchsin), which are 50—100 nm in diameter, and are of various electrondensity.

4. G-cells (gonadotropin-producing cells; FSH-cells and LH-cells are basophils, or δ-cells. Both FSH and LH are glycoproteins. Glycoproteins other than TSH suggested to be gonadotropins, were demonstrated by *Pearse* (1953), *Falin* (1961), *Mitikewich and Levina* (1965) and *Waidl* (1960). G-cells are ovoid — their granules are of variable electron density and size, about 150—300 nm in diameter. Numerous lysosomes are present within the cytoplasm, which are related to the presence of hydrolases (*Jirásek*, 1963). Both FSH and LH were demonstrated by specific radioimmunoassays to be present in a 68 day-old fetus.

5. ACTH-cells (ACTH-producing cells, γ-cells of Romeis) ACTH cells are regarded as basophils with lipoid cytoplasmic droplets. Under EM, their specific feature seems to be sparse fibers 60—80 A⁰ in diameter. The specific granules are small, less than 150 nm in diameter. According to the author's view, however, in agreement with Romeis, γ-cells, the ACTH-producing cells are big "degranulated" chromophobes. Immunoreactive ACTH is detectable in the pituitary of 7 week-old embryos (*Kaplan et al.*, 1976). ACTH-cells are evident in the tenth week (author's unpublished observations).

Chromophobes cells

Chromophobes cells of the classic histology are regarded as "undifferentiated cells, before specific granules are developed". "Big" chromophobes may be transitionally degranulated cells. Increase in big chromophobes was observed after adrenalectomy. All specific adenohypophyseal cells originate from an ectodermal, cylindrical, glycogen-rich cell of the Rathke's pouch. There is still incomplete evidence concerning whether all the cells originate from two (or more) different precursor-cells; one for the cells secreting glycoproteins sharing the α-subunit (FSH, LH, TSH), and another one for the cells secreting "pure" polypeptides (GH, PRL, ACTH).

THE NEUROHYPOPHYSIS

Until mid-gestation, the neurohypophysis comprises about 10% of the whole gland. During the second half of intrauterine life, the contribution of the neural lobe increases to approximately 25%. The neurohypophysis represents terminals for the hypothalamohypophyseal tract formed by axons from the nucleus supraopticus and nucleus paraventricularis. The nerve endings form irregular "palisades" at the border of each neurohypophyseal lobule and near the connective tissue interlobular septa, which are rich in capillaries. Among the unmyelinized fibers there are scattered glial cells, known as pituicytes. Neurosecretory substances (vasopressin AVP and oxytocin AVT) may be stained by chrome alum hematoxylin, or aldehyde fuchsin. The neurosecretory droplets are described as Herring bodies. They are present within the cytoplasm along the axons, and especially in the "palisade" terminals. Under EM, neurosecretory granules are membrane-bound, 100—300 nm in diameter.

Oxytocin and vasopressin are produced by different cells. The neurohypophysis attains its definitive structure by the end of sixth month.

The neurosecretory material appears in the ganglionic cells of hypothalamic nuclei by 20 weeks and at the neurohypophysis by 23 weeks (*Benirschke and McKay*, 1953; *Rinne et al.*, 1962).

THE HYPOPHYSEAL HORMONES

GROWTH HORMONE (GH)

hGH is a simple protein with an unbreached chain containing 190 aminoacids. The synthesis of GH was demonstrated in vitro using fetal hypophyseal tissue cultures. If ^{14}C labelled aminoacids were added to the medium, synthesis of GH was observed in the hypophysis in 9 week-old fetuses, but did not occur in eight and eight and a half week-old hypophyses. There is a steady increase in GH within the hypophysis throughout gestation (*Franchimont et al.*, 1972; *Kaplan et al.*, 1976).

The data concerning the GH content of the hypophysis and GH fetal serum concentrations are presented in Table 14 (data from *Kaplan et al.*, 1976; *Franchimont et al.*, 1972 in parentheses and Graph 14).

The concentration 8—9 ug of GH per mg of tissue is reached between 25—29 weeks and does not change thereafter. Maximal serum GH levels are reached at midgestation, approximately the 120th gestational day, decreasing thereafter. The decrease between the fourth month and term is approximately 75% (see Graph 14).

Growth hormone is not essential for normal fetal growth. The growth of an individual born without an hypophysis may be normal. Individuals affected by pituitary nanism are born with a normal birth weight.

Heterogenity of GH in the pituitary and serum GH was observed in man as well as in other mammals (*Bala et al.*, 1970; *Frohman et al.*, 1972). There are three different forms of GH known as the "little" GH (MW approximately 20,000), "big" GH (MW approximately 40,000) and the "big-big" GH (with a high molecular variable weight). *Frohman and Stachura* (1973) and *Kaplan et al.* (1976) reported that in the fetal pituitary, the "little" GH represents 85—95%, the "big" contributes 2—10%, and the "big-big" GH is often not detected.

Table 14. GH hypophyseal content, concentration and fetal serum level. (based on Franchimont et al. and Kaplan et al).

Weeks	Hypophysis μg content	Concentration μg/mg	Serum ng/ml
9−11	(1.0)		(65)
10−14	0.44±0.2	0.14	65.2±7.2
15−16	(9.9)		(72)
15−19	9.2±2.3	2.0±0.5	114.9±12.5
20−24	(52)		(119)
	59.4±11.1	3.8±0.6	131.9±21.9
25−29	225.9±40.5	9.2±3.2	(72)
			53.5±7.0
30−34	577.6±90.9	9.3±1.2	42.5±7.0
35−40	675.0±112.3	7.5±1.5	(27)
			34.6±3.3
1−30 days after birth	808		33.5±4.2
	79.1		

PROLACTIN (PRL)

The human prolactin is a simple protein, containing about 200 aminoacids. Formed by carmosinophilic cells, PRL may be detected in a very low concentration from the 10th to 20th gestational week (*Aubert et al.*, 1975). *Levina* (1968) using bioassays by 18 weeks. The secretion of PRL was demonstrated using tissue cultures at the end of fourth gestational month (*Siler-Khodr et al.*, 1974). In tissue cultures, the

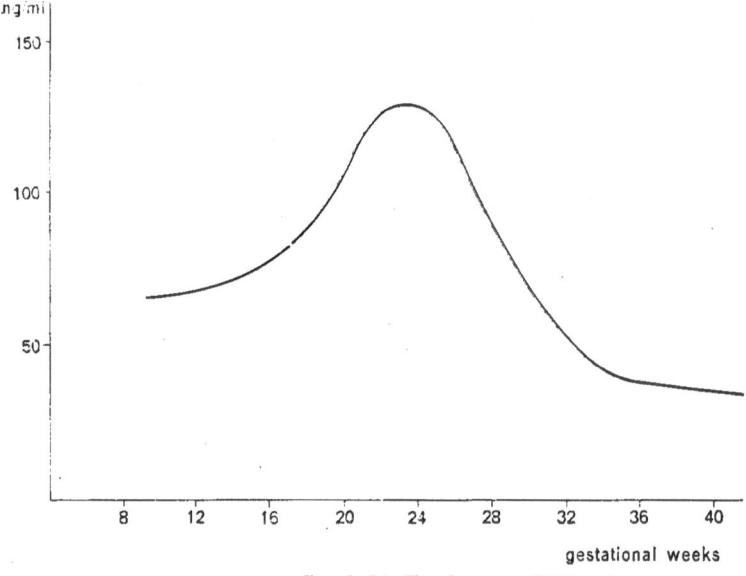

Graph 14. Fetal serum GH levels.

production of PRL remains unaffected by the administration of hypothalamic extracts to the cultivating medium and increases during several weeks of cultivation. The prolactin hypophyseal content and fetal serum concentrations are summarized in Table 15. (Data of *Aubert et al.*, 1975). Fetal and maternal serum prolactin levels are compared in Graph 15.

Table 15. PRL hypophyseal content and fetal serum level.

Weeks	Hypophysis content (ng)	Serum level (ng/ml)
10—14	4.1 ± 1.4	25.3 ± 4
15—19	14.8 ± 4.6	16.8 ± 3.5
20—24	405 ± 142 ⎱	18.1 ± 4.9
25—29	542 ± 204 ⎰	
30—34	872	208.4 ± 27.4
35—40	2039 ± 459	268.3 ± 52.2
newborn (full term)		167.8 ± 14.2

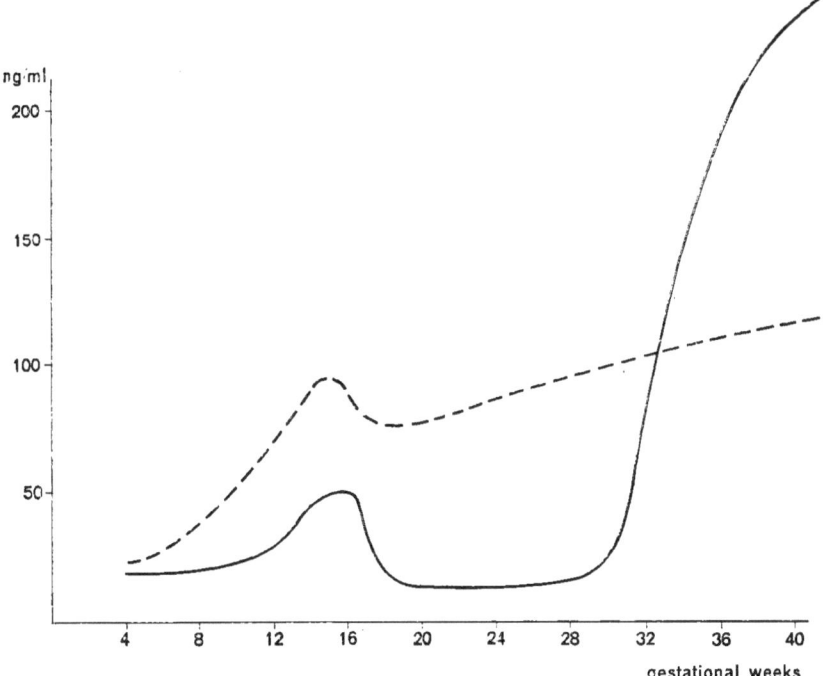

Graph 15. Fetal and maternal serum prolactin levels.
(Fetal levels full line; maternal, dashed line)

Pituitary PRL content and concentration increase sharply between 14—26 weeks of gestation. During the last trimester the pituitary concentrations remain relatively unchanged. Serum PRL level increases until birth. At birth the fetal PRL concentration is higher than the maternal. High PRL level falls to normal during the first postnatal week. Gestatioal PRL is partially of decidual origin.

Prolactin accumulates in the amnionic fluid. The highest levels (10,000 ng/ml) were found in the first trimester of gravidity and decreased thereafter. The amnionic level of PRL at birth is approximately 1,000 ng/ml (*Friesen et al.*, 1973). Electrophoretic and chromatographic characteristics of the amnionic prolactin are similar or identical to that of hypophyseal origin (*Ben-David et al.*, 1973). PRL occurs in several forms such as "little"and "big-big" (*Suh and Frantz*, 1974). "Little" prolactin contributes about 80—95% of the hormone. The role of the hormone in the developing fetus is not known.

ADRENOCORTICOTROPIN (ACTH)

ACTH is a simple polypeptide formed by 39 aminoacids, M. W. approximately 4,500. Immunoreactive ACTH is detectable in the fetal pituitary by seven weeks after fertilization (nine weeks of gestation). Secretion of ACTH is detected at 12 weeks. The concentration of pituitary ACTH rises throughout mid-gestation, and after the 26th week remains steady. The fetal serum levels are maximal between 12—19 weeks, decreasing thereafter. In newborns the ACTH levels are significantly higher than in older children and adults. There is a temporary increase around birth.

The ACTH pituitary concentration and fetal serum level are summarized in Table 16 and Graph 16.

The negative feedback between cortisol and ACTH becomes operative before week 20 of gestation.

MELANOTROPIN (MSH)

Melanotropin is a polypeptide occuring in two forms, α and β. The human hypophysis does not contain either of them. The material reacting with β-MSH antisera is either related to the similarity of the amino acid sequence (between the 8th and 20th amino acid) in ACTH and β-MSH or to the presence of β-lipotropin (β-LPH). β-lipotropin (β-LPH) is a large molecule consisting of 91 amino acids and is biologically inactive. This molecule probably gives rise to ACTH, β-MSH, enkephalins and endorphins (*Li, Chung*, 1976). Enkephalins and endorphins are involved in the modulation of mood, behavior and pain sensitivity.

HYPOPHYSEAL GLYCOPROTEIN HORMONES

The three hypophyseal glycoprotein hormones, TSH, FSH and LH, are similar. Their molecules are composed of two subunits, α and β. The α-subunit is identical not only in TSH, FSH and LH, but also in hCG. The molecular structure of TSH, FSH and LH and hCG molecules are determined by two genes each. However, the genetic coding of the α-chain is identical in all of them. The β-chain is related to their specific activities (*Pierce et al.*, 1971; *Vaitukaitis et al.*, 1972). The presence of free subunits

Table 16. ACTH hypophyseal content, concentration and fetal serum level

Week	Pituitary content	Concentration related to mg	Serum level	
			pg / ml	Weeks
(1) 8	0 mU	0 mU		
9—10	1.0—1.55 mU	6.5—9.0 mU		
11—16	8.3—11.0 mU	11.6—20.0 mU		
17—19	27.3—4.3 mU	12.3—2.4 mU	249 ± 65.7	12—19
(2) 20—22	75.3—3.5 μg	30.9—2.0 μg		
23—25	440—84 μg	92.2—18.2 μg	234 ± 29.0	20—34
full term	1561 μg	256 μg	143 ± 7.0	35—42
(delivery)	1526—82 μg	117.0—10.8 μg		
1—7 days			120—8.3	1 (postnatal)

(1) according to *Pavlova et al.*, 1968
(2) according to *Winters et al.*, 1974

in addition to intact hormones has been demonstrated in the serum, the pituitary and the placenta. The predominance of the α-subunit secretion was demonstrated in tissue cultures from human fetal hypophysis (*Franchimont and Pasteels*, 1972) and in homogenates of the pituitaries (17—19 weeks) and in the fetal serum (*Kaplan et al.*, 1976).

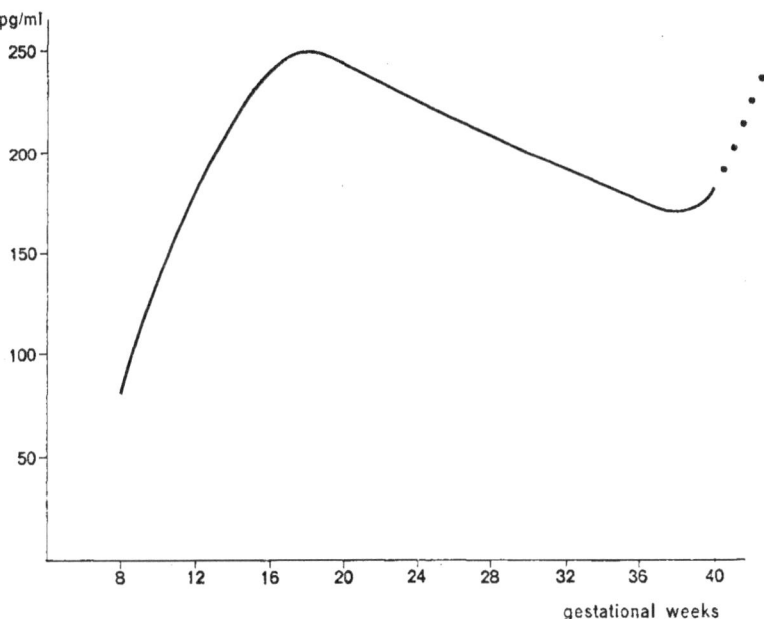

Graph 16. Fetal serum ACTH levels.

Nesither α nor β subunits has any intrinsic bioactivity. Recombination of α and β-subunit is necessary for the specific effect of the hormone (*Rayford et al.*, 1972; *Catt et al.*, 1973).

The clearance rate of the subunits is more rapid than of the intact hormone (*Pepperell et al.*, 1975).

THYROTROPIN (TSH)

The molecular weight of the complete hormone molecule, composed of α and β-subunit, is about 28,000. The sialic acid content of TSH is about 1%. Immunoreactive TSH is present both in the fetal pituitary and in fetal serum by 12—13 weeks of

Table 17. TSH fetal serum levels (based on Fisher et al., 1970).

Week	TSH serum μU/ml
11—18	2.4 ± 0.14
22—34	9.6 ± 0.93
38—40	8.9 ± 0.93
38—40	8.9 ± 0.93

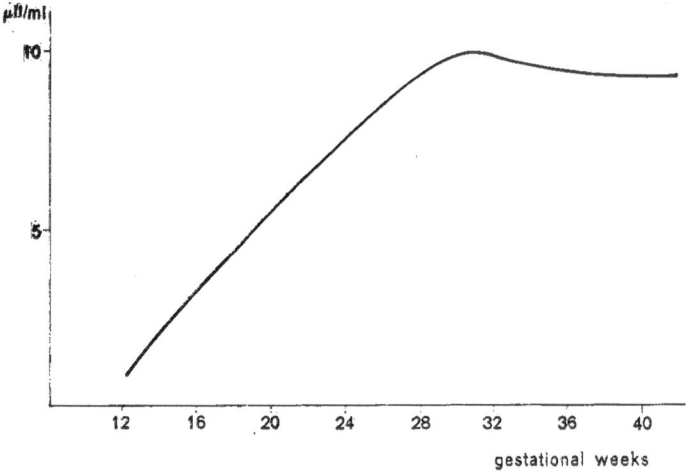

Graph 17. Fetal serum TSH levels.

gestation. Pituitary TSH is detectable between 8—10 weeks (*Fukuchi et al.*, 1970; *Fischer*, 1972). Fetal TSH serum levels are seen in Table 17 (according to *Fischer et al.*, 1970) and in Graph 17.

The concentration of TSH remains low until 16 weeks, increasing to weeks 28 and decreasing slightly thereafter. These data suggest that the negative feedback between T_4—TSH secretion is established at the end of the second trimester. Secretion of TSH is controlled by the hypothalamic TRF. Within 30 minutes after delivery TSH rises from levels of 9.5 to 86 uU/ml (*Fischer and Odell*, 1969) and is followed by neonatal thyroid hyperactivity.

The transplacental passage of TSH is very limited (*Kearns and Hutson*, 1963; *Dussault et al.*, 1972).

HYPOPHYSEAL GONADOTROPINS, FSH AND LH

Both folliculostimulating (FSH) and luteinizing (LH) hormones appear in the fetal hypophysis at eight weeks. Both hormones are glycoproteins consisting of α and β subunits. FSH contains 5% sialic acid, LH about 1%.

Immunoreactive FSH was detected in the fetal pituitary at 68 days (*Kaplan et al.*, 1976) and increased in males throughout gestation. In females, beginning day 80, the levels of FSH are higher than in males, reaching a maximum between 26—30 weeks of gestation and declining thereafter.

The FSH fetal hypophyseal contents and concentrations in males and females are summarized on Table 18 (from *Grumbach and Kaplan*, 1974).

Table 18. FSH hypophyseal content and concentration.

Weeks	FSH content (ng)		FSH concentration ng/mg	
	males	females	males	females
10—14	1.8±0.7	7.4±5.2	0.6±0.3	1.6±0.05
15—19	13.0±4.4	315.8±216.0	5.8±2.1	49.6±32.8
20—24	51.2±18.6	3725.0±2105.9	11.5±4.4	119.5±47.0
25—29	149.5±69.1	5788.6±1460.7	2.2±0.9	101.8±
30—34		2010.2±908.3		67.7±22.2
35—40		360.0±122.2		3.1±0.9
2 months	0.6—2	1.7—53.5	5.0—5.4	15—41

The lower levels of FSH in males suggest a negative feedback between testicular androgens (testosterone) and FSH early in ontogenesis. In females, the high levels of FSH are observed during periods in which oogonia multiply and start their meiotic prophase. The levels decline as soon as a considerable number of primary and growing follicles become differentiated in the late fetal ovaries (probably in consequence of ovarian androgen production).

In the LH, there is a sharp increase in hypophyseal LH content from weeks 19—25 in both sexes. The content of LH is higher in females than in males. In males, the maximal LH concentrations are found between 20—24 weeks. In females, maximal concentrations are reached between weeks 26—28. In infants the LH content and concentrations are similar in both sexes during the first two months. LH fetal hypo-

143

physeal contents and concentrations are given in Table 19. Fetal LH serum levels are presented and male and female LH levels are compared in Graph 18.

Levina (1968) using less sensitive FSH bioassays, detected FSH in female fetuses six weeks earlier than in males, by 13—14 weeks in females and by 19—20 weeks in males. She also described a decrease in FSH concentration after 20 weeks of pregnancy.

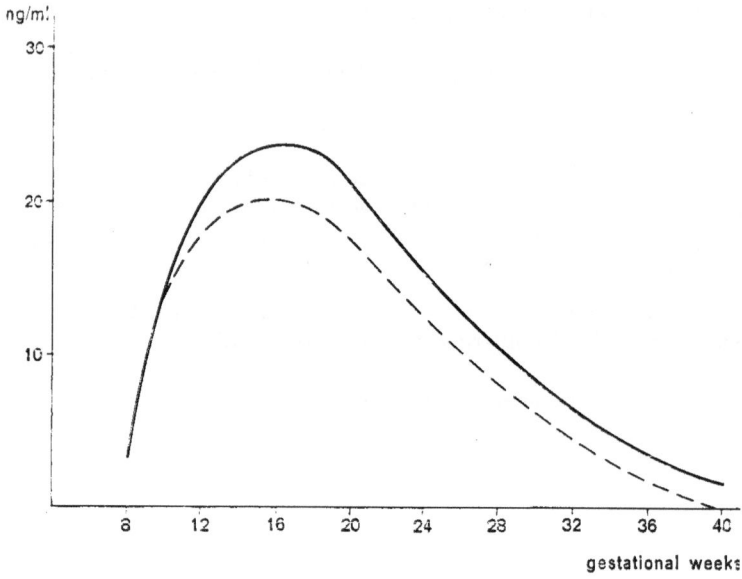

Graph 18. Fetal serum LH levels (in females full line, in males dotted line).

Table 19. LH hypophyseal content and concentrations (data by *Kaplan and Grumbach*, 1976).

Weeks	LH content (ng)		LH concentration (ng/mg)	
	males	females	males	females
10—14	21.0—11.6	88.2—44.2	3.3—1.2	32.7—9.1
15—19	165.3—56	797.0—274.7	39.2—19.2	153.1—57.3
20—24	489.4—148.3	3940.0—1846	114.5—57.1	129.9—35.6
25—29	1222.0—389.6	4938.8—1128.4	22.3—5.2	75.4
30—34		2353.5—1165.5		42.1—17.4
35—40	1590.2—484.8		15.0—4.9	
2 months	5.4—5.0	4.5—5.9	54.3—43.9	34.5—107.5

144

VASOPRESSIN (AVP)

The physiologic role of vasopressin (AVP; arginine vasopressin) is the retention of water within the body. The stimuli for the vasopressin secretion come from osmo- and baroreceptors stimulated by hyperosmotic blood plasma or by a decrease in blood volume. Both AVP and AVT (arginine vasotocine) are synthesized in the supra- optic and paravenctricular hypothalamic nuclei by separate cells. At the site of synthesis, the hormones are bound to neurophysins by noncovalent bonds. When AVP and AVT are discharged by exocytoses, the bonds split and free octapeptidic hormone and free neurohypophysin enter the circulation. Mammalian development occurs in an osmotically well-balanced medium provided by the maternal mechanism. AVP and AVT were found in the human fetal pituitary by 12 weeks (*Kaplan et al.*, 1976). Pituitary concentration of AVP is lower than AVT. In late gestation the concentra- tion of AVP is higher. In newborns the pituitary AVP content is 350—400 mU (*Heller and Zaimis*, 1949).

CEREBRAL NEUROENDOCRINE COMPLEX AND HYPOTHALAMIC FEED — BACK SYSTEMS

The basic organization of the CNS becomes evident early in ontogenesis at the stage of neural groove before the neural tube closes. On the cerebral anlage, the prosen- cephalic, the mesencephalic and the rhombencephalic areas are recognized in early somite embryos 22—25 days of age. As the neural tube closes, starting from the level of somite seven, the cerebral vesicles are formed. The anterior neuropore closes in 26—28 somite embryos, 26—28 days old. The differentiation of prosen- cephalon into telencephalon and diencephalon becomes evident as soon as the optic cups appear. The telencephalic vesicle becomes evident at 37—40 days (11 mm embryos, S. H. XVI), hemispheres and olfactory bulbs at 42—44 days (14 mm embryos, S. H. XVII). Within the diencephalon on the lateral side of the third ven- tricle, the hypothalamic sulcus extends up to the attachment of the optic stalk. The hypothalamic sulcus represents a forward continuation of the sulcus limitans. The hypothalamic sulcus separates the hypothalamus from the thalamus and an- other shallow epithalamic sulcus separates the epithalamus.

The thalamus grows much more rapidly than the epithalamus and hypothalamus. This growth is related to the development of thalamic nuclei and medial and lateral metathalamic geniculate bodies. The thalamus is a relay center for visual (lateral geniculate body), auditory (medial geniculate body), tactile, pain, and other proprio- ceptive impulses on their way to the cerebral cortex.

Within the hypothalamus, the neuroblasts of the mantle zone differentiate into the nuclei at the end of the second month and during the third month. On the ventral side of the hypothalamus the mamillary bodies and the tuber cinereum to which the hypophyseal stalk is attached, become evident during the third month. Hypothalamic nuclei are classified topographically. The anterior group includes the preoptic nucleus, the anterior hypothalamic nucleus, the suprachiasmatic nucleus, the supraoptic nucleus and the paraventricular nucleus. Within the tuber cinereum, the ventromedial, the dorsomedial, the arcuate nucleus and the lateral tuberal nuclei are distinguished. The posterior group includes the mamillary, the posterior hypothalamic, the supramamillary and the tuberomamillary nuclei.

Hypothalamic nuclei are interconnected and receive imput from the brain stem and from the hemispheres. The forebrain structures connected with the hypothalamus are known as the "limbic system". According to the neurotransmitter released, three different neuron systems are recognized: the norepinephrine, the serotonin and the dopamine system. The norepinephrine system includes the reticulothalamic tract, the serotonin system is represented by the rhaphe neurons and the dopamine system forms the tuberohypophyseal tract. Homeostatic neurons of the hypothalamus are peptide forming. According to the site of action, they are called neurohypophyseotropic (octapeptidic, producing AVP and AVT) and adenohypophyseotropic (peptidic, producing somatostatin, corticotrophin releasing factor, thyrotropin releasing factor and gonadotropin, or luteinizing hormone releasing factor.

Neurohypophyseal hormones are formed by the magnocellular system. Adenohypophyseotropic hormones are produced by the parvicellular neurosecretory system. Most of the neurons are located in different hypothalamic nuclei of the "hypophysiotropic area" of *Szentagothai* (1968). The area comprises the mediobasal hypothalamus. The formation of the nuclei is finished by 18 weeks of gestation. The axon terminals develop during the next two weeks (19—20 weeks). The hypophyseal portal system develops during the third and fourth month. Primary and secondary portal plexuses are interconnected by 20—21 weeks.

VASOPRESSIN AND OXYTOCIN

Oxytocin and vasopressin are produced in the perikarya (pl. of perikaryon) of neurons of the paraventricularis and supraopticus nuclei (magnocellular system). Each hormone associated with a carrier protein, hypophysin, is transported in a membrane-bound complex by the way of an axon, and is released by axon terminals (*Robinson*, 1965). The supraopticohypophyseal tract, originating from both nuclei, enters the hypothalamic median eminence. Some neurons terminate in the palisade zone of the eminence, most of the neurons enter the palisades of the neurohypophysis.

VASOPRESSIN FEED — BACK SYSTEM

Vasopressin acts on the distal convoluted tubule of the kidney, regulating the reabsorption of water. Following dehydration, the blood volume falls and the plasma becomes hypertonic. The volumoreceptors and osmoreceptors activate the vasopressin output. Vasopressin increases the water permeability of the cells in the distal convoluted tubules, water is reabsorbed and hypertonic urine is excreted. After a water load, the blood volume rises, plasma becomes hypotonic, vasopressin falls, permeability of the distal convoluted tubule decreases and hypotonic urine is excreted. A vasopressin stimulatory factor acting between the volumo- and osmoreceptors and neurosecretory neuron was proposed but remains unknown.

Intrauterine fetal dehydration does not occur. The newborn has the ability to respond to a water load (*Smith*, 1959), or to hypertonic saline (*Fisher et al.*, 1963). Immature renal function are blamed for the decreased urine concentration ability in newborns. The vasopressin feed — back system and aldosterone-, renin-, angiotensin systems are closely related.

Somatostatin (SRIF)

Immunoreactive somatostatin was demonstrated in the hypothalamus and cerebral hemispheres in human fetuses from 10—22 weeks (*Kaplan, Grumbach and Aubert, 1976*). There is a linear serum SRIF increase with gestational age. The levels are 7.3 pg/mg an tenth week rising to approximately 40 pg at the 22nd week. Using immunohistochemical methods, the release of somatostatin was localized in the axon terminals in the median eminence.

SOMATOSTATIN AND STH FEED — BACK SYSTEM

Early in gestation, STH and SRIF secretion seem to be autonomous. It is not known if STH has any influence on the SRIF synthesis. In midgestation, the production of both STH and SRIF is intense. In the last trimester of gestation, SRIF restrains the production of STH, and STH falls until a steady dynamic equilibrium between STH and SRIF production is achieved. This type of relation between a hormone and its releasing or inhibitory factor may be divided into four different phases: (1) an autonomous secretion (basal) (2) an unrestricted secretion (reaching maximal values) (3) a restricted secretion (falling from a maximal to a balanced level and (4) a balanced secretion. Somatostatin has been found to cause a decline in plasma glucose and insulin and glucagon secretion (*Yen et al.*, 1973; *Yen et al.*, 1974).

PROLACTIN FEED — BACK SYSTEM

No specific PRL RF has been isolated. In anencephalic fetuses, the levels of PRL are comparable with normal, suggesting that in the prenatal period no PRL RF is required. There is good evidence that the hypothalamic dopamine system is a strong stimulator of pituitary PRL release. The existence of such a feed — back mechanism is not known in human fetuses. The unconjugated estrogens (17 β-estradiol, estrone, estriol) promote both the synthesis and release of PRL. The rise in fetal PRL late in gestation may be related to the increased circulating estrogens (*Aubert et al.*, 1975).

CRF AND ADRENOCORTICOTROPIN FEED — BACK SYSTEM

The existence of CRF is accepted although the isolation and characterization of this substance has not been achieved. There is some evidence that serotonin is involved in CRF secretion. There is evidence of the dependence of the prenatal growth of the adrenal cortex of the ACTH secretion. In the last trimester, however, the fetal serum ACTH is falling, while the cortisol is rising. The feedback between ACTH production and circulating cortisol is present as early as 9—10 weeks of gestation. In general, the low level of circulating cortisol stimulates the CRF synthesis and release into the hypophyseal portal system, and ACTH secretion takes place. The high level of circulating cortisol suppresses the CRF release and the circulating ACTH falls. In addition to the ACTH stimulation, there is a relationship between the increasing total body weight, the growth of the adrenal and the DHA and DHAS synthesis and secretion. The equilibrium between ACTH secretion and cortisol production is established postnatally, after involution of the DHA and DHAS producing fetal zone of the adrenal cortex. The secretion secretion of DHA and DHAS reappears in four or five year-old children and preceeds the onset of puberty.

TRF AND TSH FEED — BACK SYSTEM

TRF was found in the human fetal hypothalamus as early as in the 10th week of gestation (*Kaplan, Grumbach and Aubert, 1976*). TRF production is localized in the median eminence, and in lesser amount in the periventricular, dorsomedial, ventromedial and the arcuate nuclei. In various mammals, only 20—30% of TRF is present in the hypothalamus. The remaining 70—80% is found in the hemispheres, thalamus, mesencephalon, pons, cerebellum and spinal cord. In human anencephalics, a large amount of TRF was found in the cerebellum. The TRF hypothalamic content varies from 0,64—184 ng (between 10 and 22 weeks). *Winters et al.* (1974) detected TRF in the brain of an 32 day-old embryo. TRF was present in prosencephalon and rhombencephalon. Recently, TRF was reported to be present also in the placenta (*Shambaugh et al.*, 1978). A comparison of the presence of TRF and the production of TSH suggest that in early gestation there is probably an autonomous secretion of both TRF and TSH, followed by a parallel TRF-TSH increasing phase between weeks 16 and 28. The equilibrium is established around week 30 of gestation. After delivery, there is a short parallel increase due to both "birth stress" and environmental temperature drop, resulting in a so-called "neonatal thyroidal hyperactivity". The gestational equilibrium is related to the development of the "sensitivity" of hypophyseal TSH-cells to TRF stimulation, and to the sensitivity of both TRF-producing cells and TSH-cells to thyroxin. Estrogens in levels comparable to those in late pregnancy increase TSH response to TRF.

LH RF AND FSH, LH FEED — BACK SYSTEMS

LH RF is formed in the anterior hypothalamus (in the interstitial nucleus of the stria terminalis) in the periventricular nucleus and in the arcuate nucleus near the tuber cinereum. LH RF-producing neurons are ovoid or fusiform, about half the size of magnocellular vasopressin secreting neurons (*Barry, 1976*). LH RF granules are 75—90 nm in diameter and are transmitted into the portal system by the palisade nerve terminals in the median eminence. In the median eminence, long and branched ependymal tanycytes extend from the ependymal layer lining the infundibular recess of the third ventricle to the surface of the median eminence contacting the capillaries of the portal system. The neuron terminals of the neuroendocrine peptidergic neurons contact the capillaries between the tanycytes. Serotonin (5-HT), dopamine (DA) and norepinephrine-(NE) producing neurons are involved in the control of LH RF secretion. Norepinephrine appears to be stimulative and DA restrictive.

LH RF was found in the CNS of a 32 day-old embryo and in the hypothalamic area in embryos and fetuses 8—24 weeks of age. The levels of LH RF were 4—65 pg/mg of wet tissue (*Winters et al.*, 1974). *Kaplan, Grumbach and Aubert* (1976) found in 10—22 week-old fetuses that serum LH RF concentration is 0.27—13.1 pg/ml. The hypothalamic LH RF content varied from 208—4300 pg with no correlation to age or sex. Because of the substantial differences in steroid production between fetal testes and ovaries during the prenatal development, the sexes are considered separately. In males, androstenedione and testosterone synthesis by the testicular Leydig cells begins at the end of the eight conceptional week. From the beginning the secretion is under the influence of hCG. The binding of hCG is related to the differentiation of the Leydig cells. The lower levels of FSH and LH found in males beginning at 10 weeks of gestation already suggest a functional feed back at this period. Testosterone diminishes secretion of LH RF in male fetuses. An increase in FSH and LH production should be positively correlated with LHRF production.

In tissue cultures, testosterone inhibits the LH RF-mediated LH release, but potentiates the LH RF-mediated FSH release (*Drouin and Labrie*, 1976).

After birth, the hCG and LH influenced population of the testicular Leydig cells completely disappears (such as the fetal zone of the adrenal cortex), and LHRF as well as FSH and LH production fall to basal levels. A new feed-back system becomes established during puberty.

In females, the high levels of FSH and LH until midgestation reflect an unrestrained secretion of LH RF and both FSH and LH. Maximal concentrations of FSH and LH in female fetuses are achieved at the same time between weeks 25—29. At this period, the LH RF secretion becomes inhibited either due to the increased hypothalamic sensitivity or to the increased fetal androgen level (mostly of ovarian origin) or to both these mechanisms. The early testosterone production in males is the basic difference in the gonadotropin feed-back in the two sexes.

After the negative feed-back control of FSH and LH becomes established (weeks 25—29), there is a negative phase of LH RF, FSH and LH secretion. An intersting fact, however, is that in perinatal ovaries, follicular growth and maturation proceeds for a certain period, in spite of falling gonadotropins. This probably is caused by the pre-programmed steroidogenic capacity of the differentiated thecal cells. At birth the FSH levels are higher in females than in males. The LH levels are the same. In contrast to the ovarian follicular maturation, there is no maturation of spermatogonia during prenatal or perinatal period.

After birth, during the first half of the first year, LH RF, FSH, LH and sex steroids fall to basal levels. A new feed-back equilibrium becomes established at puberty.

STEROID SENSITIVE AREAS OF THE BRAIN

Steroid hormones are involved in the development of the brain regulating the pattern of gonadotropin secretion and influence behavior (to a certain degree). Two kinds of closely related steroid brain receptors have been identified: testosterone and estrogen receptors. Specific progesterone binding sites were never found in the CNS. Regarding testosterone, the testosterone taken by various brain areas is always converted to estradiol which can be recovered from the nuclear fraction (*McEwen*, 1976). The differences between males and females are consistent with the hypothesis that during a limited period in ontogenesis a specific estrogen-binding protein is present which does not bind testosterone. Estrogens are bound to this protein which makes them unable to enter the neurons. In contrast, testosterone, which is not bound to the protein, enters the target brain neurons, and is converted to estrogens within the neurons thus influencing their differentiation.

Steroid-binding neurons with estrogen receptors are numerous in the hypothalamus in an area extending from the preoptic region to the caudal portion of the nucleus arcuatus. Within the telencephalon, the nucleus amygdalae and stria terminalis bind estrogens. 60—80% of adenohypophyseal cells contain steroid-binding proteins similar to those found in peripheral tissues. Some scattered steroid binding may be present even in the cerebral hemispheres.

Pulsatile or tonic gonadotropin release in adults is dependent on early testosterone exposure of the hypothalamus. The critical period related to the gonadotropin release pattern includes the first nine postnatal days in rats. In rats, the tonic gonadotropin release is achieved either by androgen or by estrogen treatment during the critical postnatal period. The effect of early steroid exposure in the human has been reviewed by *Money* (1973).

The hypothalamus is able to form catecholestrogen (2-hydroxyestron and 2-hydroxy-estradiol-17β) which may serve as a link between estrogens and catecholamines influencing neuronal activity (*Ball et al.*, 1972; *Paul and Axelrod*, 1977).

PHYLOGENESIS OF THE HYPOPHYSIS

The hypophyseal phylogenesis remembers the ontogenesis. The Rathke's pouch extending from the floor of the oral cavity to the diencephalon represents the adeno-hypophysis in sharks. In Teleosts and in Amphibia, the adenohypophysis is formed by a solid cellular cord. A similar cord connecting the adenohypophysis and the oral cavi-ty is present in some birds and some mammals. The remnant of the cavity of Rathke's pouch remains preserved in some vertebrates (including man) during their entire life as a slit separating the anterior and the middle portion of the adeno-hypophysis. In Cyclostomes, the hypophysis develops in relation to the nasal sacs. From the phylogenic point of view, the primitive adenohypophyseal secretion was probably released into the pharynx and easily reached the thyroid primordium and subsequently the gut. In amphibians and in all higher vertebrates, the adeno-hypophysis has three parts: distalis, tuberalis, intermedia. The pars tuberalis is not present in fish, in some reptiles and in lizards. In poikilotherms, where skin color changes according to the environment, the MSH secretion is related to optic stimuli. The neurohypophysis is a part of the CNS. The hypothalamic neuro-secretion represents a very old phylogenetic mechanism related to circadian rhythms, sexual irritation and conservation of water within the body. A hypothalamic infundibulum may be recognized in fish and amphibians. In fish, the infundibulum is represented by the saccus vasculosus. The saccus vasculosus represents an evagination from the floor of the third ventricule, whose wall is formed by special supportive cells (tanycytes) and ciliated neuroepithelial cells. The cilia protrude into the third ventricle. The outer surface of the saccus vasculosus is extremely rich in vascular plexuses. The exact function of this organ remains to be established. The neurohypophysis is present only in Dipnoi and Tetrapodes. A fascinating comparative study of the phylogenic evolution of gonadotropin structure and function was contributed by *Licht et al.* (1977). They concluded that two separate gonadotropins are a primitive characteristic of tetrapods. If a second gonadotropin should not be found in some of them, that would represent a secondary evolutionary loss rather than a primitive character. Even in fish, there is evidence of two gonadotropins which are homologous to the mammalian FSH and LH.

Biochemical findings of a high degree of structural conservatism among different species of FSH and LH are sometimes in contrast to the lack of their biochemical activities in some species. The differences, however, are related to their peripheral binding. Evolutionary differences exist in their control of gonadal metabolism, and the same hormone may play a different role in different tetrapods. Although two gonadotropins are present, their peripheral gonadal action may be very similar or the same. In reptiles, FSH binds to Leydig cells stimulating the testosterone secretion, and in the reptilian ovary, FSH and LH stimulate progesterone formation in the same tissue. There is probably the same receptor for both gonadotropins.

In Amphibians, FSH and LH have specific actions in urodels and anurans.

The phylogeny of tetrapods, as emerged from the study of *Licht et al.* (1977) is summarized in Graph 19.

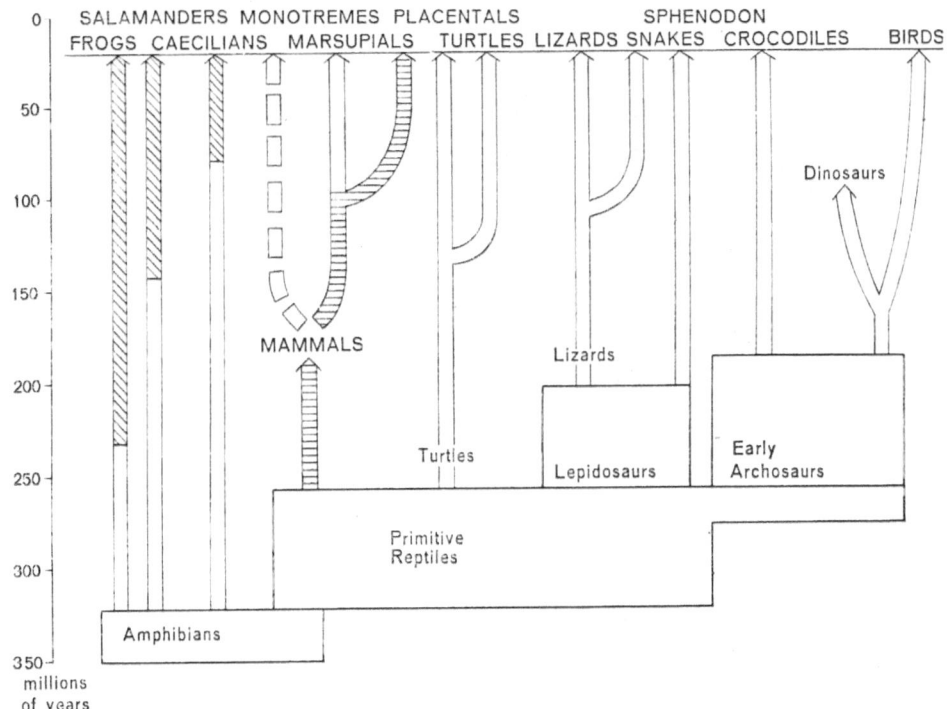

Graph 19. Phylogenesis of tetrapods (according to Licht et al. 1977).

PATHOLOGY

HYPOPHYSEAL APLASIA

A complete hypophyseal aplasia is a rare feature related to panhypopituitarism. Data on four babies born without hypophyses are summarized in Table 20.

It is evident that the presence of the hypophysis is not nesessary for embryonal development of any particular organ. In the absence of hypophysis, total body weight might be normal. The weight of the adrenals is about 8% of the normal in the 700 g fetus and 5% of normal newborn weight. This small adrenal is related to the absence of the definitive zone, except the glomerulosa, and to hypoplasia

151

Table 20. Organ weights in hypophyseal aplasia (in g).
Data from: *Blizzard and Alberts* (1954), *Edmonds* (1950), *Brewer* (1957) *and Reid* (1960).

Total body weight	700	1970	3750	3900
Adrenals	0.21	0.25	<1.0	0.53
Thyroid	—	0.08	<1.0	0.35
Gonads	"normal testes"	ovaries 0.18	"small testes"	"small testes"
Liver	40	75	—	140
Kidneys	7.3	12.0	—	20
Heart	—	—	—	25
Brain	porencephaly	porencephaly	normal	normal

of the fetal zone. The weight of the thyroid is slightly less than normal. Gonads
are mentioned as being small in most cases. The weight of the kidneys and liver
is reduced to 60—70%. The weight of the heart, mentioned only in one case, was
normal.

PITUITARY DWARFISM

Pituitary dwarfs are ateleiotic (proportions of the body are normal). The condition
becomes evident early in childhood. Three different types are recognized (*McKusick*,
1976).

Pituitary dwarfism I (Sexual ateleiotic dwarfism), isolated growth hormone deficiency.

Pituitary dwarfism II (Laron type), the abnormality is limited to growth hormone,
the levels of the hormone are rather high. An abnormal GH, or GH-insensitivity
are supposed.

Pituitary dwarfism III (Panhypopituitarism): A syndrome consisting of hypopituitary dwarfism, hypoplasia of the optic nerves and malformation of the prosencephalon were described by *Kaplan, Grumbach and Hoyt* (1970).

ANENCEPHALY

Common features: the cerebral hemispheres and the diencephalon are missing. They
are replaced by a vascularized connective tissue, known as the area cribrovasculosa.
The defect of the brain reaches different levels. Sometimes mesencephalic remnants,
pons and cerebellum are present. The medulla oblongata is found in most of the
cases. Desmogenic bones (calvarium) are missing. Chondrogenic parts of the skull
(chondricranium) are present. Anencephaly is accompanied by craniorrhachischisis
is some cases. Spina bifida and anencephaly are regarded as one entity. The optic
and auditory apparatus are developed. The trunk and extremities are normal in
most of the cases. Anencephaly is a frequent malformation with a striking geographic
variation (1 : 1000—1 : 105 in Southern Wales). The sex ratio is MI : F 3—7
(*Shulman*, 1973). The defect is considered to result from a nonclosure of the anterior
neuropore (around day 26 of development). A secondary rupture of the brain vesicle

cannot be ruled out in some cases. Cerebral tissue in contact with the amnionic fluid degenerates. If polyhydramnios does not develop in the last trimester gestation is prolongued. Maximal, well-documented pregnancy length with an anencephalic fetus is 385 days (*Liggins*, 1973). Anencephaly is incompatible with life. The risk of familial reoccurence is 5%.

Prenatal diagnosis of anencephaly is possible by checking the amnionic level of α-fetoprotein by ultrasound, by rtg and by low estriol levels in the maternal urine. Endocrinologic studies in anencephaly were reported by several authors (*Grunt and Reynold*, 1978; *Hayek et al.*, 1973; *Grumbach and Kaplan*, 1973; *Allen et al.*, 1974).

The adenohypophysis is always present, the weight being reduced to approximately 50%. The neurohypophysis and pars intermedia are absent in most of the cases. GH-cells, PRL-cells, TSH-cells, G-cells and ACTH-cells were identified (*Satow et al.*, 1972). The hormonal serum levels (ng/ml) in anencephalic fetuses after birth are summarized and compared to normals in Table 21.

Table 21. Pituitary hormones serum levels (ng/ml) in anencephalics and normal newborns.

Hormone	Anencephaly	Normal	Comment; in anencephaly
STH	7	33.5	significantly lower
PRL	65 — 283	167.8 — 14.2	similar
TSH	undetectable in most	8.9 uU	less than 1%, high sensitivity to TRF
FSH	<1	360.5 in females	less than 1%, insensitivity to LHRF
LH	<1	42 — 17	less than 1%, insensitivity to LHRF

STH in anencephalics is low and remains low after arginine infusion, or insulin-induced hypoglycemia in most of the cases. The insulin response following arginine infusion is low, and the glucose tolerance may be diabetic in character (*Grunt and Reynolds*, 1970; *Allen et al.*, 1974; *Grumbach and Kaplan*, 1973).

PRL: comparable data between anencephalics and normals indicate that PRL secretion is independent of hypothalamic, and in general telencephalic development.

ACTH level is very low (5% of normal) in anencephaly; however, it may rise after vasopressin infusion (*Hayek et al.*, 1973).

TSH is undetectable in most anencephalics. TRF administration, however, causes a brisk rise in secretion (*Hayek*, 1973). Thyroidal function in anencephalics seems to be sufficient, probably as a consequence of the TSH activity of hCG or placental TRH.

FSH and LH: low levels of both gonadotropins stress the importance of the LHRF for their secretion. The normal masculinization of the external genitalia in anecephalic males suggests that hypophyseal gonadotropins are not essential for testosterone production in the first trimester of gestation. The undescended testes found in anencephalic males, hypoplastic ovaries in females and hypoplastic external genitalia in both sexes, suggest the role of pituitary gonadotropins in the perinatal period. Administration of LHRF does not raise FSH or LH level in anencephalics, suggesting probably that a longterm stimulation by LHRF is required before the response of the adenohypophyseal G-cells is achieved.

DOUBLING OF THE HYPOPHYSIS

Doubling of the hypophysis is a very rare anomaly, considered as the mildest form of anterior duplication (diprosopia). Two lateral eyes and a median eye, and double mouth and nose may be present in some very rare cases.

LEPRECHAUNISM (DONOHUE SYNDROME)

Common features: short gestational period, birth weight approximately 2,600 g. Large ears and lips, large hands and feet, sexual precocity. Altered carbohydrate metabolism with hypoglycaemia. Hyperplasia of pituitary basophils and pancreatic islets (β-cells) were reported (*Rogers*, 1966). Hyperplasia of testicular Leydig cells in males, and multiple ovarian follicular cysts in females were noticed. Sex ratio M1 : F3. Affected individuals are insensitive to exogenous insulin.

CHAPTER 7

THE EPIPHYSIS (PINEAL GLAND, PINEAL BODY)

The pineal gland originates as an evagination from the roof of posterior diencephalon recognized first at 35—38 days (7—9 mm, S. H. XV). The primordium is very distinct in 37—44 day-old embryos (10—14 mm, S. H. XVII). In 44—50 day-old embryos (13—17 mm, S. H. XVIII), the neuroblasts migrate outward from the ependymal zone to form a segregated layer and become arranged into a follicular-like pattern. The minute interculleular spaces within these neuroepithelial follicles do not connect with the lumen of the epiphyseal evagination (*Streeter*, 1948). This tissue forms the anterior solid lobe of the epiphysis. In embros 50—60 days-old (20—35 mm, S. H. XX—XXIII), the pineal neuroblasts are arranged in glandular-like cords and tubules. During the next period of epiphyseal development, the posterior hollow pineal stalk, the trabecular comissure can be recognized, and posteriorly, the posterior comissure is found.

Differentiation of neuroblasts into pinealocytes, and differentiation of spongioblasts into ependymal cells and neuroglial cells occur after 20 weeks of development. The pinealocytes form irregular lobules separated by connective tissue septae, derived mostly of meningeal mesenchyme originating from the neural crest. Concrements (acervulus cerebri) are not found prenatally. Pinealocytes are irregular cells with numerous processes ending at the border or within the interlobular septa. The terminals of the processes are thickened and contain dense bodies and vesicles. Pineal sympathetic innervation originates from the superior cervical ganglia. Nerve fibers together with cytoplasmic processes and terminals are found close to the perivascular spaces.

The blood to the epiphysis is supplied by small arterioles from the posterior chorioid plexus and is drained by small vessels entering the vena cerebri magna (of Galen). Two kinds of hormones are formed by the epiphysis: indoleamins and peptides. Melatonin is the best known representative of the first group, and arginine vasotocine (AVT) of the second group. NE and 5-HT are precursors of melatonine. NE is formed and released at the nerve edings. 5-HT and AVT are formed by the pinealocytes.

Circadian rhythms of melatonin secretion are generated postnatally by diurnal changes in the release of noradrenaline. Noradrenaline stimulates the β-receptors which results in an increased synthesis of serotonin N-acetyltransferase by mediation of cAMP system. The increased activity of N-acetyltransferase (during the night) diminishes the concentration of 5-HT and increases N-acetylserin. Hydroxyindole o-methyltransferase converts consequently N-acetylserotonin to melatonin. The biological clock, modulated by light, is present in the hypothalamus near the suprachiasmatic nucleus (*Axelrod*, 1974). In rats, melatonin inhibits ovulation by preventing LH release. In tissue cultures of human ovaries melatonin increases synthesis of progesterone by the corpus luteum cells and increases incorporation of acetate into androstenedione (*MacPhee et al.*, 1975). Pineal extracts from 4—6 month-old human fetuses contain AVT which exhibits an antigonadotropic activity (*Pavel et al.*, 1973).

The phylogenesis of the pineal gland is fascinating because the pineal body is homologous to the retinal primordium of the parietal (median) eye of early vertebrates. In ostracodermsand crossopterygiens such an eye was universally present, but was always much smaller than the paired eyes. The parietal eye opening is not found in sharks. In early terrestrial animals and in early amphibians and reptiles the parietal eye was present. In the Triasic period the eye disappeared. The eye is present in lampreys, in Sphenodon and in some lizards underneath the parietal skin. In lampreys, there are two median eyes — the epiphyseal and the paraphyseal; the epiphyseal is dominant. Although the light-perceptive function became lost during phylogenesis, and the retinal primordium of the pineal eye has been transformed into the pineal gland, light perception still influences the circadian rhythm of pineal function.

CHAPTER 8

PHARYNGEAL DERIVATIVES

The endodermal complex of pharyngeal endocrine glands and lymphatics includes: the thyroid gland, the parathyroid glands, the palatine tonsils and the thymus. The development of these organs is related to the phylogenic changes in the branchial

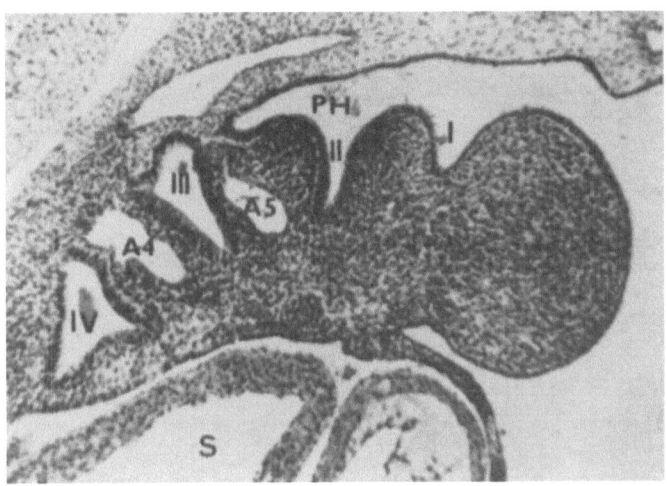

Fig. 90. Parasagittal section of pharynx of a 5 mm embryo (35 days, S. h. XIII). I, II, III, IV — endodermal portions of pharyngeal pouches I—IV, A4, A5 — third and fourth aortic arches, PH — pharyngeal cavity, S — the heart cavity.

area after the lungs have developed and the gills have lost their respiratory function. The early pharyngeal area comprises the branchial arches and pouches (Fig. 90). In human embryos, the pharyngeal pouches appear as furrows closed by bilaminar ecto-endodermal branchial membranes located between the pharyngeal arches. The branchial membranes never rupture. From the ectodermal parts of the pouches, only a part of the first one is preserved, converted into the external auditory meatus and into the external layer of the tympanic membrane. Ectodermal parts of the other pouches disappear. The endodermal pouches develop into the pharyngo-tympanic tube, the tympanic cavity and the internal layer of the tympanic membrane (first pouch), the tonsillar recessus and the palatine tonsil (second pouch), the parathyroid glands (dorsal parts of the third and fourth pouches), the thymus (ventral part of the third pouch) and the lateral thyroidal primordia (ventral part of the fourth pouch considered as the fifth pouch, or the ultimobranchial body, by some).

THE THYROID

The thyroid originates from the endodermal proliferation of the primitive pharynx. There are three primordia contributing to the gland: one medial (the main primoridum) and two lateral. The specific area of thyroidal endoderm of the main primordium can be recognized in 26 day-old, 25 somite embryos (S. H. XII).

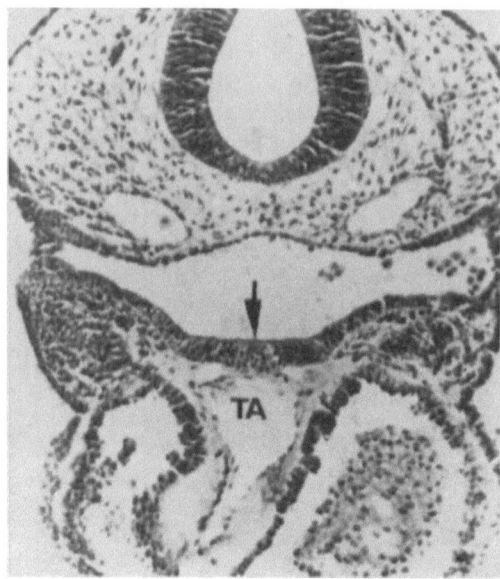

Fig. 91A. Special thyroidal epithelium in the middle portion of the pharyngeal floor (arrow) representing primordium of the medial thyroid. The epithelium contacts the endothelium of the arterial truncus. Embryo 3,5 mm lomg (26 days, S. h. XII). TA — arterial truncus.

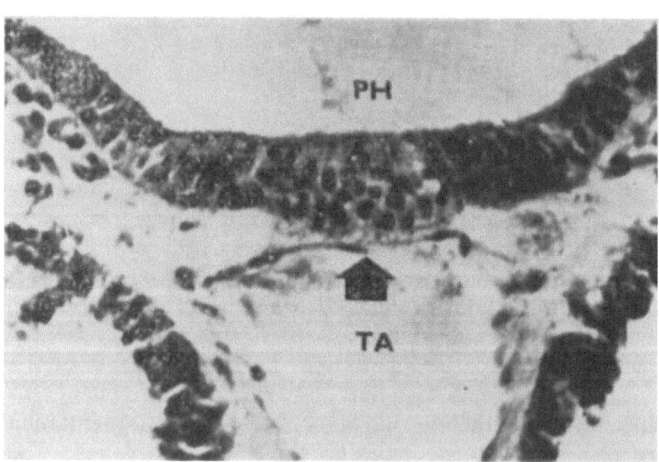

Fig. 91B. Detail from the previous picture showing adhesions between the epithelium of the medial thyroidal primordium and the endothelium of the arterial truncus. PH — pharynx, TA — arterial truncus.

The thyroid area is localized at the midline of the pharyngeal floor, between the first and second pharyngeal arch. The endoderm of the medial thyroid contacts the endothelium of the arterial truncus prior to its bifurcation into the two aortic arches (Figs 91A, 91B). In the area of contact, the endodermal epithelium becomes cylindrical and gives rise to a spherical evagination (27—28 somite embryos, 26 days) (Fig. 92). The proliferating epithelium fills the evagination, which becomes bilobed (Figs. 93, 94). The formation of the two lobes is related to the two aortic arches.

Fig. 92. Spheroid lumenized invagination of the medial thyroid (arrow) in contact with the arterial truncus branching into two aortic arches. Embryo 3,5 mm long, 28 somites (28 days, S. h. XII).

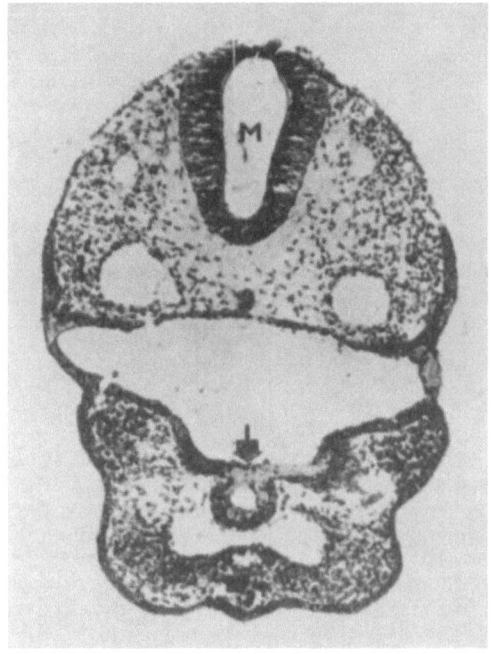

As the pharyngeal arches grow, the distance between the pharyngeal floor and the arterial truncus increases and the medial thyroid primordium descends. The primordium is attached to the foramen caecum of the tongue by a solid cellular thyroglossal duct (cord) (35—38 days, 7—9 mm embryos, S. H. XV. Fig: 95).

The thyroglossal cord disintegrates and gradually disappears. The place of the lingual attachment of the thyroid may be recognized in some individuals as a foramen caecum linguae. In most newborns, it is impossible to find the foramen caecum. The distal part of the thyroglossal cord persists as a pyramidal thyroid lobule, which is present in all fetuses after the third month and disappears later in most of them. The main (medial) primordium contributes two-thirds to three-fourths of the definitive gland.

The lateral thyroid primordia appear in 42—44 day embryos (12—15 mm, S. H. S. H. XVII) in the medioventral area of the endodermal fourth pharyngeal pouch. Some consider this area as fifth pharyngeal pouch. This area, located ventrally and medially to the primordium of the parathryroid IV, is also known as the ultibranchial body (*Sugiyama et al.*, 1959; *van Dyke*, 1959; *Kingsbury*, 1939). In embryos 50—55 days-old, the endodermal ultimobranchial epithelium fuses with the epithelial cords

159

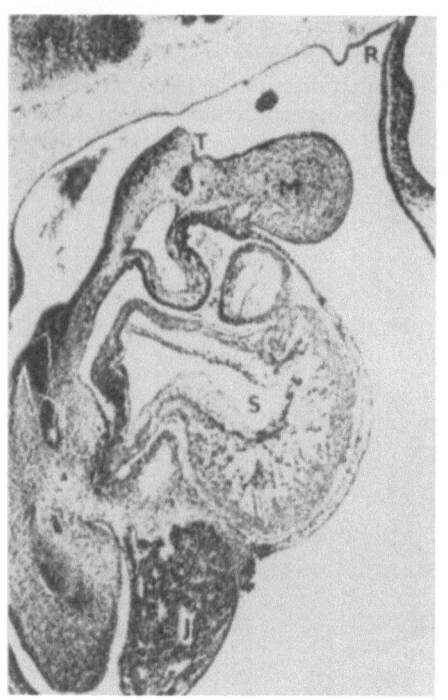

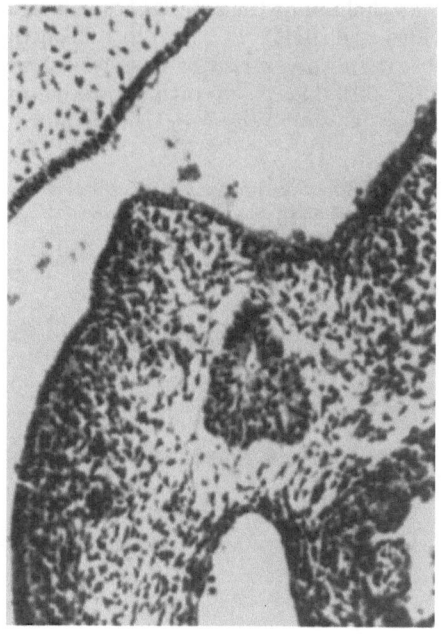

Fig. 93. Sagittal section of a 5 mm embryo (34 days, S. h. XIII). T — medial thyroid primordium detached from the arterial truncus, M — mandibular arch, R — Rathke's pouch. S — heart, J — liver

Fig. 94. Epithelium of the medial thyroid primordium (stage of diverticulum).

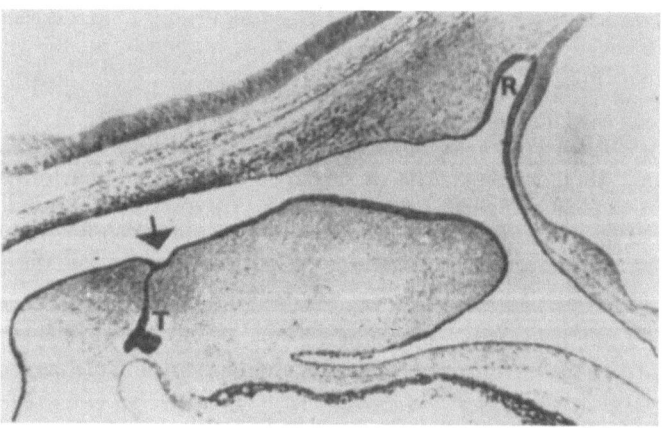

Fig. 95. Bilobed medial thyroid primordium connected by the thyreoglossal duct (cord) with the foramen caecum (arrow) of the future, tongue. R — Rathke's pouch.

160

and lamellae of the medial thyroid primordium (Fig. 96). The border between the two primordia may be recognized dorsally and medially to the common carotid artery. In embryos ca. 55—60 days-old (25 mm, S. H. XXII—XXIII), all the three primordia (one medial and two lateral) are completely fused. In the absence of the medial thyroid, the lateral primordia fail to develop. The parathyroid IV is attached to the lateral primordium of the thyroid. The parathyroid III is bound to the thymic primordium. The thymus in humans, in contrast to some other mammals, originates exclusively from the third pharyngeal pouch. The various endodermal areas of the pharyngeal arches are easy to identify in 17—25 mm embryos (50—55 days, S. H. XX—XXII) according to a variable amount of glycogen and other P. A. S. positive material.

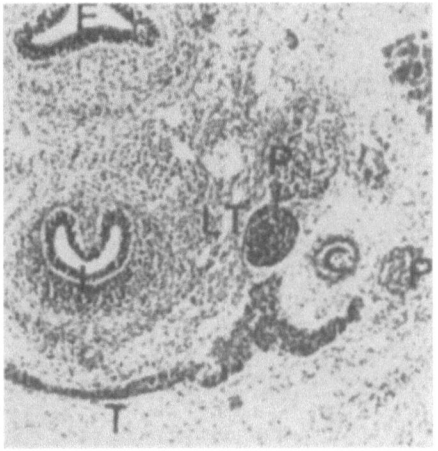

Fig. 96. Transverse section through the neck of a 25 mm embryo L — larynx, LT — lateral thyroid primordium connected with the parathyroid IV, T — medial thyroid primordium, C — arteria carotis communis, E — esophagus, P — parathyroid.

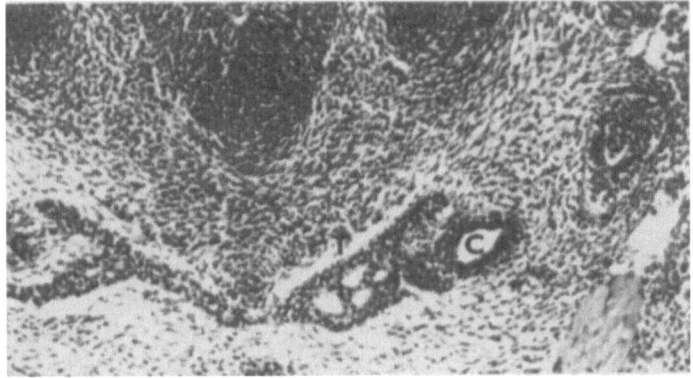

Fig. 97. Epithelium of the thyroid (T) in a 18 mm embryo (40 days, S. h. XVI — lamellar stage). C — arteria carotis communis.

161

HISTOGENESIS AND GROWTH

Jirásek (1963, 1977) distinguished the following stages of human thyroid development: 1. endodermal, 2. lamellar unpolarized, (Figs 97, 98) 3. lamellar polarized 4. follicular, (Fig. 99). *Shepard et al.* (1964, 1967) distinguished a pracolloid beginning coloid and follicular-growth phase. Both classifications are compared in table 22.

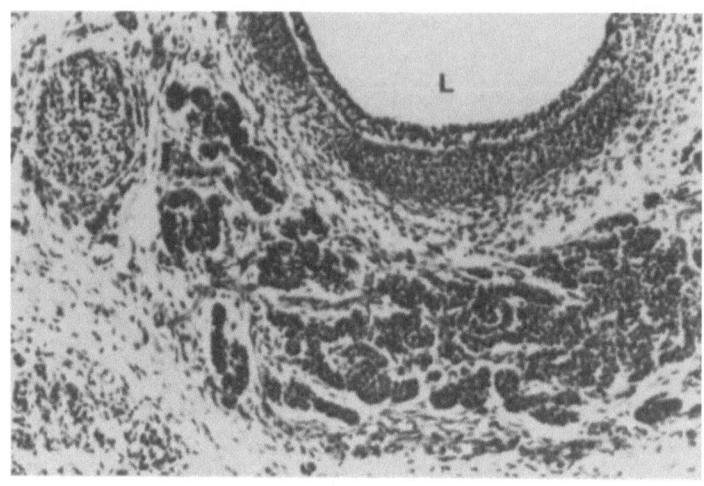

Fig. 98. Epithelium of the thyroid in a 30 mm embryo (56 days, S. h. XXIII) — lamellar stage. P — parathyroid glands, L — larynx

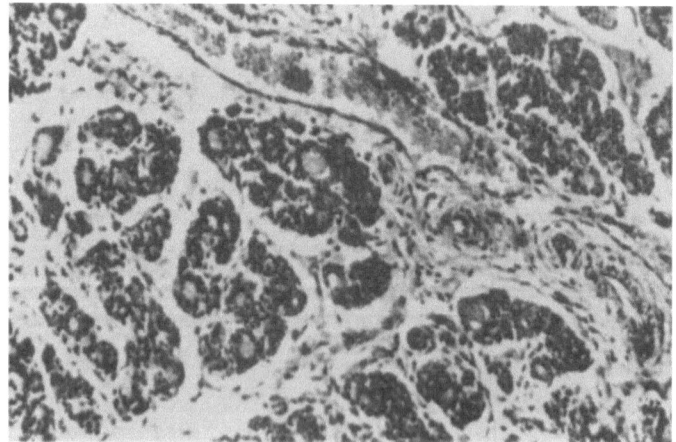

Fig. 99. Thyroid in a fetus from fourth month. Follicular stage.

Table 22. Stages of prenatal thyroid development.

Jirásek (1977) stages	Embryo age and stage	Shepard (1964, 1967), stages	Embryo age in days	Remarks
1. Endodermal	25–35d (XII–XIII)	–	–	TG appears
2. Lamellar unpolarized (prefollicular)	36–60 (XIV-XXIII)	1. Precolloid	47–72	TG present
3. Lamellar polarized (early follicular)	9 weeks	2. Beginning colloid	73–80	T_4 appears
4. Follicular	10 weeks and more	3. Follicular growth	80+ and more	TSH in serum

During the endodermal stage, the epithelium of the thyroid invagination is single layered cylindrical, formed by glycogen-rich polarized cells. Alkaline phosphatase is present in the apical portion of the cells, α-naphtylesterase is absent.

Proliferating endodermal epithelium forms solid cellular cords and lamellae. All the thyroid tissue in 7–40 mm embryos has a lamellar character. The lamellae are formed of glycogen-rich cylindrical or polyedric cells. No alkaline phosphatase, acid phosphatase or esterase are present. During the ninth week in fetuses 35–40 mm long, polarization of cells becomes evident. The cells, especially in the lateral parts of the thyroid, lose glycogen and, consequently, the acid phosphatase and non-specific heat resistant esterase appear in T-cells in an apical localization. In embryos 60 to 65 mm long, first follicles are differentiated, and P. A. S. positive colloid becomes evident within the follicles.

The vascularization of the connective tissue septa around lamellae and follicles begins in 40–50 mm long fetuses (9th or 10th week).
The growth of the thyroid gland (not the formation of the primordium) depends on TSH stimulation. The weight increase of the fetal thyroid gland is summarized in table 23 and on graph 20.

Table 23. Total body weight of the fetus and the weight of the thyroid.

Total body weight in g	Age in weeks	Weight of the thyroid in mg
below 75	(12–13)	20–30
75–149	(14–15)	30–150
150–299	(16–17)	150–180
300–500	(18–24)	ca 250
500–1000	(25–30)	ca 600
ca 3000	(40)	1000–2000

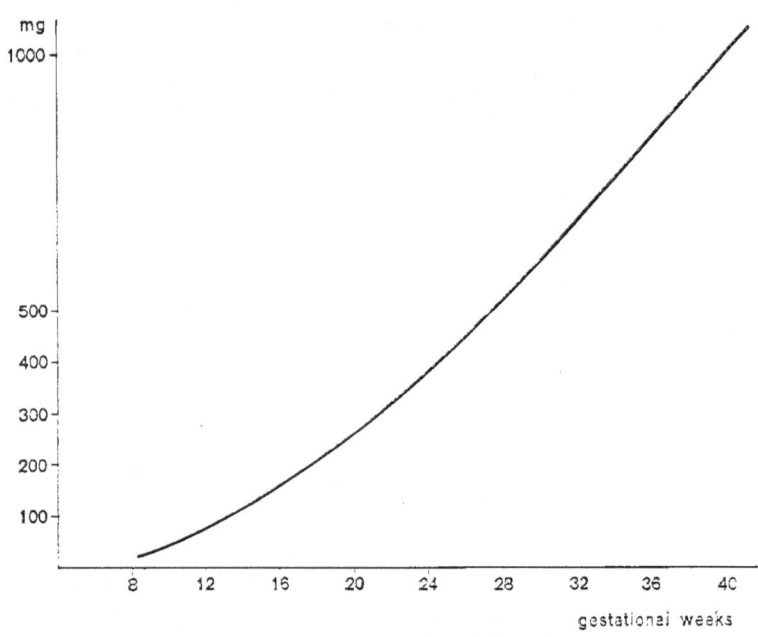

Graph 20. Weight of the fetal thyroid.

THYROIDAL HORMONES

The thyroid gland produces two kinds of hormones: iodized thyronines and calcitonin. The thyroxin (T_4) and triiodothyronine (T_3) are produced by the T-cells. Calcitonin is synthetized in C-cells.

T-cells are endodermal in origin and exhibit the thyroglobulin synthesis as a basic feature. Thyroglobulin is a large glycoprotein with a molecular weight of approximately 660,000. Thyroglobulin appears sometimes during the formation of the evagination of the medial thyroid. Thyroglobulin is formed in the polysomes and ribosomes scattered in the cytoplasm. During the prefollicular phase of thyroid development, thyroglobulin synthesis is very limited. Thyroglobulin is present in small bristle-coated vesicles (as revealed by EM).

During the cell polarization, tight junctions, desmosomes and gap junctions appear between adjacent cells sealing clusters of cells into the follicular epithelium. A well developed Golgi complex becomes localized between the nucleus and the apical part of the cytoplasm. Microvilli are formed projecting into the early follicular cavity. Bristle-coated pits between the microvilli suggest secretion of thyroglobulin into the follicular cavity. Extracellular thyroglobulin is subjected to iodination. Iodination requires oxidation of iodide by the thyroperoxidase. Thyroperoxidase is formed in polarized T-cells by rough endoplasmic reticulum and is secreted into the lumen of the follicles. The iodination of thyroglobulin occurs extracellularly exclusively. Iodized thyroglobulin droplets are ingested by pseudopods of follicular T-cells and subjected to hydrolysis. Lysosomes containing acid phosphatase and protease fuse in the apical cytoplasm with phagosomes containing colloid and form phagolysosomes. Colloid is

164

digested into thyronins. Iodinated thyronins (MIT, DIT) couple to form T_3 and T_4. T_3 and T_4 and a small quantity of unhydrolysed thyroglobulin pass into the blood. T_1 and T_2 are deiodinated and reused by the T-cells separately for thyroglobulin synthesis and iodination.

TSH stimulates the T_3 and T_4 synthesis by the activation of the cAMP cycle. TSH is bound to the specific receptors on the cell membrane of T-cells. The β-subunit of TSH is believed to be involved in the binding, whereas the α-subunit stimulates the adenyl cyclase. TSH, in addition to the increase of T_3 and T_4 secretion, increases the iodine thyroid uptake.

From the T-cells, T_3 and T_4 pass into the blood by diffusion. In blood, there are three circulating thyroxine-binding proteins: Thyroxine-binding globulin (TBG), thyroxine-binding prealbumin (TBPA) and albumin. Approximately $75-80\%$ of T_3 and T_4 are bound to TBG.

Regarding the peripheral effects of thyroid hormones, two hypotheses have been presented. The first (Ismail-Bergi, Edelman, 1970) considers that thyroxine is involved in the energy supply for the maintenance of low intracellular sodium and high intracellular potassium related to the function of the membrane bound Na-K ATPase. This enzyme generates ATP from ADP and requires oxygen. The Na-K ATPase utilizes about 45% of the body's total caloric output. The second hypothesis (proposed by *Tata and Widnell*, 1963) is based on the demonstration of T_3 specific binding in the cell nucleus (*Oppenheimer et al.*, 1974). T_3 nuclear receptors bind specifically to DNA and suggest the T_3 role in facilitating the transcription of DNA. It is possible that T_4 is related primarily to the Na-K ATPase activation, and T_3 facilitates the transcription of DNA.

THYROID FUNCTION IN THE HUMAN FETUS

Thyroglobulin is synthesized by the medial thyroidal primordium as early as 30 days of development. Concentration of iodine begins at $10-12$ weeks of gestation and the DIT, MIT, T_4 and T_3 synthesis begins at the same time. The hypophyseal TSH was demonstrated by 12 weeks in the fetal serum (*Shepard*, 1967; *Fisher et al.*, 1970; *Fukuchi et al.*, 1970; *Greenberg et al.*, 1973).

The fetal thyroid gland T_3 and T_4 contents and T_3, T_4 and free T_3, T_4 serum levels are shown in table 24, the mean serum levels in table 25 (according to *Fisher et al.*, 1973). Fetal T_4 and FT_4 levels are low between $11-18$ weeks and increase from week 22 until term (Graph 21). The T_3 and T_4 levels are low, increasing with the gestational age (Graph 22). The T_4/T_3 and FT_4/FT_3 ratios are high. These data are consistent with a relative fetal T_3 deficiency.

The high fetal T_4/T_3 ratio indicates either that the fetus cannot convert T_4 to T_3 in a "sufficient" manner, or that not enough T_4 is present for this conversion. In fetal sheep, the peripheral production of T_3 is low (*Chopra et al.*, 1975). The TSH regulation of thyroid function and the development of TSH feed back has already been discussed (see hypophysis, TSH). TSH is suppressible in term fetuses by increasing serum T_4 concentration without a change in T_3 levels (*Fisher et al.*, 1977). There is a positive feed back between TSH and T_4 until 30 weeks of gestation and in early postnatal life. The T_3 and T_4 levels peak ca. 2 hours after delivery. The final equilibrium between TSH and T_4 is reached at one month postnatally.

Table 24. T_4 and T_3 thyroid contents per gland (according to Fisher et al., 1973.

	Content per gland		
Weeks	Gland. weight mg	$T_4\,\mu$g	$T_3\,\mu$g
13—15	22—30	0.06—0.40	0.01—0.025
16—20	11—109	0.05—3.24	0.01—0.120
21—24	—	—	—
25—30	315	2.8	0.220
31—34	565	3.0	0.150
35—40	—	—	—

Table 25. Fetal T_4, FT_4, and FT_3 serum levels (according to Fisher et al., 1973).

Weeks	$T_4\mu$g%	FT_4ng%	T_3ng%	FT_3pg%
13—15	2.0—2.4	1.6—1.9	15.	102
16—20	2.9—3.1	1.0—2.3	15.	95—122
21—24	4.2	2.7	15.	105
25—30	5.6—14.0	2.2—5.2	15—33	32—162
1—34	5.6—14.0	2.0—3.9	15—66	69—224
35—40	11—17	3.6—6.1	52—126	187—315

Recent findings suggest that a third hormone 3, 3,'5' T_3, or RT_3 is significant for the fetus (*Chopra et al.*, 1975). This hormone is produced (97%) by peripheral deiodination of T_4. Serum RT_3 increase is parallel with T_4 levels and both are relatively high in the fetal serum. RT_3 is also high in amnionic fluid (*Bergman et al.*, 1976), and could be used for the prenatal diagnosis of fetal hypothyroidism. The fetal TBG and TBPA levels were reported by *Grunberg et al.* (1970). The levels at mid-gestation are comparable with those found at term.

PLACENTA AND FETAL THYROIDAL FUNCTION

The trophoblast is involved in iodine transport from the maternal to the fetal compartment. Beginning at 10—12 weeks of development, iodine concentrates in the fetal thyroid. If radioactive iodine is administered to women more than 10—12 weeks pregnant, concentration of radioactive iodine in the fetal thyroid follows immediately. There is no justification for radioactive iodine administration during pregnancy (*Hamilla et al.*, 1961; *Beierwaltes et al.*, 1963).

In euthyroid mothers, there is practically no transplacental passage of TSH, T_4 and T_3. There is no correlation between maternal and fetal serum TSH, T_4 and FT_4 at any time during gestation (*Fisher et al.*, 1973). The fetal serum TSH levels are higher from week 20 until term than the maternal (4—5 uU/ml). Free maternal thyroxine serum levels decrease during pregnancy (from approximately 30 ng/l to 4.2 ng/l).

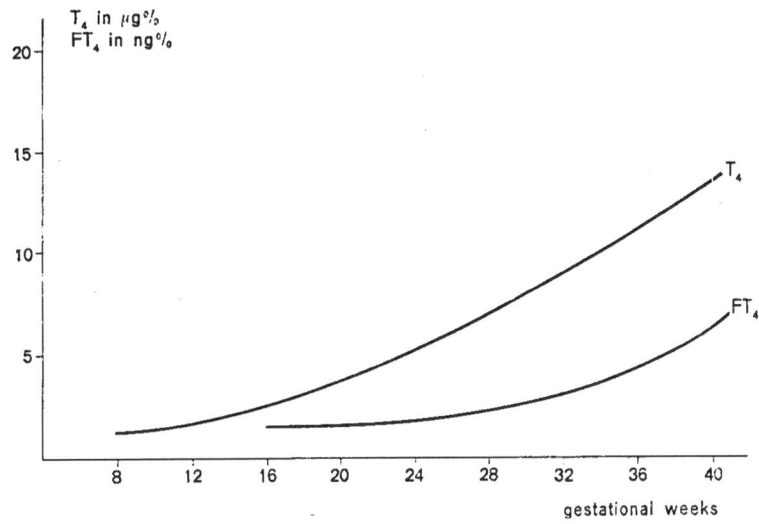

Graph 21. Fetal serum T_4 and FT_4 levels (T_4 in $\mu g\%$. FT_4 in ng%)

The fetal serum levels become higher than maternal 3—4 weeks before delivery. Even under conditions of a high maternofetal difference, the placental T_4 and T_3 transfer is very limited in both directions.

Thyroid agenesis results in hypothyroidism which may be easily detected at birth. Anti-thyroid drugs do cross the placental barrier and result in fetal hypothyroidism accompanied by a TSH rise leading to fetal thyroidal enlargement. Anti-thyroid

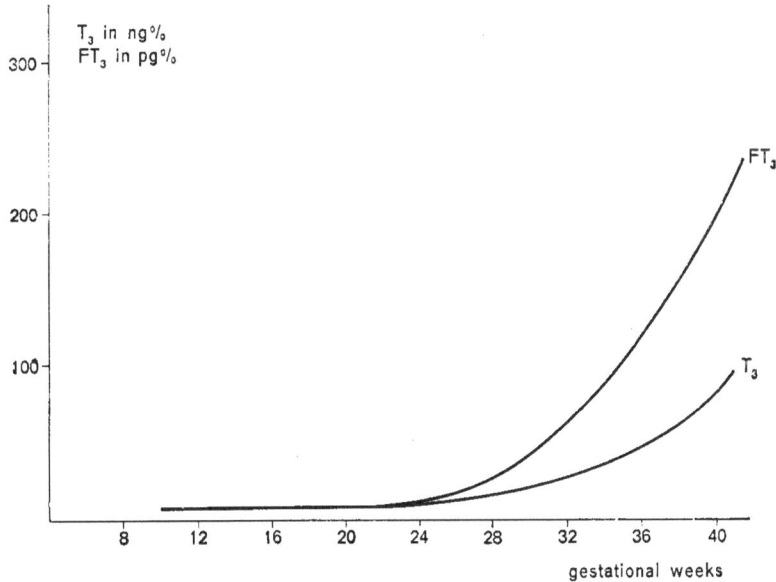

Graph 22. Fetal serum T_3 and FT_3 (T_3 in ng%, FT_3 in pg%).

drugs, if administered to the mother after delivery, are secreted in milk. In severe maternal thyrotoxicosix, the doses of propylthiouracil should not exceed 200 mg per day (*Selenkow et al.*, 1973). The placental barrier is permeable for the long acting thyroid stimulating globulins (LATS). In hyperthyroid mothers, LATS may influence the fetal thyroid.

CALCITONIN

Calcitonin is a peptide containing 32 aminoacids, M. W. approximately 3500, produced by the thyroidal C-cells. Most of the cells are enclosed in the epithelium of the follicles, some are in isolated groups within the septa between the follicles. C-cells may be found in an extrathyroidal localization, such as parathyroids, mediastinum, and even liver. C-cells originate from the neural crest, invade the endodermal epithelium of the ventral part of the fourth pharyngeal pouch "fifth pouch", (ultimobranchial body) and join the medial thyroidal primordium (*Pearse and Polak*, 1971). They take up catecholamines, or convert precursors to catecholamines, and store them together with calcitonin.

Under EM, the typical structural features of C-cells are small membrane-bound secretory granules 1000−1800 Å in diameter, which are formed from the lamellae of the Golgi complex. Rough endoplasmic reticulum is extensive.

Calcitonin lowers plasma calcium by inhibiting bone resorption by osteoclats. Calcitonin is bound to specific plasma membrane receptors and activates the adenylcyclase. The phosphodiesterase increases and calcium is released from the cells. Calcitonin does not pass the placental membrane (*Garel et al.*, 1965).

The role of calcitonin in the fetus is not known. Osteopetrosis is regarded as a condition resulting from defective resorption of bone by osteoclasts. There is a unique observation of four children affected by osteopetrosis who were born to a woman affected by a medullary calcitonin-producing carcinoma of the thyroid with stromal amyloidosis. This woman had five unaffected children in addition. The plasma calcitonin was high in the mother, but low in two unaffected children. This observation suggests an autosomal dominant inheritance of the disorder.

PHYLOGENESIS

The development of the thyroid gland is related to the accumulation of iodine. In invertebrates, monoiodothyronin and dioiodothyrosine and traces of thyroxine were identified in some corals, annular vermins and molluscs (*Gorbman*, 1959). Most of the iodine is protein-bound; present within the calcified material. Thyroxin was detected in the sweetwater living mollusc Musculinum and in various insects. These findings are not surprising because iodination of proteins followed by hydrolysis occurs spontaneously if proteins are incubating with iodine without any enzymes present (*Reineke*, 1949). In invertebrates, the presence of thyroxine or iodinated thyronins, is without any metabolic significance. The only structure present in invertebrates which could be compared to the thyroid is the so-called pharyngeal tooth, also containing scleroprotein bound iodine.

In Amphioxus, an exocrine tubulous gland is present in the pharyngeal floor known as the endostyle. This gland contains a protease which is able to hydrolyse iodized proteins (*Clements and Gorbman*, 1955).

In Amniocoetes, during metamorphosis into a lamprey, the exocrine endostyle becomes detached from the pharynx and breaks up into thyroid follicles. The exocrine gland changes into endocrine. The product of the exocrine secretion (thyroglobulin) accumulates within the follicles, becomes reabsorbed, hydrolyzed and is released into the blood. In this way, the thyroid's secretory function as an exocrine gland and the resorptive function of the gut epithelium become unified.

In Chlamydoselachia (sharks), the duct of the thyroid gland is preserved, breaks through the basihyal cartilage and opens into the pharynx. The persistent remnants of the thyroglossal duct are frequently found in mammals including man. In sharks, thyroidal follicles are present along the ventral aorta and afferent branchial arteries. In some fish, the thyroid is enclosed by pronephric remnants. In Elasmobranchials, the thyroid is adjacent to the aortic bifurcation near the origin of the first and second branchial artery. In Amphibians, the thyroid is located near the mandibular angle, covered by the mylohyoid (interhyoid) muscle. In reptiles, turtles and some lizards, there is a single thyroid without any lobes. In most snakes, the thyroid is in the vicinity of the aortal arch; in birds, at the tracheal bifurcation. In all mammals, the thyroid is bilobed and is in a pretracheal position. The lobes are connected by an isthmus. Thyroidal hormones are involved in general tissue metabolism. They influence the growth, body temperature, neural development, internal ear development and reproductive function. In Amphibians, they control metamorphosis.

C-cells originate from the neural crest, and immigrate the endoderm of the fifth pharyngeal pouch. In fish, amphibia, reptiles and birds, calcitonin is secreted by a separate ultimobranchial gland. Ultimobranchial glands are paired, located beneath the esophagus.

PATHOLOGY

THYROID DUCT REMNANTS OR CYSTS

Thyroidal remnants are found near the midline in an area extending from the radix of the tongue over the hyoid bone to the sternum. They move at swallowing. Cysts originating from the thyroglossal duct (70% of cases exhibiting thyroidal remnants) are lined by endodermal epithelium, sometimes multi-layered squamous, stratified cylindrical or respiratory in type, or even signel-layered cylindrical resembling the epithelium of the stomach or gut (Sade and Rosen, 1968). They are filled with a mucinous fluid. A marked lymphatic infiltration is always present around the cyst. Adjacent thyroidal tissue is found in ca. 30% of the cases of cysts. Ectopic thyroidal tissue, present at the foramen caecum of the tongue, is known as the struma lingualis. Lingual thyroid may be the only thyroid tissue present within the body. Therefore, if a surgical removal is proposed, the check up by radioiodine is necessary. Thyroid remnants are rare. Sex ratio, M1 : F1.

THYROID APLASIA AND DYSGENESIS

Thyroid aplasia is related to the rare sporadic agoitrous cretinism (Andersen, 1969). In 80% of children exhibiting an excessive hypothyroidism, some thyroidal remnants are found (thyroid dysgenesis). Common features of an untreated hypothyrosis of several months duration are macroglossia, large belly, hypotonia and sparse and dry hair. The newborns are lethargic, fail to thrive and suffer from obstipation. They breath loudly because of laryngeal and pharyngeal myxedema. Mental retardation becomes evident early in infancy. Fetal hypothyroidism, if suspected, may be diagnosed prenatally by checking the amnionic TSH, T_4 and RT_3 levels. In newborns, the T_4 serum concentrations <7 ng/dl and TSH<100 uU/ml suggest thyroid aplasia or dysgenesis (*Dussault et al.*, 1976; *Klein et al.*, 1976). Familial aggregation of athyrotic cretinism was observed. Maternal antibodies were blamed for the destruction of the fetal thyroid in some cases (*Blizzard et al.*, 1960), and may be implicated in familial cases.

CONGENITAL GOITER AND HYPOTHYROIDISM

Thyroglobulin synthesis defects (classification according to McKusick)

Common features: goiter, hypothyroidism, normal or high radioiodine uptake. Familial occurrence was reported (*Riddick et al.*, 1969). Abnormal biosynthesis of thyroglobulin was discussed by *Stanbury* (1972).

Type I (iodine accumulation, transport or trapping defects)
  Defect in intracellular concentration of iodine common to thyroid, salivary glands and gastric mucosa (*Stanbury and Chapman*, 1960; *Stanbury*, 1972).

Type II A (severe organification defect)
  The iodination of thyrosine is unpaired because of lack of peroxidase activity in the thyroid cells. Enzyme activity may be restored by the addition of hematin contributing to the prosthetic group of peroxidase. *Valenta et al.* (1971) provided direct evidence of defective peroxidase in a patient with congenital goiter and hypothyroidism. Accumulated thyroidal iodide is promptly released by perchlorate.

Type II B (partial organification defect)
  associated with congenital deafness (Pendred syndrome) is related to a defect in iodinase. Cases without deafness were also reported (*Furth et al.*, 1967).

Type III (coupling defect)
  The defect in coupling of iodothyrosyl into iodothyronine hormones may result from an abnormal thyroglobulin. The "coupling enzyme" is hypothetical. The proof of the defect is to be made by the absence of iodothyronines in biopsy specimens of the thyroid (*Alexander and Burrow*, 1970).

Type IV (deiodinase defect)
  There is a general iodothyrosine deiodinase defect in many tissues including the thyroid in most of the cases. Some cases may be limited to the thyroid only (*Kusakabe and Miyake*, 1964).

Type V (plasma iodoprotein defect)
  There is a large amount of an albumin-like iodoprotein in the serum of the affected patient. The thyroglobulin in the thyroid follicles is replaced by iodinated albumin-like protein (*Lissitzky et al.*, 1967).

THYROTROPIN INSENSITIVITY

This defect was supposed in a patient with congenital hypothyroidism with high levels of biologically active TSH (*Stanbury et al.*, 1968).

ISOLATED TSH DEFICIENCY

Patients exhibit cretinism and low, or absent, TSH. If TRH is administered, no increase in TSH is found (*Miyai, et al.*, 1971).

SYNDROME OF THYROID APLASIA, CUTIS VERTICIS GYRATA AND MENTAL RETARDATION (*Akesson*, 1965).

Five affected males in three families of two generation were described. X-limited autosomal dominant inheritance is probable.

PENDRED SYNDROME (hereditary goiter and deafness)

Perceptive deafness, sometimes associated with defective vestibular function is found in all cases. Euthyroid or hypothyroid goiter is present. The thyroid shows a deficient organification of iodine (thyroid hormonogenesis type II B defect). McKusick suggested that a peroxidase deficiency may be related to both cochlear and thyroid defects. Deafness may be present at birth, goiter may develop until the second decade. A mild mental retardation is found in some cases (related probably to the treatment of hypothyroidism), growth is unaltered in most cases. Severe dysplasia of thyroidal epithelium is always present, and may be mistaken for a carcinoma. *Doel* (1973) demonstrated deafness in mice born to females treated with propylthiouracil during pregnancy.

The frequency of Pendred's syndrome in Great Britain is estimated as 1 : 14,300 (*Fraser*, 1965). If both parents are affected, the condition is inherited in all their children.

SIPPLE SYNDROME
(Medullary thyroid carcinoma, phaeochromocytoma and parathyroid disease).

Familial occurrence of medullary thyroid carcinoma associated with phaeochromocytoma and some other endocrine neoplasias represent a disorder linked to the cells originating from the neural crest.

CHAPTER 9

THE PARATHYROID GLAND

Parathyroid glands, two pairs usually being present in humans, are endodermal pharyngeal derivatives. A primordial stage, a separation stage and a definitive stage were distinguished during their development (*Norris*, 1937). Primordia of the

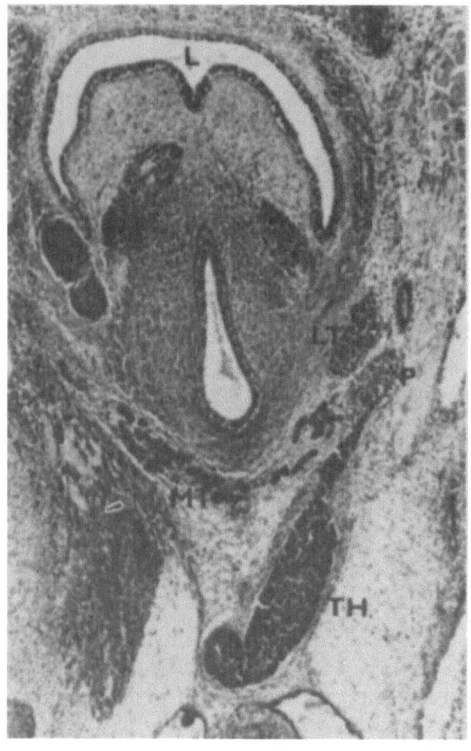

Fig. 100. Cervical area in a 30 mm long embryo (58 days, S. h. XXIII). Parathyroid III (P) detaches from the thymus (Th). LT — lateral thyroidal primordium, MT — medial thyroid.

parathyroid glands are recognizable in 9—12 mm embryos (S. H. XVI, 38—42 days-old) in the dorsal area of the IIIrd and IVth endodermal pharyngeal pouch. They are formed by cylindrical glycogen-rich endodermal cells. The proliferating cells fill the branchial pouch they originate from, forming a solid cord or nodule. During this stage, the parathyroidal nodules are invaded by capillaries (S. H. XVIII, XIX, 45—50 days), and are detached from the pharyngeal endoderm (separation stage) (Fig. 100). During detachment, the cellular cords connecting the parathyroids with the pharynx are known as the pharyngobranchial ducts. Fragmentation of the parathyroid epithelium may occur during the stage of separation resulting in the formation of accessory parathyroids. The parathyroids, III derived from the IIIrd pouch, become detached in 17—22 mm embryos (S. H., XIX, 48—51 days), the parathyroid IV (from the IVth pouch) become detached from the thymic primordium in 25 to 30 mm embryos (54—60 days, S. H. XXII, XXIII).

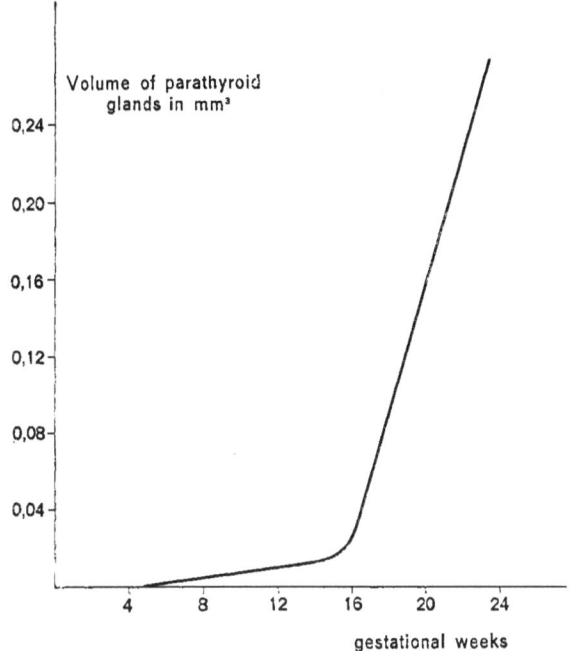

Graph 23. Growth of fetal parathyroid gland (according to Norris, 1946).

The definitive parathyroidal structure showing epithelial cords and interposed capillaries is attained at 10—12 weeks (*Boyd*, 1950; *Politzer and Hann,* 1935; *Norris,* 1937, 1946).

Growth of the parathyroid gland was measured by *Norris* (1946). Because in young embryos it is impossible to separate parathyroids anatomically, their volume was measured from histological sections. The growth proceeds slowly until the end of week 14. Thereafter, a marked acceleration is observed which exceeds the total body weight increase of the fetus (see graph 23). At birth, the diameter of the parathyroid glands is approximately 1—2 mm.

CELLS OF THE PARATHYROID (PTH CELLS)

The endodermal cell exhibiting alkaline phosphatase in apical localization, becomes converted into a clear primordial parathyroidal glycogen-rich cell without any alkaline phosphatase activity (Figs. 101, 102). The first clear PTH-cells

173

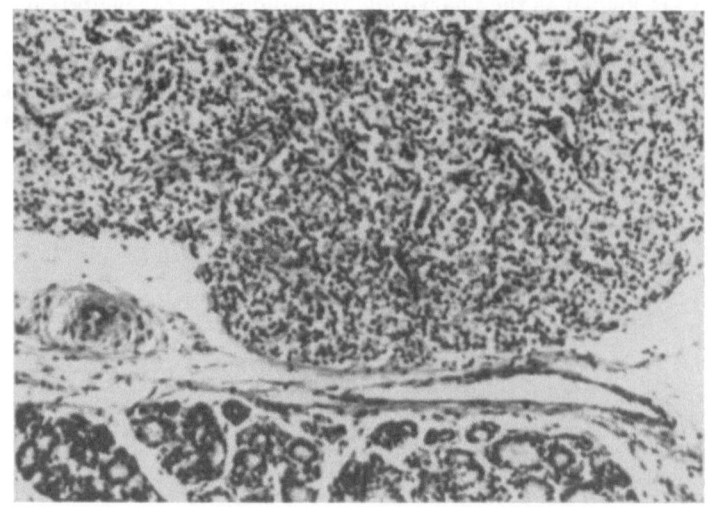

Fig. 101. Parathyroid of a four month old fetus, adjacent to thyroid (lower portion of the picture).

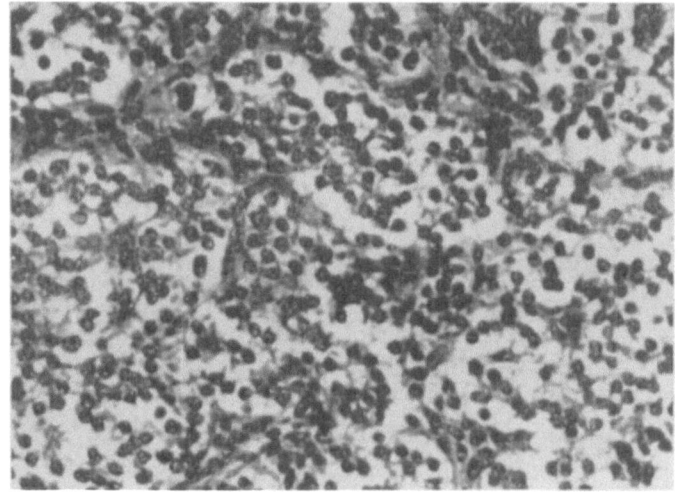

Fig. 102. Uniform clear cells of a fetal parathyroid.

become differentiated during the separation of the parathyroids from the pharynx. *Norris* (1946) distinguished vesicular cells (appearing in the IIIrd month), clear cells, dense cells and dark cells. All of them, however, are functional varieties of one basic PTH-producing cell. Primordial and vesicular cells are predominant in fetal parathyroids. No oxyphil cells are present. Oxyphil cells appear at puberty. They were reported, however, as an exception in a three year old child (*Gilmour*, 1937). Their number increases with advancing age. Under EM, the PTH-cell (chief cell) has a well developed rough endoplasmic reticulum and Golgi zone. Abundant cytoplasmic glycogen is found in primordial cells before the cells enter the secretory cycle. Coated

174

granules containing PTH, comparable to argyrophilic granules seen by light microscopy, are present not only in the cytoplasm, but also inside the mitochondria. Lipid droplets of unknown significance may be present in some cells. The cellular membranes of adjacent cells connect by desmosomes. The function of the human parathyroid begins at the end of the third month. Human parathyroids from 12—13 week old fetuses produce bone resorption if cultivated in contact with parietal rat bones on a chicken chorionallantois (*Scothorne*, 1964).

PARATHORMONE (PTH)

Parathormone is a single-chain polypeptide of 84 aminoacids, M. W. around 8500 (*Hawker et al.*, 1966). The hormone regulates the extracellular concentration of calcium. Increase in extracellular calcium suppresses and decreased calcium stimulates both hormone secretion and synthesis. The isolation of specific parathormone coding m-RNA followed by translation of the m-RNA in heterologous cell-free systems, showed that about 15—20% of the biosynthetic activity is devoted to the synthesis of bigger hormones: the pre-proparathyroid hormone (in a very small quantity) and the proparathyroid hormone. The pre-proparathyroid hormone is a polypeptide of 115 aminoacids containing the sequence of proparathyroid hormone. Proparathyroid hormone contains 90 aminoacids, 84 of them forming the sequence of parathormone (*Habener and Potts Jr.*, 1978). The prohormone-specific hexapeptide bond (between arginine and serine) is highly sensitive to cleavage by trypsin. Prohormone is about 10% as active as PTH in the bone citrate decarboxylase assay (*Hamilton et al.*, 1971 a).

Pre-Pro PTH is the initial product synthetized on ribosomes. The conversion of Pro PTH occurs during transport of the polypeptide into the cisternae of the rough endoplasmic reticulum. 20 minutes after synthesis of Pre-Pro PTH, Pro PTH reaches the Golgi zone and is converted to PTH. PTH is stored in secretory granules until released into circulation in response to the fall of the extracellular calcium (*Habener et al.*, 1977). Transcriptional (synthesis of m-RNA) rather than translational events are involved in the regulation of the hormone synthesis. High concentrations of extracellular calcium stimulate and low concentrations inhibit intracellular PTH degradation (*Chu et al.*, 1973). If PTH secretion is exogenously suppressed, acid hydrolases containing lysosomal bodies appear in the parathyroid cells and digest PTH-containing granules. The increase of extracellular calcium after PTH release is related to the Ca release from bones, tubular Ca^{2+} absorption in kidneys and increased Ca^{2+} absorption by the gut. Adenyl cyclase and c-AMP mediates the peripheral action of PTH and Ca controlled PTH production. Biological PTH, degradation takes place in kidneys. Osteoclasts releasing anorganic as well as organic bone substances are the main PTH target during fetal life. PTH is effective only if vitamin D is present. In D-avitaminosis, the parathyroids hypertrophy, but the bone calcium release is limited. Excretion of calcium by the breast has to be considered in breast feeding women. PTH influences both absorption and excretion of magnesium. Hypocalcemia is resistant to vitamin D treatment if hypomagnesaemia is present at the same time.

Parathormone does not cross the placental barrier. In newborns, the plasma PTH levels are 251 ± 63 pg/ml. In the mother, 267 ± 45 pg/ml. Plasma Ca levels at delivery in newborns are 5.16 ± 0.24 mEq/l and in mother, 4.54 ± 0.24 mEq/l (*Lequin et al.*, 1970).

PHYLOGENESIS

Parathyroids are present in amphibians. No comparable structures are known in fishes. Their development is related to the transition from an aquatic to a terrestrial life. During this period when the gill-type respiration changed to the pulmonary one, the regulation of the calcium level became important.

In different species, the number as well as the position of the parathyroids is variable. In most amniotes, including man, there are two pairs of parathyroids. In some snakes and some tetrapods, there are three pairs derived from endodermal pouches two, three, and four. In some animals, only one pair of parathyroids is present.

CALCIUM HOMEOSTASIS IN PREGNANCY

The normal adult plasma Ca levels are $8.8-10.3$ mg/100 ml. Approximately 47.5% of this amount represents free ionized Ca^{2+}, 46% is protein bound, 1.6% forms $CaHPO_4$. 1.7% ionized Ca-citrate the rest are unidentified Ca complexes. At the end of pregnancy. the maternal calcium rises to 11.9 mg/100 ml and the fetal calcium level is 12.5 mg$\%$.

The ionized Ca fraction, which is biologically the most important, is exchanged across the placental membrane. All the calcium for the fetus comes from the mother. Calcium is deposited into the fetal skeleton beginning at $10-11$ weeks of gestation. There is an intense exchange of calcium ions between the blood plasma and the organs. The skeleton of the newborn contains approximately 30 g calcium. Daily calcium intake to provide a positive calcium balance during the last trimester of pregnancy is estimated at $1-2$ g (*Duggin et al.*, 1974). The fetal daily requirement at the end of gestation is approximately 250 mg.

CALCIUM AND CELLULAR FUNCTIONS

The level of extracellular ionized calcium (1.2 mmol) exceeds the intracellular level measured within the cytosol. The cytosol Ca concentration is estimated as $0.12-0.012$ mmol. The intracellular estimates are highly inaccurate because of difficulties with the protein binding. The gradient between extracellular and intracellular calcium suggests a calcium pump. Blood coagulation depends on the presence of extracellular calcium ions. Ionized calcium influences the permeability of the cellular and mitochondrial membranes. Increased levels of extracellular calcium decrease the permeability of cellular membranes; decreased extracellular calcium, increases the cellular membranes permeability. In hypercalcaemia, the tubular reabsorption of sodium is decreased leading to polyuria, resistence to AVP and loss of ability to concentrate urine.

In hypocalcaemia, an increased cellular permeability to Ca^{2+} and calcium release at the terminals of splanchnic nerves, increases the secretion of catecholamines by the adrenal medulla. In nerve fibers, the depolarization of the membrane and ATP efflux occur. The ATP synthesis falls and the resting potential of the cell membrane of the neuron diminishes. The low calcium level stimulates the split of energy-rich ATP bounds. The action of most protein hormones is inhibited in the absence of Ca^{2+}, even though ability to increase or decrease cAMP is unimpaired.

The changes in the cellular membranes permeability are related to the calcium binding by phospholipids. In addition, calcium forms chelates and is able to bind phospholipids and ATP. The affinity between Ca^{2+} and ATP is one thousand times bigger than the affinity to AMP.

Calcium is accumulated within the mitochondria. The energy required for accumulation is released from ATP. Much less energy is required for the maintenance of the Ca^{2+} gradient between the mitochondria and the cytoplasm than for the intramitochondrial Ca^{2+} accumulation. The transport of calcium into mitochondria does not require the presence of phosphate. The transport of phosphate requires the presence of bivalent kations, predominantly calcium. Bivalent katitons are concentrated by mitochondria. The transport of bivalent kations varies in different tissue and is changed by parathormone, cortisol, estrogens and vitamin D. In contrast to the plasma membranes, increase in ionized calcium increases the permeability of mitochondrial membranes. Magnesium seems to stabilize mitochondrial membranes permeability and the electron transport coupled with oxydative phosphorylation.

MAGNESIUM

Magnesium is involved in activities similar to that of calcium. Magnesium regulates the activity od many enzymes, such as those involved in the synthesis and hydrolysis of ATP, isocitric dehydrogenase, carboxylase, pyruvateoxidase, alkaline phosphatase and influences the ribosomal synthesis of peptides. The effects of magnesium are antagonistic to thyroxin. The factors involved in the regulation of magnesium levels are largely unknown. Increased levels of parathormone decrease the serum levels of magnesium.

PHOSPHATES

The regulation of the serum phosphates and calcium are closely related. Most of the phosphates are bound together with calcium within the bones in the form of a hydroxyapatite $[Ca^{2+}_{10-x}(H_2O^+)_2{}^+ \cdot (PO_4)_6 (OH^-)_2]$. Within the serum, most of the phosphates is in ionized form as HPO_4^{2-} (approximately 0.5 mmol/l)l About $15-20\%$ of serum phosphates are protein bound. Phosphates are of basic importance for every living cell. They are present in DNA and RNA molecules and together with adenine and guanine contribute the macroenergy bonds. They participate in the glucose metabolism. In the form of phospholipids, they are involved in the molecular structure of membranes.

Anorganic pyrophosphates are genetically related to the inhibition of calcium and phosphate precipitation from oversaturated solutions. In vivo, they prevent precipitation and dissolving of the hydroxyapatite. In ossification, the bone pyrophosphatase splits pyrophosphates and, because of the decreased level of pyrophosphate, hydroxyapatite is deposited. Precise proper regulation of serum calcium and phosphorus favors mineralization of bones without producing calcification of the soft tissues.

In bone resorption, the pyrophosphate inhibition increases the dissolving of the bone mineral. Alkaline phosphatase is one of the pyrophosphatases.

CITRATE

The main source of serum citrate are the bones. The citrate level increases after administration of parathormone and vitamin D. Estrogens and glucocorticoids decrease the citrate level. Citrate is converted to isocitrate in the tricarboxylic acids cycle by the NAD-dependent isocitrate dehydrogenase. Mitochondria represent an organelle which is influenced by bivalent kations, parathormone and vitamin D. The changes in the mitochondrial membrane permeability in response to Ca^{2+} and Mg^{2+} concentrations are related to changes in citrate oxidation. In addition, Mg^{2+} stimulates and Ca^{2+} inhibits the mitochondrial isocitrate dehydrogenase activity.

PATHOLOGY

Maternal hyperparathyroidism always jeopardises the pregnancy outcome. Neonatal tetany is observed in children born to hyperparathyroidic mothers. In one such case reported, both maternal as well as fetal PTH were elevated. The fetal elevation in PTH was regarded as a result of hypomagnesaemia related to a relative endorgan refractoriness to PTH (*Montelone et al.*, 1975).

In a survey (*Ludwig*, 1962) of 34 pregnancies in 23 hyperparathyroid women, the outcome was the following: antenatal fetal death in 7 cases (30.4%), death of the newborn in 2 cases (9%). Neonatal tetany in all living children. No disturbances in ossification or cystic bone dysplasia. Hypoparathyroidism in three brothers born to a hyperparathyroid woman was described by *Buchs* (1961).

Infantile hypercalcaemia was observed (*Lightwood*, 1952) in artificially fed babies and was considered to be due to extensive intake of vitamin D.

OSTEODYSPLASIA CYSTICA GENERALISATA

Osteodysplasia cystica generalisata with a diffuse enlargement of the parathyroids was observed in a fetus born to a mother with hypoparathyroidism (*Gerloczy and Farkas*, 1953).

ABSENCE OF PARATHYROIDS AND THYMUS (Di George Syndrome)

Absence of parathyroids and thymus is a rare congenital anomaly involving the structures derived from the IIIrd and IVth endodermal pharyngeal pouches. Affected children have low set ears, a peculiar appearance and immune deficiencies (*Di George*, 1968).

HYPOPARATHYROIDISM

Familial early hypoparathyroidism associated with hypomagnesaemia was described by *Niklasson*, 1970.

ERRORS IN PARATHORMONE SYNTHESIS

Errors in parathormone synthesis giving rise to an inactive hormone were proposed, but are insufficiently documented (*Nusynowitz and Klein*, 1973).

ALBRIGHT'S HEREDITARY OSTEODYSTROPHY

Includes both pseudohypoparathyroidism and pseudo-pseudohypoparathyroidism.

Common features:

The syndrome becomes evident after birth, the metacarpal and metatarsal bones are short, long bones are thickened, cataracts are present, calcification of the basal ganglia and ectopic bone formation is observed. Epileptiform seizures, sometimes lethal, occur. Hypocalcaemia and hyperphosphataemia are evident. Combinations of Albright's osteodystrophy, hypothyroidism and hypogonadism are common. The affected individuals are insensitive to PTH (*Williams and Seriver*, 1973). In pseudohypoparathyroid patients, the PTH does not raise the urinary cAMP. In pseudopseudohypoparathyroid patients, the PTH administration produces a rise in urinary cAMP, but there are no changes in the Ca^{2+} level. Sex ratio is M 1 : F 2, the disorder seems to be X-linked dominant, or sex-influenced autosomal dominant. Both disorders may be present in the same family. The possibility of passing from the pseudo- to the pseudopseudo state during the life of the affected patient was suggested (McKusick). Turner's syndrome patients sometimes show Albright's hereditary osteodystrophy; however, the two conditions are not to be confused.

CHAPTER 10

ENTEROENDOCRINE CELLS AND PANCREATIC ISLETS

Enteroendocrine cells are scattered in the epithelium of the stomach and small intestine. They produce polypeptidic enterohormones known as gastrin, secretin and cholecystokinin-pancreozymin (CCK-PZ). Gastrin occurs in two forms, gastrin I and gastrin II, both have a molecule with 17 aminoacids and differ in one aminoacid. Gastrin is the most potent activator of gastric acid. Secretin principally stimulates the water and bicarbonate secretion by the pancreas. The sequence of 14 of the 27 amino-acids contributing the molecule of secretin is identical to that in glucagon. Chole-cystokinin-pancreozymin (CCK-PZ). polypeptides with an identical molecule contai-ning 33 aminoacids, stimulate the secretion of pancreatic enzymes and contractions of the gall bladder.

The gastrin producing cells are present in the gastric and duodenal mucosa as well as in the pancreatic islets in four month old fetuses (*Lomský and Jirásek*, unpublished). The function of the enterohormones in the prenatal period remains unknown.

In addition to enterohormones, somatostatin (tetradecapeptid) was found in a suprisingly high concentration in the stomach and in pancreatic islands. Somato-statin inhibits glucagon, and gastrin secretion.

THE PANCREAS

The pancreas has two parts, the exocrine, secreting enzyme-rich pancreatic digestive juice into the duodenum; and the endocrine, involved mainly in the regulation of glycaemia.

DEVELOPMENT

The pancreas originates from two endodermal evaginations formed from the duo-denum (Fig. 103). The first one, the dorsal pancreatic primordium, which appears in 35—38 day-old embryos (6.5—8.5 mm, S. H. XV) is located opposite and slightly cranial from the hepatic evagination. The dorsal pancreatic primordium grows into the dorsal mesoduodenum to the left vitelline vein. The ventral pancreatic pri-mordium appears close to the hepatic evagination in 38—42 day-old embryos (8—12 mm, S. H. XVI) and grows into the ventral mesoduodenum. The opening into the duodenum is common to the hepatic and ventral pancreatic primordium. The rotation of the duodenum in 40—44 day embryos (12—14 mm, S. H.) leads to the apposition of the ventral to the dorsal primordium and both pancreatic primordia fuse. Only a part of the definitive pancreatic head originates from the ventral primordium. The remaining part of the head, the corpus and the cauda are formed from the dorsal primordium. As the fusion occurs, the main ducts of both

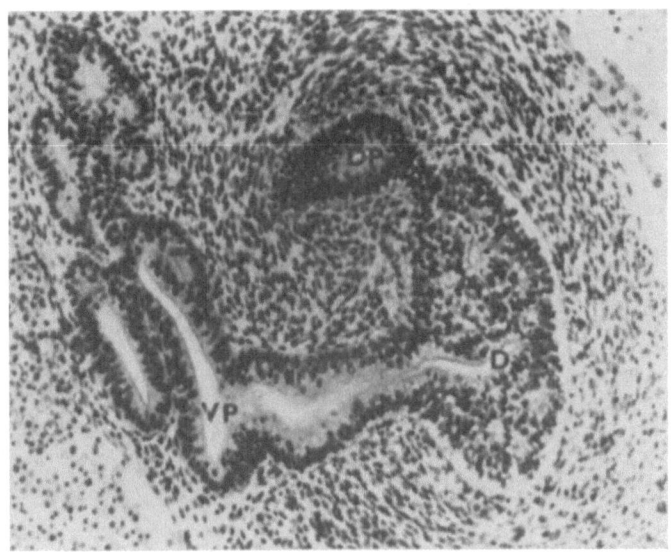

Fig. 103. Dorsal (DP) and ventral (VP) pan creatic primordia growing from duodenum (D). Embryo 14 mm (42 days, S. h. XVII).

parts join together. The proximal portion of the main duct of the definitive pancreas is formed by the main duct of the ventral primordium, the distal portion by the distal part of the main duct of the dorsal primordium. The proximal part of the main duct of the dorsal primordium undergoes regression in most cases. If persisting, the dorsal duct is known as the accessory duct of the pancreas (*Liu and Potter*, 1962; *Neubert*, 1927).

The pancreatic primordium is formed by branched tubules lined with a simple endodermal cylindrical epithelium (Fig. 104). The endodermal cells are glycogen rich, the supranuclear cytoplasm is pyroninophil, and in the apical localization, alkaline phosphatase is present. The alkaline phosphatase disappears as the glandular tubules become branched. The differentiation of the exocrine and endocrine tissue becomes evident at the end of the ninth week in 40—50 mm long embryos (*Ferner and Stockenius*, 1951; *Landau and Lugibihl*, 1967; *Pearse*, 1903). The organophosphate resistant non-specific α-naphtylesterase (peptidase) may be used as a marker enzyme for the exocrine tissue. Glycogen is the characteristic feature of the epithelium of the fetal pancreatic duct and the absence of glycogen and organophosphate resistant naphtylesterase is a characteristic of the development of endocrine islets (*Jirásek*, 1965). The endocrine tissue in 9 and 10 week old fetuses forms cords arranged in nodules attached to the pancreatic ducts (Fig. 105). This connection is gradually lost and the islets are separated (first at the beginning of week ten). At the same time, capillaries are formed between the cords of the pancreatic islets.

CELLS OF THE PANCREATIC ISLETS

The pancreatic islets contain at least four different types of cells. A-cells produce glucagon, B-cells insulin and the D-cells are heterogenous. Some of the D-cells

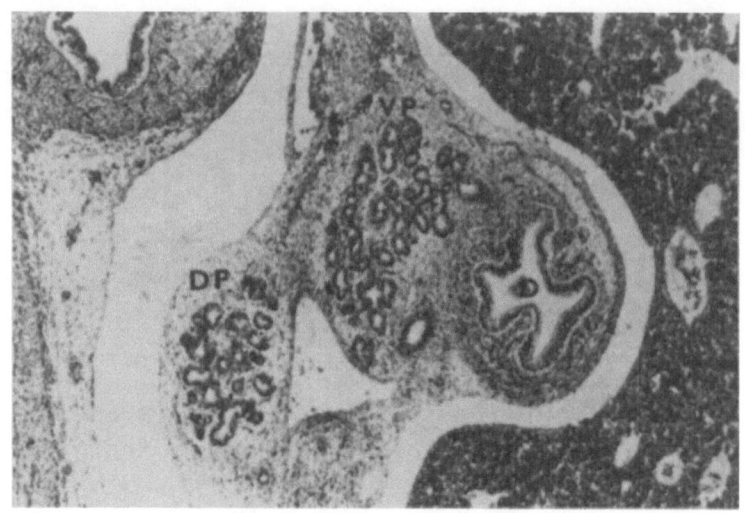

Fig. 104. Branching glandular tubules of pancreatic primordium in a 25 mm embryo ·(52 days, S. h. XXI). D — duodenum, VP — venral ptancreas, DP — dorsal pancreas.

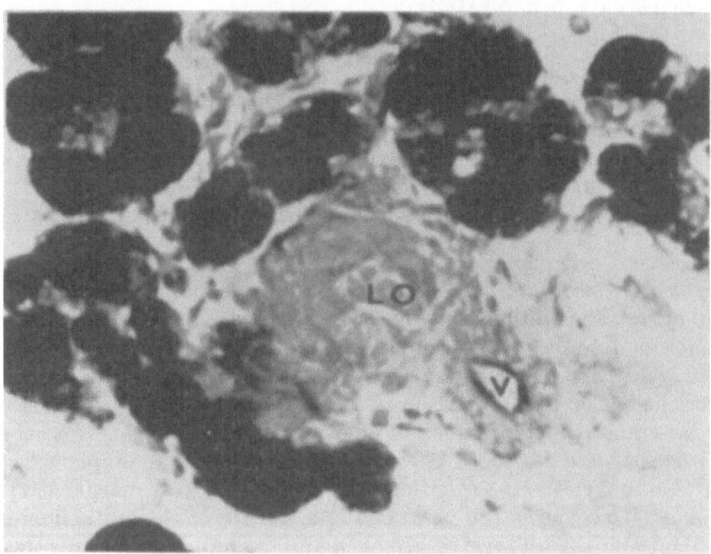

Fig. 105. Differentiation of a pancreatic islet, which is still connected with a pancreatic duct. Peptidase stain. The enzyme is present in the exocrine cells and in the apical portion of the epithelium lining the duct. (V)-pancreatic islet - LO.

are involved in the production of somatostatin (SRIF), some in the production of gastrin. Both gastrin and SRIF-producing cells represent specific cellular types with different granules (*Goldsmith et al.*, 1978). SRIF-producing cells are adjacent to A-cells. Gastrin-producing cells are scattered in the islets. The SRIF-producing cells may be of neuroectodermal origin. At birth, B-cells represent approximately

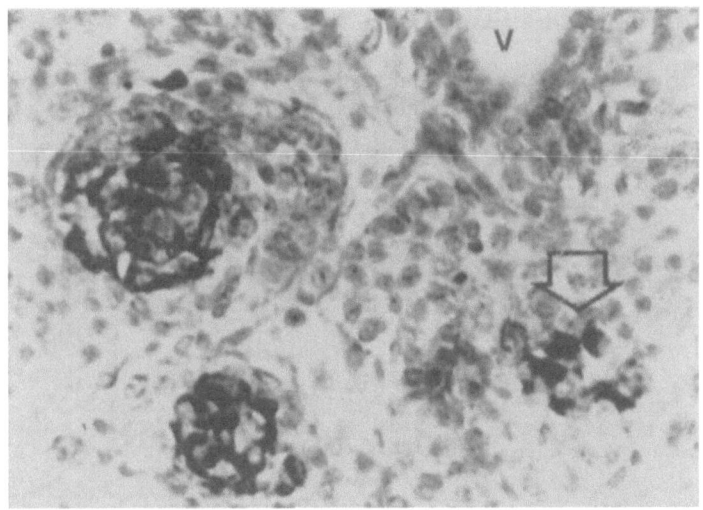

Fig. 106. β-cells in pancreatic islets stained by aldehyd-fuchsin. 14 weeks old fetus. The arrow points on the differentiating β-cells in an islet which is not detached from the duct (V).

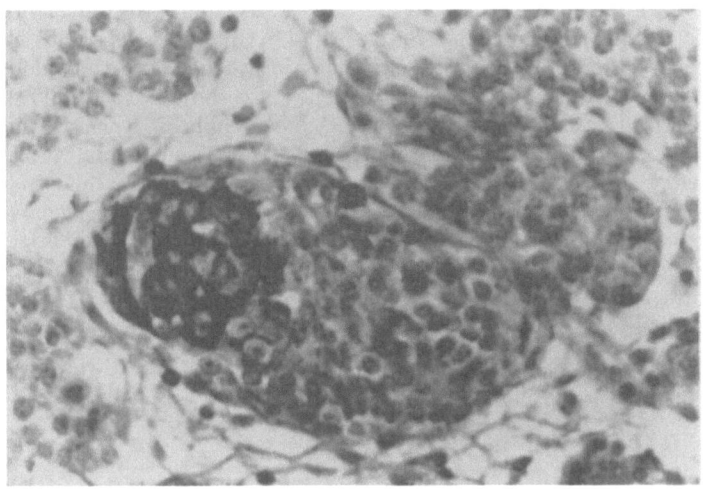

Fig. 107. Polar stage of pancreatic islet. The β-cells are concentrated at one side of the islet 14 weeks old fetus.

60%, A-cells 30%, D-cells (gastrin-cells, SRIF cells and possibly others) 10% of the islet tissue. According to the arrangement of A and B-cells within the fetal pancreatic islet, a bipolar stage (week 13—14) (Figs. 106, 107) at which the A-cells are at one and the B-cells at the other side, a mantle stage (weeks 15—25) at which the A-cells are mostly at the periphery of the islet and a disperse stage are distinguished. At the disperse stage in most islets after 25 weeks of development, the A and B-cells are intermingled.

B-CELLS AND INSULIN FORMATION

Insulin is formed in the B-cells from proinsulin which represents the "big form" of the hormone. Proinsulin (84 aminoacids) consists of the insulin A and B chains

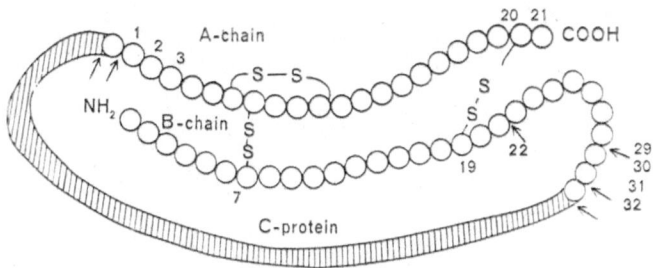

Fig. 108. Structure of human proinsulin. Arrows indicate sites of tryptic cleavage.

linked by a polypeptide segment (30—35 aminoacids), known as the C-protein (C-connecting, Fig. 108.)

The proinsulin chain is formed by ribosomes of rough endoplasmic reticulum. The conformation of the molecule depending on the correct pairing of disulphide bonds between the A and B chain, occurs within the cisternae of the endoplasmic reticulum. Proinsulin is transported into the vesicles of the Golgi complex and is condensed into membrane-coated granules. These granules are identical to the aldehydfuchsine positive granules of the light microscopy. They are roundshaped 200—400 nm in diameter, electron translucent with a distinct lucent halo underneath their limiting membrane. A crystaloid of various angular forms is present in many of them. The proteolytic enzymes cleaving proinsulin at specific sites where A and B insulin chains join the C-peptide, are probably localized in the granules, or their membranes (*Rubenstein et al.*, 1977). After hydrolysis, insulin and C-peptide are retained together within the secretory granules and subsequently released in equimolar amounts by exocytosis into the circulation. Zinc which is usually found associated with insulin, has a role in insulin storage or release.

The first B-cells may be identified in the human pancreatic islets at 10 weeks.

A-CELLS AND GLUCAGON

Glucagon is produced predominantly by A-cells. Some A-cells are found in an extrapancreatic localization. Glucagon, a single-chain protein with 29 aminoacids (M. W. 3600) is synthetized in the ribosomes of the rough endoplasmic reticulum and passes into the Golgi cysternae, where glucagon becomes incorporated into the granules. The granules of the A-cells are round 200-400 nm in diameter with a dense core and a paler halo underneath the membrane of the granule. A-cells exhibit formalin-induced fluorescence suggesting occurrence of catecholamines.

D-CELLS (D-G-CELLS; D-SRIF-CELLS)

Two types of D-cells can be distinguished by EM or immunohistochemistry: D-G-cells with big secretory granules producing gastrin (*Lomský et al.*, 1969) and D-SRIF-cells

184

with small granules producing SRIF (*Orci and Unger*, 1975; *Dubois*, 1975; *Goldsmith*, 1975). Granules in both types of D-cells are difficult to fix. If O_sO_4 fixation is used, the granules are swollen, vacuolated and broken in most cases.

D-G-cells (gastrin producing) are polyedric or oval, the Golgi complex is located opposite to the vascular pole of the cell, the granula are big 300—450 nm, uniquely gray, the material they contain is apposited to the membrane of the granule. A halo underneath the membrane is never seen. D-G-cells are present in the pancreatic islets in four month old fetuses (*Lomský and Jirásek*, 1976). D SRIF-cells (somatostatin producing) are much smaller, they are 150—175 nm in diameter, uniquely gray, without any halo underneath their membrane. D SRIF-cells are always apposed to A-cells. SRIF suppresses insulin, prolactin and growth hormone and lowers glycemia (*Yen et al.*, 1974). Some D cells exhibit a formalin-induced fluorescence related to catecholamines similar to the A-cells.

PANCREATIC ISLETS PHYLOGENY

The exocrine as well as endocrine parts of the pancreas were originally represented by cells enclosed in the duodenal mucosa. In Amphioxus insulin, glucagon and gastrin-containing cells are present in the anterior part of the mid-gut scattered among enterocytes (*van Noorden and Pearse*, 1976). Insulin-like material is present in the enterocytes. In all higher animals, at least in their adult forms, insulin-producing cells are separated from the intestine. In Amniocetes, the insulin-producing cells are in the intestine near the junction with the esophagus, becoming isolated during amniocetes metamorphosis into a lamprey. Then they are embedded within connective tissue. In myxinoids, the islets form lobules near the liver, surrounding the distal part of the gall duct. The lobules are composed of B-cells and an additional cell type. No A-cells are found. In some myxinoids, follicles of unknown function are present in the endocrine pancreas. However, myxinoids do produce enteroglucagon. The A-cells remain in the intestine later than the B-cells. (*Epple and Lewis*, 1973.)

In gnathostomes, the islets develop in association with the exocrine pancreas. The association between islets and exocrine pancreas guarantees a quick transport of the hormone into the liver without any dilution in the gut, or with the blood of the gut.

In addition to their role in the intermediary metabolism, pancreatic islets are involved in some fish in the osmoregulation. The metabolic islets function, however, prevails in all tetrapods. In birds, there is an increased importance of glucagon, while in mammals, the insulin is of basic importance.

Insulin is a phylogenetically old polypeptide, far more wide-spread than glucagon The structure of the insulin molecule seems to have been remarkably stable during evolution (*Falkmer and Ostberg*, 1976). Biochemical data strongly suggest a common origin for both the gastro-intestinal and islet hormones from one or more large precursors (*Thompson*, 1975). It seems that enterohormones and islet hormones originally had only a local effect, influencing the gut resorptive and secretory functions locally near the area of their origin. After the liver and exocrine pancreas became separated from the gut, the pancreatic islets were also isolated and the islet hormones and enterohormones became secreted into the blood.

INSULIN AND ITS METABOLISM

Insulin is the main hormone regulating glycaemia. The fetal pancreatic insulin content concentration and serum level are given in table 26. Fetal serum insulin levels are presented in graph 24.

Table 26. Insulin content and concentration within the human fetal pancreas and fetal serum insulin concentration (according to *Pronina and Sapronova*, 1976 and *Spellacy et al.*, 1973).

Age of the fetus in Weeks	Pancreas		Serum level μU/ml
	content μU	concentration mU/mg	
8 — 9	1.5 ± 0.4	0.33 ± 0.08	—
10 — 11	9.7 ± 1.2	0.53 ± 0.05	—
12 — 14	54.0 ± 11.8	1.0 ± 0.22	—
15 — 16	238.0 ± 35.5	2.0 ± 0.31	2.35 ± 0.5
17 — 18	336.9 ± 43.8	1.8 ± 0.31	7.7 ± 2.5
19 — 21	449.0 ± 124.0	2.0 ± 0.25	4.2 ± 1.5
22 — 24	1181.7 ± 263.1	3.8 ± 0.82	4.5 ± 1.4
25 — 27	2288.0 ± 500.0	3.8 ± 0.17	7.6 ± 2.2
28 — 32	10337.0 ± 3515.0	10.1 ± 2.65	34.1 ± 14.1

Insulin lower glucose, free fatty acids and free aminoacids in the blood, in liver and muscles. In adipose tissue, insulin promotes glycogen synthesis and fat synthesis. Insulin also stimulates protein synthesis. Insulin is an anabolic hormone necessary for energy storage. Its secretion increases after feeding and decreases in response to fasting. Glucose is the first and principal factor promoting insulin secretion and also stimulates insulin synthesis. A hypothesis was proposed that glucose may act on a receptor site at the B-cell membrane to stimulate insulin release. An intracellular intermediate produced in the course of glucose metabolism within the B-cell may be responsible for the activation of the adenyl cyclase — cAMP system leading to insulin synthesis. Calcium is essential in insulin secretion (*Curry et al.*, 1968). Aminoacids also stimulate insulin secretion, and insulin is partly related to the secretion of pancreozymin (*Marks and Samols*, 1970). Pancreatic islets are rich in autonomic nerve terminals. The vagus inhibits, and epinephrine and norepinephrine stimulate insulin secretion. Dopamine stimulates both insulin and glucagon release (*Leblanc, Abu-Fadil, Lachelin and Yen*, 1977).

The feedback of insulin secretion is asserted by both glucose and aminoacids. If their levels are elevated, insulin secretion elevates and the formation of glycogen and protein increases. If the glucose and aminoacid levels drop, the secretion of insulin diminishes. The circulating insulin is destroyed in the liver and kidneys.

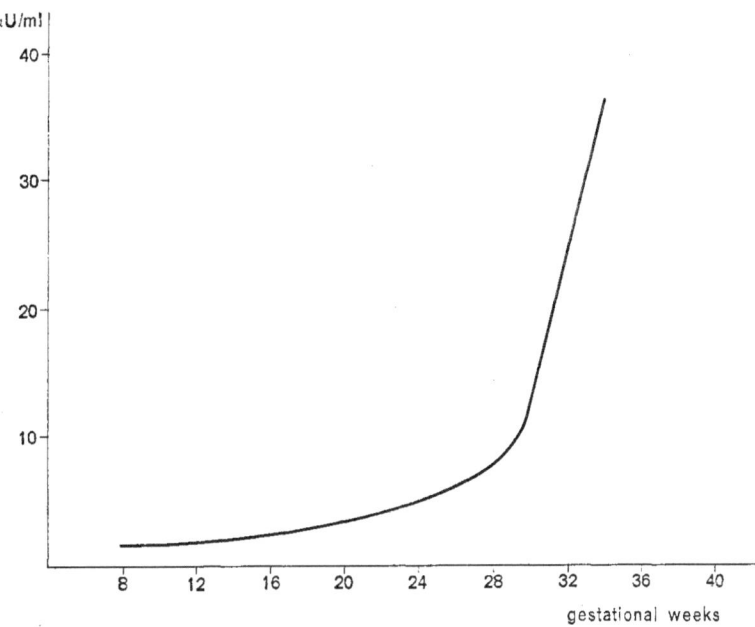

Graph 24. Fetal serum insulin level μU/ml.

GLUCAGON AND ITS METABOLISM

Similar to insulin secretion, secretion of glucagon depends on the circulating glucose concentration and aminoacids concentration, particularly alanine. Hypoglycaemia and hypoalaninaemia increase glucagon secretion. Elevation of glycaemia reduces glucagon secretion. Glucagon is regarded as a catabolic hormone. Glucagon stimulates hepatic glycogenolysis and activates proteolysis and lipolysis. As a consequence of lipolysis, ketogenesis and gluconeogenesis increase. Glucagon increases the hepatic cAMP. Glucagon is destroyed in many tissues, principally in the liver and kidneys. Glucagon was found in 50 day old human embryos (*Schaeffer et al.*, 1971). The balanced glycaemia is maintained by the opposing actions of insulin and glucagon (*Felig et al.*, 1976). Catecholamines are involved in the regulation of balance between insulin and glucagon secretion between B and A-cells in the pancreatic islets. Epinephrine and norepinephrine stimulate glucagon secretion and inhibit insulin secretion. Dopamine increases the secretion of both insulin and glucagon, and there is some evidence that this effect is mediated by somatostatin. *Orci et al.*, (1975) demonstrated tied and gap junction between the islets cells and proposed their role in the coordination in the secretory activities of different cells.

GLYCEMIA IN PREGNANCY AND DIABETES

Neither insulin nor glucagon pass the placental barrier. In pregnant women, pancreatic islets experience hypertrophy; hyperinsulinemia and insulinresistance are evident (*Yen, et al.*, 1971, *Yen*, 1973).

187

During the first trimester of pregnancy, the hypoglycemic effect of insulin is similar to that seen in non-pregnant women, or is slightly elevated.

MODIFICATION IN LIPID METABOLISM IN PREGNANCY

During the second and third trimester of pregnancy, the free fatty acid levels are increased (*Blecher et al.*, 1964). At the same time, glycerol is released. The release of free fatty acids by lipolysis in the maternal adipose tissue occurs regardless of glucose or insulin. This mechanism represents a unique metabolic system covering the needs of energy within the maternal organism to the expense of fat. The glucose and the aminoacids are saved for the development of the fetoplacental unit. The placental hormones, hCS and estrogens, are involved in the regulation of mechanisms metabolically favoring the developing fetus.

MATERNAL DIABETES AND THE DIABETIC FETOPATHY

Both main pancreatic hormones, insulin and glucagon, are involved in the pathogenesis of diabetes (*Unger*, 1976). In the hypertrophied islets of juvenile diabetics the number of A-cells and SRIF-cells are increased (*Orci et al.*, 1976), however, there is evidence that insulin is the determining factor for glucose utilization (*Felig et al.*, 1976). In pregnant women, diabetes has been classified in various terms such as: prediabetes, gestational diabetes, overt diabetes, etc. Prediabetes: the diagnosis is suspected if the women develop diabetes sometime after pregnancy begins and delivers a baby of more than 10 pounds. The diagnosis is made in retrospect.

Gestational diabetes: during pregnancy, the glucose tolerance is abnormal, but reverts to normal after delivery.

Overt diabetes: is evident clinically and is confirmed by the fasting glycaemia.

DIABETIC FETOPATHY

Glucose passes the placental barrier by a facilitated diffusion. Ketoacidosis in the pregnant diabetic woman threatens the fetus. None of the pancreatic hormones pass the placental barrier. However, the insulin antibodies, if present, may pass in some cases. Although catecholamines are inactivated within the trophoblast (by monoamine oxidase and catechol-o-methyltransferase), some still may pass (*Morgan et al.*, 1972).

Infants of diabetic mothers are large and heavy. Their average body weight, if the maternal diabetes was not compensated, exceeds by about 1000 g the average weight of a normal full-term infant. The excessive weight is related to the maternal hyper glycaemia (*Osler*, 1965), and is due to the accumulation of fat and visceromegaly of heart and liver (*Cole*, 1975). The body water is decreased to 70% of the total body weight (78% in normal newborns). This lowering affects more extracellular than intracellular fluids. The head is relatively small; the brain is of a normal size.

Maternal hyperglycemia causes fetal hyperglycemia and hypertrophy of the fetal pancreatic islets. The number of β-cells is increased. In some cases eosinophilic infiltration of the islets was found. A striking relation was reported between the hypertrophy of pancreatic islets and the birth weight (*Cardell*, 1958). The heart contains a large amount of glycogen. In the liver and the spleen, hematopoesis is found. The differentiation of the kidneys corresponds to the "true" age of the fetus and not to his weight. Pathologic changes are not evident in the hypophysis, the thyroid or the adrenals. The placenta is big and heavy. The villi contain more cytotrophoblasts than normal and in the stroma, Hofbauer cells are present at term. These features are usually characteristics for an immature placenta. Non-specific degeneration such as edematous villi, angiopathies and placental infarcts are frequently seen. The diabetic fetopathy becomes evident after 28 weeks of pregnancy. Intrauterine death shortly before delivery occurs in some diabetic fetuses without any reason for the death being evident.

After delivery, hypoglycemia occurs in about 50—70% of infants born to diabetic mothers. Higher blood calcium in pregnant diabetics is reflected in the fetus leading to neonatal hypocalcemia in some cases (*Cole*, 1975).

The high infant mortality is usually associated with respiratory distress syndrome due to lung hyaline membranes or (and) pulmonary atelectases. Miscarriage in diabetic mothers is more frequent. The incidence of congenital anomalies in diabetic fetuses is approximately three times the normal rate. The anomalies involve mostly the cardiac and skeletal systems and seem to be related to the maternal ketoacidosis early in pregnancy. Hydramnion is frequently encountered in pregnant diabetics. Diabetes does not seem to be a single entity. Genetic factors are obvious, but the mode of inheritance is obscure. Children of diabetic fathers, if the maternal pregnancy glycemia has been normal, have a normal birth weight. The probability of diabetes in the child is increased if both parents are diabetics. If a sibling is affected, the probability for another sibling is approximately 25%. Juvenile diabetes mellitus may be related to a gene closely linked to HLA-D which has a 50 per cent penetrance (*Rubinstein etl al.*, 1977).

TRANSIENT NEONATAL DIABETES MELLITUS

This rare condition is characterized by polyuria, polydypsia and dehydration. There is hyperglycemia, glucosuria and low birth weight. The disorder is transient and disappears spontaneously.

EXOMPHALOS-MACROGLOSSIA-GIGANTISM SYNDROME
(EMG syndrome, Beckwith-Wiedemann syndrome)

Common features: birth weight over 4000 g in most cases, macroglossia is present in about 75% of cases, omphalocele is frequent. Hypoglycaemia in the newborn period is marked, and is resistent to insulin, but does respond to hydrocortison. Hypoglycaemia is a frequent cause of death. Serum insulin is increased, sometimes polycythemia is present. At autopsy, visceromegaly hyperplasia of the pancreatic islets, adrenocortical cytomegaly, hyperplasia of the testicular Leydig cells in males and ovarian thecal cells in females and dysplasia of the renal medulla are found. Nephroblastomas were reported in several cases.

The syndrome is rare, the pathogenesis is unknown.

PANCREATIC AGENESIS

Pancreatic agenesis is a very rare condition, characterized by a severe growth retardation (1200—1500 g full-term), poor adipose tissue and muscle development. No insulin is present. The cases, including two born in the same family from a consanguinous parents were reported by *Dourow and Buyl-Strouvens* (1969) and by *Sherwood, Chance and Hill* (1974).

NEONATAL HYPOGLYCAEMIA, HYPERINSULINISM AND ABSENCE OF PANCREATIC ALPHA-CELLS

was described by *Gotlin and Silver* (1970) and by *McQuarrie et al.* (1950).

CHAPTER 11

AMNIONIC FLUID AS A HORMONAL COMPARTMENT

Amnionic fluid fills the amnionic sac. In early embryonal life, during the first five weeks, amnionic fluid represents a transudate of maternal plasma. As the fetal circulation and the chorion develop, the amnionic liquor becomes a transudate of

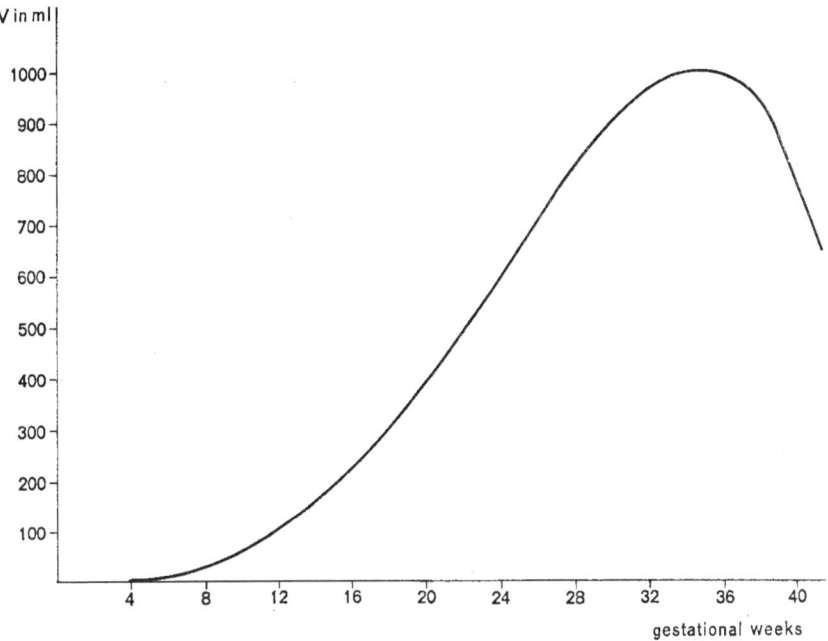

Graph 25. Volume of amnionic fluid in normal pregnancies.

the fetal bloods (weeks 6—12). Later on, the surface ectoderm of the embryo differentiate into the epidermis, becoming impermeable, and the fetus swallows amnionic fluid and contributes urine. As the fetal kidneys ripen, the urine becomes more and more hypotonic. The swallowing of the liquor in the third trimester is considered to be ca. 500 ml daily (*Abramovich*, 1970). The volume of the amnionic fluid increase is estimated at 25 ml from week 11 to 15, and 50 ml from week 15 to 28. At the end of the fourth month, the volume is estimated at 150—250 ml; at 20 weeks, approximately 400 ml; at 24 weeks approximately 500 ml; at 30 weeks approximately 900 ml and at 35 weeks 1000 ml (graph 25). At the end of week 40 (the end of gestation), the average amount is about 650 ml. The osmolarity of the amnionic fluid decreases with increasing age and with increasing contribution by the fetal urine, dropping from $275-280$ mOs at gestational weeks $4-12$ to approximately 270 at week 20, 265 at week 30, 255 at week 35 and 250 at week 40. Osmotic damage of the amnionic epithelium is considered as one of the principal fetal factors timing the delivery (*Jirásek*, 1977).

The increased amount of amnionic fluid is known as the polyhydramnion, the decreased amount as the oligohydramnion. Oligohydramnion is found in fetal renal agenesis (Potter's syndrome), after fetal intrauterine death if the delivery does not follow for three or more days, in toxemic pregnancies and in prolonged pregnancies (more than 41 weeks of gestation). Polyhydramnion is associated usually with the fetal inability to swallow, or absorb the amnionic fluid. This occurs in alimentary tract obstructions such as: esophageal atresia, duodenal atresia, gut atresia, or in severe disturbances of the central nervous system — in some anencephalics and hydrocephalics. Fetal cells are released (desquamated) into the amnionic fluid from the amnion, skin, buccal and vaginal mucosa and from the urinary tract. The cells are used for the cytological, cytochemical and cytogenetical diagnostics of genetic disorders. The checkup of the chemical composition of the amnionic fluid permits evaluation of the severity of fetal hemolytic anemia (bilirubin in Rh isoimmunization), or evaluation of the fetal lung maturity related to the danger of the respiratory distress syndrome (lecithin-sphingomyelin ratio), or diagnosis of various metabolic disorders.

HORMONES

The hormones in the amnionic fluid reflect some basic parameters of the fetal metabolism. They permit an early diagnosis of the fetal sex and hypothyroidism. Prenatal diagnosis of the adrenogenital syndrome and anencephaly is also possible by hormonal checkups.

ESTROGENS

More than 90 percent of the amnionic estrogens are represented by conjugated estriol (*Troen et al.*, 1961), the remaining by conjugated and free estrone and estradiol 17β. The free hormones are probably passed from the placenta, the conjugated hormones from the fetus. In the amnionic fluid, 80 percent of the estriol is present as estriol glucosiduronate, and an additional 15 percent, approximately, as estriol sulphate. The free estriol and the estriol sulphate are rapidly exchanged between the maternal and fetal blood compartments. Estriol glucosiduronate accumulates within the amnionic fluid and passes into the maternal compartment very slowly. Amnionic estriol does correlate with maternal urinary estriol excretion (*Berman et al.*, 1968; *Klopper and Biggs*, 1970), however, the range of values is wide and a single determination is of limited value. Amnionic estrone and estradiol do not change too much from 12 weeks to term. Estrone concentration is $2.5-4.4$ ng/ml. Estradiol concentrations decline slightly from $9-20$ weeks and rise to term. The levels are about 5.6 ng/ml at week 10, 3.2 ng/ml at week 20 and $11.5-17.2$ at term (*Warne et al.*, 1978). There are, however, broad variations (see graph 26). Amnionic estriol concentration is about $4.6-14.6$ ng/ml between weeks $12-20$, rising to $200-500$ ng/ml at term (see graph 27). Low amnionic estriol levels are found in patients with hydramnions. In pregnancies with anencephalics, the levels reported were $22-440$ ng/ml (*Schindler*,

1972). Low levels were also found in pregnancies with hypothyroid babies and Down's syndrome babies (*Huhtaniemi and Vikho*, 1971). There are no sex differences. Amnionic estetrol levels follow basically the levels of estriol (*Sciarra et al.*, 1974).

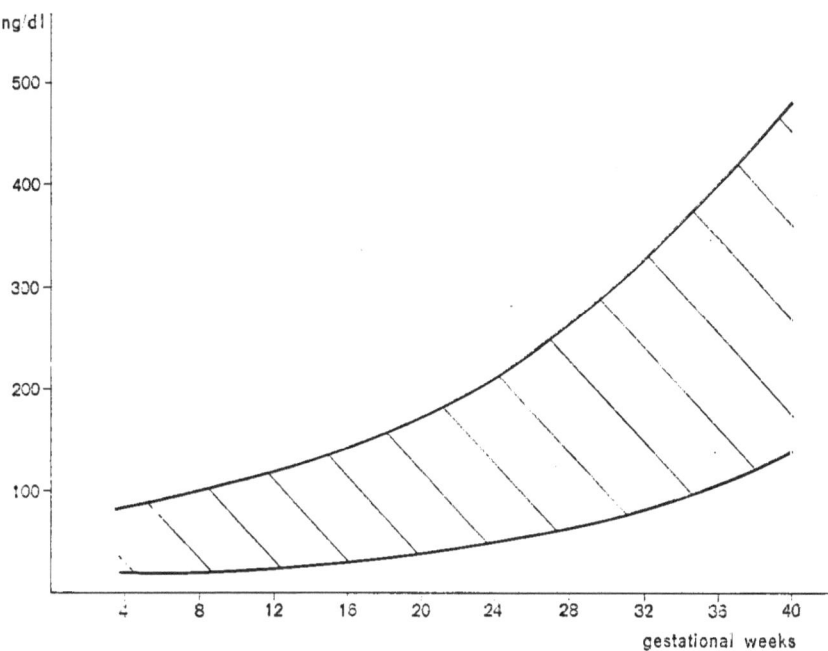

Graph 26. Free amnionic E_2 levels (no sexual differences).

PROGESTERONE

Amnionic fluid progesterone is derived from the fetal circulation. Its amnionic level falls as the conversion of progesterone to corticoids in the fetal adrenal increases. The mean level of progesterone at 14 weeks is 55 ng/ml and at term, 26 ng/ml (*Johansson and Johansson*, 1971). A sharp decrease occurs shortly before delivery.

PREGNANEDIOL

Pregnanediol, a metabolite of progesterone which is present in conjugated form as a glucosiduronate, is derived mostly from fetal urine. Its amnionic level is 1.5 to 5 ng/ml at term. About 12 ng/ml of amnionic fluid pregnanediol is in the sulphate form (*Schindler*, 1972).

DEHYDROEPIANDROSTERONE (DHA) AND 16-HYDROXY-DHA

Although the concentration of DHA and 16-OH-DHA within the fetal blood is approximately equal, the concentration of 16-OH-DHA in the amnionic fluid is 100 times higher than that of DHA (*Schindler and Siiteri*, 1968). The amnionic level of DHA at week 15 varies between 0.5—10 ng/ml and does not change until term (see graph 28). The amnionic level of 16-OH-DHA is about 800 ng/ml. 16-OH-DHAS amnionic concentration is low, DHAS almost zero (*Warne et al.*, 1978).

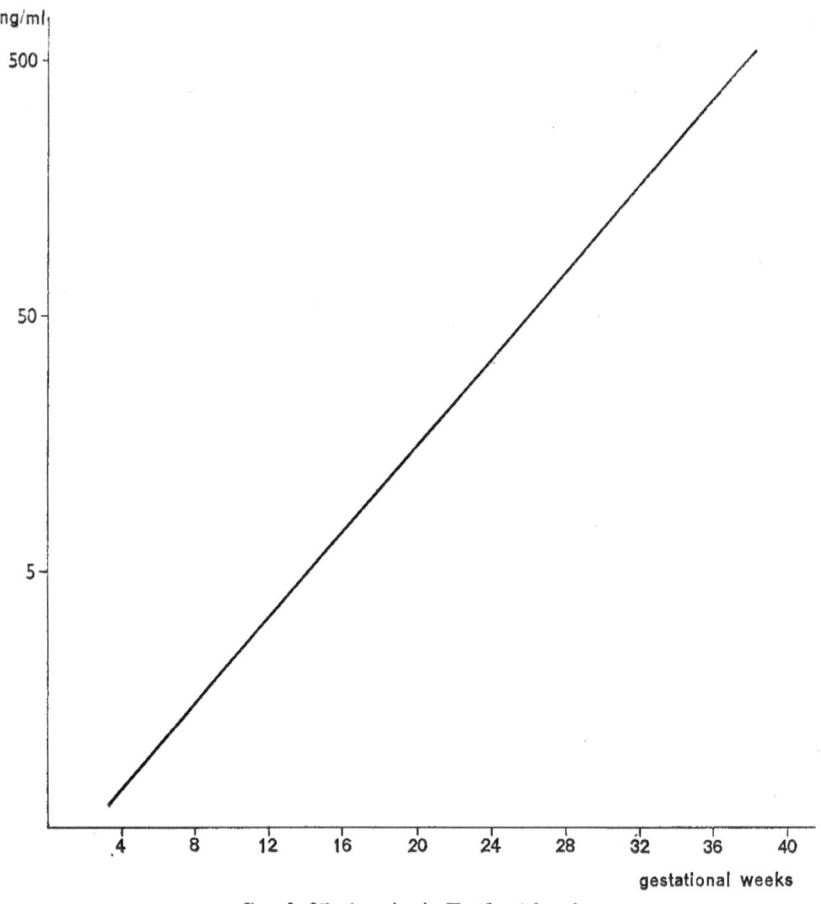

Graph 27. Amnionic E_3 (free) level.

TESTOSTERONE AND DIHYDROTESTOSTERONE

Testosterone in the amnionic fluid reflects its fetal production and between weeks 11—22 of gestation permits fetal sex determination with a reliable accuracy in most cases (*Giles et al.*, 1974) (See graph 29). In midgestation, amnionic fluid testosterone levels are 165.2 ± 15.4 pg/ml in pregnancies with a male fetus and 27.6 ± 2.6 pg/ml in pregnancies with a female fetus. In late pregnancy, there is a considerable overlap between fetuses of both sexes (*Judit et al.*, 1976; *Warne et al.*, 1977; *Dawood and Saxena*, 1977). Practically, if the amnionic fluid testosterone between weeks 11—22 is more than 80 pg/ml, there is more than a 95% chance that the fetus will be male. If the amnionic testosterone level at the same period, between weeks 11—22, is less than 50 pg/ml, the fetus will be female. There is some overlap in levels ranging from 50 to 80 pg/ml. The sex determination may be strengthened by a check of

194

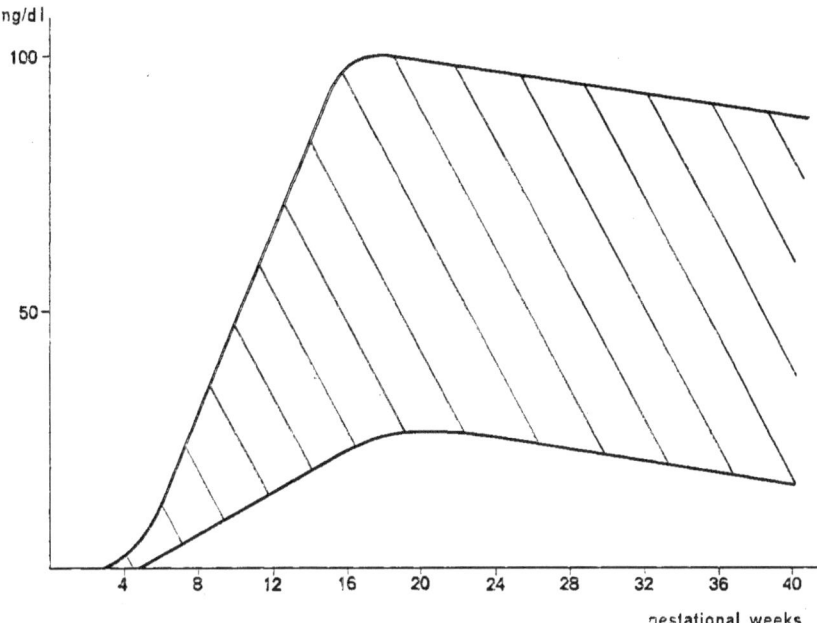

Graph 28. Free amnionic DHA levels (broad variation, no sexual differencies).

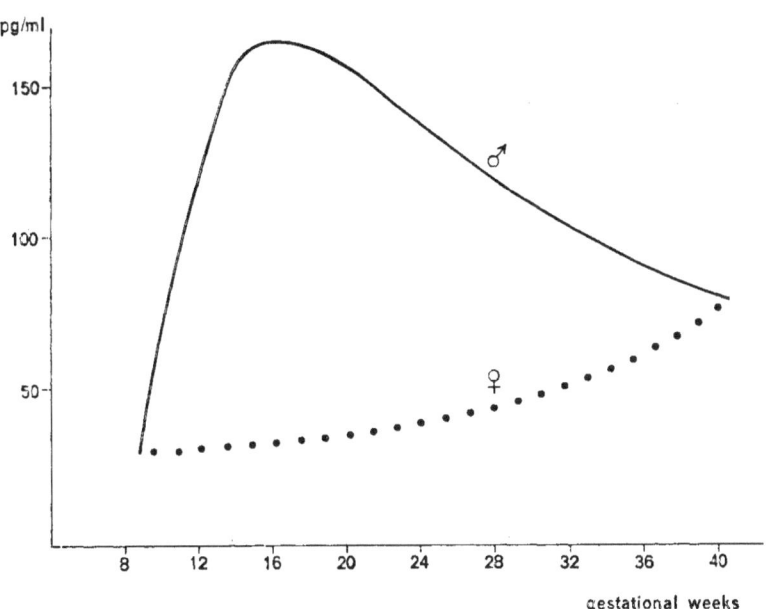

Graph 29. Amnionic testosterone levels.
Males full line, females dotted line

14

amnionic FSH. Amnionic dihydrotestosterone levels are low, mostly not detectable.

PREGNANETRIOL

In congenital adrenal hyperplasia with 21-steroid hydroxylase deficiency, amnionic pregnanetriol and 17-ketosteroids are increased (*Jeffcoate et al.*, 1966; *Nichols*, 1970). Normal levels of 17-ketosteroids are 25—40 μg/l at term, and that of pregnanetriol, 23—46 μg/l (*Abramovich and Wade*, 1969). In adrenal 21-steroid hydroxylase deficiency, the levels of 17-ketosteroids were approximately 100 μg/l, and pregnanetriol levels from 91—106 μg/l were found.

CORTISOL

There is a significant correlation between amnionic fluid cortisol and umbilical plasma cortisol (*Murphy et al.*, 1975). The cortisol level rises from 5 ng/ml at 10—15 weeks to about 10 ng/ml from 25—35 weeks. A sharp rise was observed in the last two weeks

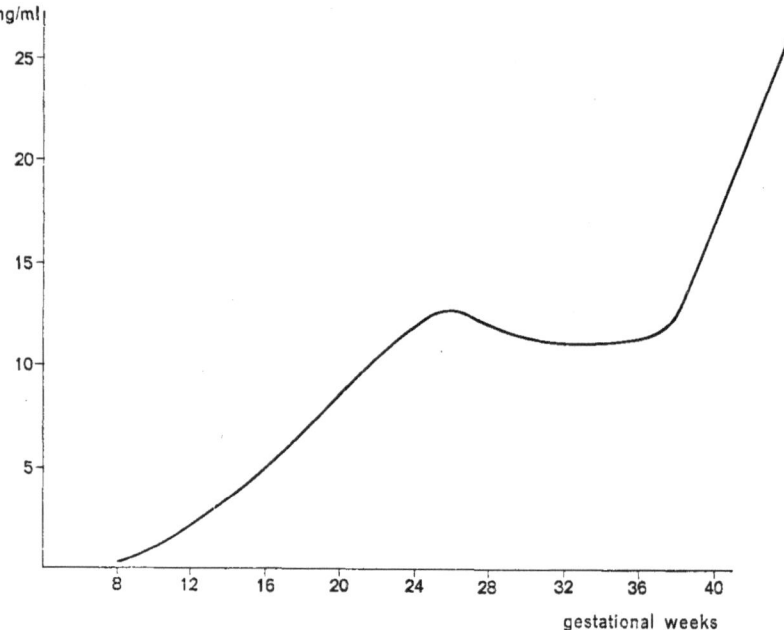

Graph 30. Amnionic cortisol levels.

preceding labor when the cortisol levels reach more than 30 ng/ml (see graph 30). In pregnancies with anencephalics, cortisol levels were low, about 12 ng/ml at term, however, even lower levels were observed in "postmature" infants and some infants of diabetics (*Brazy et al.*, 1978).

hCG

The concentration of hCG in fetal plasma is much lower than that in amnionic fluid, however, amnionic fluid hCG concentration is lower than that in maternal serum.

196

There is an increase from the seventh week of gestation, reaching peak values around the thirteenth gestational week. Thereafter, there is a marked decrease and during the second half of pregnancy, the levels 0.12—1.2 I.U. per ml are found. In the old measurements, the interference of hypophyseal LH did not allow for distinguishing

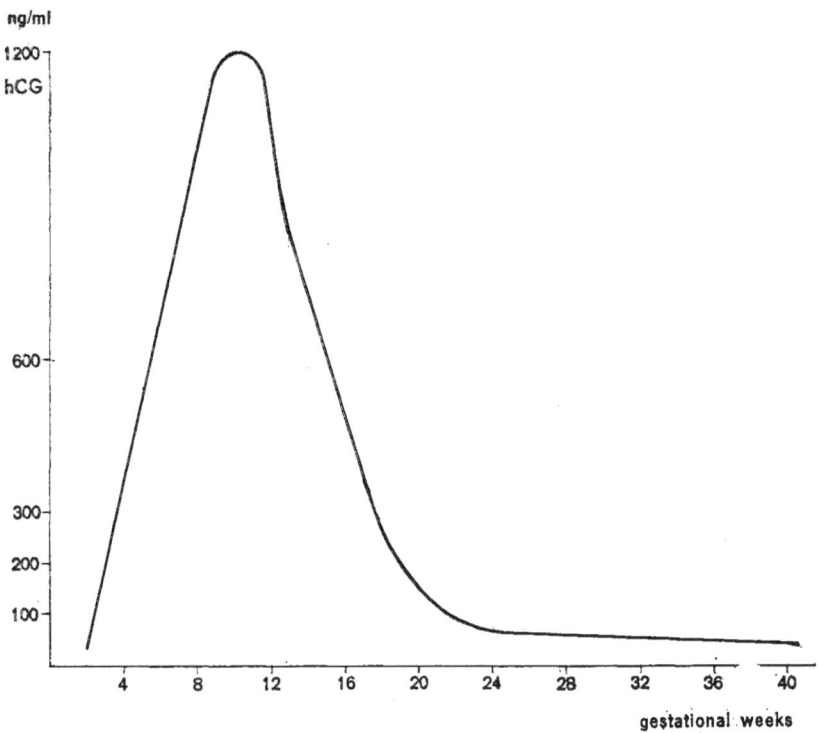

Graph 31. Amnionic hCG levels.

between the two hormones. hCG amnionic levels at 12 weeks are 933—1139 ng/ml, at 12—20 weeks, 589—783 ng/ml and at 32—40 weeks, 42—57 ng/ml (*Clements, Reyes, Winter and Faiman,* 1976) (graph 31).

hCS (CHORIONIC SOMATOMAMMOTROPIN)

The amnionic hCS concentration rises from approximately 0.4 µg/ml at twelve weeks to approximately 70 µg/ml at 32—35 weeks and then decreases to approximately 0.45 µg/ml found at term. The increasing metabolism of amnionic fluid hCS could account for the falling amnionic hCS at the end of pregnancy.

FSH

Amnionic FSH levels are similar to fetal serum levels. In female fetuses, the levels between weeks 12—20 are significantly higher than in males. Maximal levels are present around week 16. Practically, if the FSH level in the amnionic fluid from 12—20 weeks pregnancy exceeds 0.4 ng/ml, there is a good probability that the fetus

14*

will be female. If the levels are lower, the prognosis is uncertain. At birth, the FSH levels are low (*Clements et al.*, 1976). At 12—20 weeks, the levels in females are 0.6±0.1 ng/ml and in males, 0.1±0.02 ng/ml. At term, the levels are 0.1 ng/ml to 0.4 ng/ml overlapping in both sexes (see graph 32).

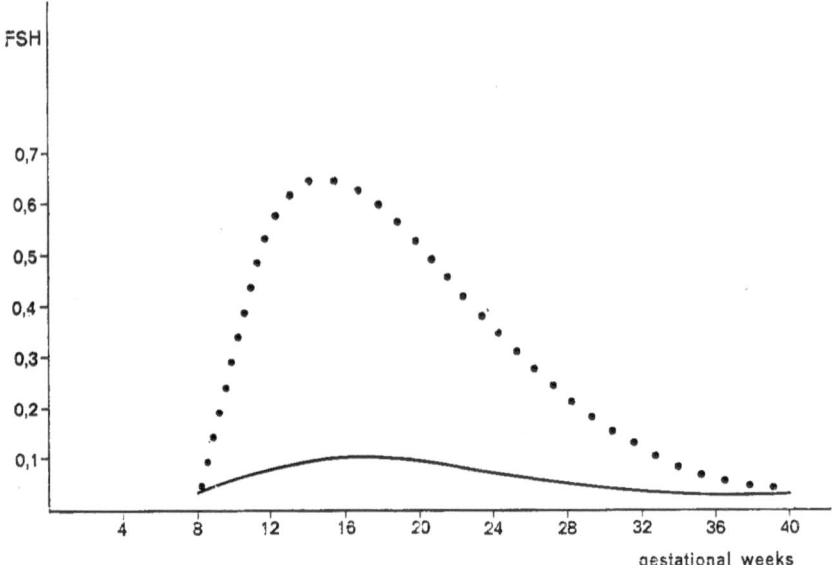

Graph 32. Amnionic FSH levels in males and females. Males full line, females, dotted line. FSH in ng/ml.

LH

Marked sexual differences exist in LH amnionic levels between weeks 12 to 20. In female fetuses, the amnionic LH levels in midpregnancy (week 12—20) are 10.8±1.1 ng/ml, whereas in male fetuses, the levels are much lower, 3.5±0.5 ng/ml. At term, however, there are no differences between males and females. In males, the levels are 0.6±0.8 ng/ml and in females 0.4±0.4 ng/ml (see graph 33). Amnionic LH may be used between weeks 12—20 to diagnose the sex of the fetus (*Clements et al.*, 1976).

TSH

Amnionic TSH level determination might be helpful for the diagnosis of fetal thyroid disorders. Maximal levels are reached at 22 weeks, declining slightly thereafter.

PROLACTIN

Amnionic prolactin levels increase between 12—16 weeks of gestation and then decline until term. At 16—17 weeks, the levels range from approximately 500 to 9000 ng/ml. At term the levels are 100—500 ng/ml (*Ben David et al.*, 1973; *Clements, Reyes, Winter and Faiman*, 1977).

Amnionic fluid PRL concentration consistently exceedes fetal serum levels. No sexual differences were noticed. Prolactin is not consistently detectable in the fetal pituitary until approximately 15 weeks of gestation. The amnionic pattern of prolactin concentration differs from the pattern seen in either the fetal or maternal serum in

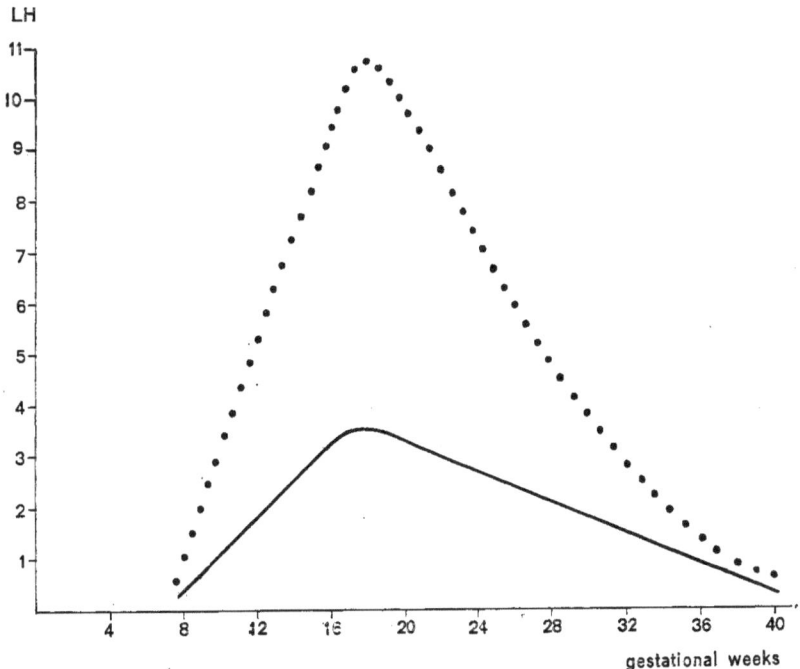

Graph 33. Amnionic LH levels in males and females. Males full line, females dotted line. LH in ng/ml.

which concentrations rise gradually throughout gestation. The amnionic PRL level seems to be correlated with the cytotrophoblastic development of the fetal membranes and with the development of decidua. The role of prolactin in lung maturation was stressed (*Hauth et al.*, 1978).

ACTH

ACTH levels in the amnionic fluid increase until approximately 20 weeks, decreasing thereafter. If very low levels of ACTH (ca. 20 pg/ml) are present, anencephaly is the most common reason. High levels of ACTH may be helpful in the diagnosis of congenital adrenaly hyperplasia. Normal ACTH amnionic levels are related to fetal serum levels. They are higher in mid-pregnancy (ca. 230 ng/ml at week 20) than at term (ca. 200 ng/ml).

hGH

Amnionic growth hormone concentration rises from 10 ng/ml at 20 weeks to 30 ng/ml at term and reflects the production of hGH by fetal hypophysis. hGH determination might be valuable in fetuses where pituitary developmental disorders are suspected. (*Spellacy et al.*, 1973.)

199

OXYTOCIN

Amnionic oxytocin in late pregnancy varies from 150−800 pg/ml (*Seppala et al.,* 1972). The highest values were found in amnionic fluids most heavily contaminated with meconium.

EPINEPHRINE AND NOREPINEPHRINE

Amnionic epinephrine and norepinephrine concentrations were reported by *Zuspan et al.* (1970, 1973). In late pregnancy, the values were 0.51−7.13 ng/ml for norepinephrine and 1.36−15.13 ng/ml for epinephrine.

INSULIN

Amnionic insulin levels increase as pregnancy advances. There is, however, a wide scattering of values from 2 μ units/ml to 25 μ units/ml. The increase is positively related to the weight of the fetus (*Spellacy et al.*, 1973).

Survey of amnionic, fetal serum and maternal serum levels of some placental, hypophyseal and steroid hormones is presented in Table 27.

Table 27. Levels of some placental and hypophyseal hormones and steroids in amnionic fluid and fetal and maternal serum.

Hormone	Fetal Levels (per ml)				Maternal Serum At term	Remarks
	Amnionic		Serum			
	Maxim. (week G)	term	Maxim. (week G)	term		
hCG	930 – 1140 ng (10)	40 – 60 ng	213 – 282 ng (10)	ca 70 ng	1000 – 1250 ng	decrease after delivery
hCS	70 μg (32 – 35)	0.45 μg l	–	0.02 μg	5 – 10 μg	decrease before delivery
PRL	500 – 3000 ng l (16)	100 – 500 ng	25 ng (12 – 14)	260 – 300 ng	140 ng	serum PRL peaks at end of 1st trimester. 2nd increase before birth.
GH	steady increase	30 ng	130 ng (22)	35 ng	5.0 ng	
ACTH	ca 230 ng (20)	200 ng	200 – 250 pg (25)	135 – 145 pg	170 – 220 pg	increase at the end of pregnancy
TSH	(22)		ca 10 μU (20 – 30)	8.5 μU	0 – 8 μU	
FSH m.	0.1 ng (12 – 20)	0 – 0.4 ng (12 – 20)	0.3ng (12 – 20)	0 – 0.6 ng	undetect.	marked sexual difference in 2nd trimester
f.	0.5 – 0.7 ng (12 – 20)	0 – 0.4ng (12 – 20)	4.0 – 6.5 ng (12 – 20)	0 – 0.6 ng	undetect.	
LH m.	3 – 4 ng (12 – 20)	0 – 1.5 ng	–	0 – 0.5 ng	undetect.	
f.	9.5 – 12 ng (12 – 20)	0 – 1.0 ng	–	0 – 0.5 ng	undetect.	
P	55 ng (14)	26 ng	300 ng	100 – 250 ng	145 – 165ng(35) 100 – 115ng(40)	falls during last. gest. month
E₁	increasing	2.5 – 4.5 ng	increasing	2 – 10	8 – 20 ng	
E₂	increasing	11.5 – 17.5 ng	increasing	4 – 6 ng	13 – 29 ng	increasing until birth
E₃	increasing	200 – 500mg	increasing	20 – 100mg	15 – 30 ng	
TEST. m·	160 – 250 pg (12 – 16)	30 – 70pg	300 – 350 pg (12 – 16)	50 – 80 pg	–	amnionic levels more than 80 pg/ml between weeks 11 –22 suggest a male fetus less than 50 pg a female fetus
f.	30 – 40 pg (12 – 16)	30 – 70 pg	ca 50 pg (12 – 16)	50 – 80 pg	–	
Cortisol	10 ng (25 – 35)	ca30 ng	increasing	30 – 40 ng	100 – 500 ng	sharp rise before birth

LIST OF ABBREVIATIONS

ACTH	corticotropin
ADP	adenosine diphosphate
AMP	adenosine monophosphate
ATP	adenosine triphosphate
ATPase	adenosine triphosphatase
AVP	arginine vasopressin
AVT	arginine vasotocine
C	conceptional age
cAMP	cyclic adenosine monophosphate
C-cell	calcitonin producing cell
CK-PZ	cholecystokinin-pancreozymin
CNS	central nervous system
CBG	corticosteroid-binding globulin
CRF	corticotropin releasing factor
DHA	dehydroepiandrosterone
DHAS	dehydroepiandrosteronesulphate
DIT	diiodothyrosine
DNA	deoxyribonucleic acid
DOPA	dihydroxyphenylalanine
E_1	estrone
E_2	estradiol
E_3	estriol
EEG	electroencephalography
FSH	follicle-stimulating hormone
FT_3	free triiodothyronine
GH	growth hormone (somatotropine)
G	gestational age
G-6-PD	glucose-6-phosphate dehydrogenase
hCG	human chorionic gonadotropin
hCS	human chorionic somatomammotropin (hPL-placental lactogen)
hCT	human chorionic thyrotropin
hMG	human menopausal gonadotropin
hPL	placental lactogen (hCS)
HSD (3) (17)	hydroxysteroid dehydrogenase
IgG	immunoglobulin G
LATS	long acting thyroid stimulating globulins
LDH	lactic dehydrogenase
LH	luteinizing hormone
LH RH	gonadotropin releasing hormone (factor)
MIT	monoiodotyronine
mRNA	messenger RNA
MSH	melanotropin
NAD	nicotinamide adenine dinucleotide
NADH	dihydronicotinamide adenine dinucleotide
NADP	nicotinamide adenine dinucleotide phosphate
NE	norepinephrine
OH-ase	hydroxylase
OH-DHAS	(16) hydroxy-dehydroepiandrosterone sulphate

202

P	progesterone
P. A. S.	periodic acid Schiff
PRL	prolactin
PTH	parathormone
RNA	ribonucleic acid
rRNA	ribosomal RNA
SDase	steroid desmolase
S. H.	Streeter's Horizon
SRIF	somatotropine release inhibiting factor (somatostatin)
T_1	monoiodothyronine
T_2	diiodothyronine
T_3	triiodothyronine
T_4	tetraiodothyronine (thyroxine)
TBG	thyroxine-binding globulin
T-cell	thyroxine producing cell
TeBG	testosterone-binding globulin
TBPA	thyroxine-binding proalbumin
TRF (TRH)	thyrotropin releasing factor (hormone)
t-RNA	transfer RNA

REFERENCES

Abramovich D. R. (1970):
Fetal factors influencing the volume and composition of liquor amnii.
J. Obst. Gynaec. Brit. Cwlth. 77, 865
Abramovich D. R. and Wade A. P. (1969):
Levels and significance of 17-oxosteroids and 17-hydroxysteroid in amniotic fluid
throughout pregnancy.
J. Obst. Gynaec. Brit. Cwlth. 76, 893
Abuid J., Klein A. H., Foley Jr. T. P. and Larsen P. R. (1974):
Total and free triiodothyronine and thyroxine in early infancy.
J. clin. Endocrin. Metab. 39, 263
Acevedo H. F., Axelrod L. R., Ishikawa E. and Takashi F. (1963):
Studies in fetal metabolism. II. Metabolism of progesterone-4-C^{14} and preg-
nenolone-7α-H^3 in human fetal testes.
J. clin. Endocrin. Metab. 23, 885
Ahluvalia B., Williams J. and Verma P. (1974):
In vitro testosterone biosynthesis in the human fetal testis. II. Stimulation by
cyclic AMP and human chorionic gonadotropin (hCG).
Endocrinology 95, 1411
Akesson, H. O. (1965):
Cutis verticis gyrata, thyroaplasia and mental deficiency.
Acta Genet. Med. Gem. 14, 200
Allen J. P., Greer M. E., McGilora R., Castro A. and Fisher D. A. (1974):
Endocrine function in an anencephalic infant.
J. clin. Endocrin. Metab. 38, 94
Alexandr N. M. and Burrow G. N. (1970):
Thyroxine biosynthesis in human goitrous cretenism.
J. clin. Endocrin. Metab. 30, 308
Alvarez H. and Caldeyro-Barcia R. (1950):
Contractility of the human uterus recorded by new methods.
Surg. Gynec. Obstet. 91, 1
Amoroso E. C. (1952):
Placentation.
in: Marshall's Physiology of Reproduction Vol. II, Chap. 15.
Parkes A. S. (ed.) London Longmans
Andersen H. J. (1969):
in. Endocrine and genetic diseases of childhood.
Gardner L. I. (ed.) Philadelphia Saunders W. B.
Armheim J. A., Meyer J., Jones H. W. and Migeon C. J. (1976):
Androgen insensitivity in man. Evidence for genetic heterogenity.
Proc. Nat. Acad. Sci USA 73, 891
Aschheim S. and Zondek B.: (1027)
Ei und Hormon, Hypophysenvorderlappenhormon und Ovarialhormon
:in Harn von Schwangeren. Klin. Wschr. 6, 1321
Attwod, H. D. and Park, W. W.: (1961)
Embolism of the lung by trophoblast.
J. Obstet. Gynaec. Brit. Cwlth. 68, 611
Atwell, W. J.: (1926)
The development of the hypophysis cerebri in man, with special reference to the

pars tuberalis.

Aner. J. Anat. *37*, 159

Atz. J. W.: (1964)

in: Intersexualiaty in vertebrates including man, Armstrong C. N., Marshall A. J. (eds), London, New York, Academik press

Aubert M. L., Grumbach M. M. and Kaplan S. L. (1975):

The ontogenesis of human hormones.

J. clin. Invest. *56*, 155

Aubert M. L., Grumbach M. M. and Kaplan S. L. (1977):

The ontogenesis of human hormones. IV. Somatostatin, luteinizing hormone releasing factor and thyrotropin releasing factor in hypothalamus and cerebral cortex of human fetuses 10–22 weeks of age.

J. clin. Endocrin. Metab. *44*, 1130

Axelrod J. (1974):

Neurotransmitters.

Sci Am. *230*, 59

Bahl O. P., Carlsen R. B., Bellisario R. and Swaminathan N. (1972):

Human chorionic gonadotropin: amnioacid sequence of the α and β subunits.

Biochem. biophys. Res. Communications *48*, 416

Baker T. G. (1963):

A quantitative and cytological study of germ cells in human ovaries.

Proc. R. Soc. Lond. (Biol.) *158*, 417

Baker T. G. (1972):

Oogenesis and ovarian development.

in: Balin H.-Glasser S (eds) Reproductive Biology Amsterdam: Excerpta Medica vol. 7

Bala R. M., Ferugson K. A. and Beck J. C. (1970):

Plasma biological and immunoreactive human growth hormone-like activity.

Endocrinology *87*, 506

Balfour F. M. (1878):

On the struture and development of the vertebrate ovary.

Q. J. Microscop. Sci *18*, 383

Ball, P., Knuppen R., Hampt M. and Brener H.: (1972)

Interactions between estrogens and catecholamines.

J. clin. Endocrinol. Metab. *34*, 736

Baltzer F. (1937):

Entwicklungs-mechanische Untersuchungen an Bonelia viridis. III. Über die Entwicklung und Bestimmung des Geschlechts und die Anwendbarkeit des Gold-schmidtschen Zeitgesetzer der Intersexualität bei Bonelia viridis.

Publ. St. Zool. Napoli *16*, 89

Bartow P., Owen D. A. J. and Graham C. (1972):

DNA synthesis in preimplantation mouse embryo.

J. Embryol. exp. Morph. *27*, 431

Barry J. (1976):

Characterization and topography of LH-RH neurons in the human brain.

Neurosci Lett. 3, 287

Bartholomew R. A. (1938):

Pathology of placenta with special reference to infarcts and their relation to toxemia of pregnancy.

J. Amer. med. Ass. *111*, 2276

Beckett R. S. and Flynn F. J. (1953):
Toxoplasmosis. Report of two cases with a clasiffication and with a demonstration of the organism in the human placenta.
New Engl. J. Med. *249*, 345

Beckwith J. B. (1969):
Macroglossia, omphalocele, adrenal cytomegaly, gigantism and hyperplastic visceromegaly.
in: The Clinical Delination of Birth Defects II. Malformation Syndromes New York National Found.

Beierwaltes, W. H.: (1964)
Genetics of thyroid disease
in: The Thyroid. Hazard J. B. and Smith D. E. (eds)
Baltimore, Williams and Wilkins Co

Beischer N. A. and Brown J. B. (1972):
Current status of estrogen assay in obstetrics and gynecology.
Obstet. Gynecol. Survey *27*, 303

Beling C. G. (1967):
Estriol excretion in pregnancy and its application to clinical problems.
in: Marcus S. C. and Marcus C. C. (eds) Advances in Obstetrics and Gynecology.
Williams and Wilkins Comp. Baltimore

Ben-David M., Rodbard D., Bates R. W., Bridson W. E. and Grumbach A. (1973):-
Human prolactin in plasma, amnionic fluid and pituitary: identity and characterization by criteria of electrophoresis and isoelectric focusing in polyacryl-amid gel
J. clin. Endocrin. Metab. *36*, 451

Benirschke K. (1956):
Adrenals in anencephaly and hydrocephaly.
Obstet. Gynec. *8*, 412

Benirschke K. and McKay D. G. (1953):
The antidiuretic hormone in fetus and infant. Histochemical observations with special reference to amniotic fluid formation.
Obstet. Gynec. *1*, 638

Benoit J. (1923):
Transformation expérimentale du sexe par ovariotomie précoce chez la poule domestique.
Compt. rend. Acad. Sci Paris 177, 1074

Berman A. M., Kalchman C. G. and Chattoraj S. C. (1968):
Relationship of amniotic fluid estriol to maternal urinary estriol.
Amer. J. Obstet. Gynec. *100*, 15

Berthezene F. M., Gorest J., Grimaud J. A., Claustrat B. and Mornex R. (1976):
Leydig cell agenesis. A cause of male pseudohermaphroditism.
New Engl. J. Med. *295*, 969

Björkman N. and Bloom G. (1957):
On the fine structure of the foetal-maternal junction in the bovine placentome.
Z. Zellforsch. *45*, 649

Björö K. (1972):
Oestriol assay in obstetric practice.
Acta Endocrinol. *161*, 69 (suppl.)

Blacker A. W. (1958):
Contribution to the study of germ cells in Anura.
J. Embryol. Exp. Morph. *6*, 491

Blandau R. J. and Bergsma D. (eds.) (1977):
Morphogenesis and malformation of the genital system.
Birth Defects Orig. Art. Series Vol. XIII No 2 New York Liss A. R.

Blandau R. J., White B. J. and Rumery R. E. (1963):
Observations on the mouvements of the living primordial germ cells in the mouse.
Fertil. Steril. *14*, 482

Blecher S. J., O'Sullivan J. B. and Freinkel N. (1964):
Carbohydrate metabolism in pregnancy.
New Engl. J. Med. *271*, 866

Blizzard R. M., Chandler R. W., Landing B. H. et al. (1960):
Maternal autoimmunization to thyroid as a probable cause of athyroic cretenism.
New Engl. J. Med. *263*, 327

Bloch E. (1964):
Metabolism of-4-C^{14}-progesterone by human foetal testis and ovaries.
Endocrinology *74*, 833

Bloch E. and Benirschke K. (1959):
Synthesis in vitro of steroids by human fetal adrenal gland slices.
J. Biol. Chem. *234*, 1085

Boe F. (1953):
Studies on the vascularization of the human placenta.
Acta obstet. gynaec. Scand. 32, suppl. 5

Bongiovanni A. M. (1964):
The adrenogenital syndrome with deficiency of 3β-hydroxysteroid dehydrogenase.
J. clin. Invest. *41*, 2086

Bongiovanni A. M. (1972):
Disorders of adrenocortical steroid biogenesis.
in: The metabolic basis of inherited disease.
Stanbury, Wyngaarden, Frederickson (eds) McGraw-Hill. New York 3rd ed.

Borell U., Fernström I. and Westman A. (1958):
Arteriographic study of the placental circulation.
Geburtsch. u. Frauenheilk. *18*, 1

Boroditsky R. S., Reys F. I., Winter J. S. D. and Faiman C. (1975):
Serum chorionic gonadotropin and progesterone patterns in the last trimester of pregnancy: relationship to fetal sex.
Amer. J. Obstet. Gynec. *121*, 238

Bourne G. L. (1962):
The human amnion and chorion.
London, Lloyd-Luke

Boyd J. D. (1950):
Development of the thyroid and parathyroid glands and the thymus.
Ann. Roy Coll. Surg. Engl. *7*, 455

Brandau H. and Lahmann V. (1970):
Histoenzymatische Untersuchungen an menschlichen Gonaden während der intrauterinen Entwicklung.
Z. Geburtshilfe Gynaekol. *173*, 233

Braunstein G. D., Vaitukaitis J., Grodin J. M. and Ross G. T. (1973):
Secretory rates of human chorionic gonadotropin by normal trophoblast.
Amer. J. Obstet. Gynec. *115*, 447

Bridges C. B. (1939):
Cytological and genetic basis of sex.
in: "Sex and Internal Secretions" (Allen E. ed.) 2nd ed. London, Baillière
Breus C. (1892):
Das tuberöse subchoriale Hämatom der Decidua.
Wien, Deuticke
Brody S. and Calstrom G. (1965):
Human chorionic gonadotropin pattern in serum and its relation to the sex of the fetus.
J. clin. Endocrin. Metab. *25*, 792
Broman I. (1911):
Normale and abnorme Entwicklung des Menschen.
Wiesbaden, Bergmann
Brown G., Brown R. and Hey E. (1978):
Fetal hyperinsulinism in rhesus isoimmunization.
Amer. J. Obstet. Gynec. *131*, 682
Brown J. J., Davies D. L., Doak P. B. et al. (1964):
The presence of renin in human amniotic fluid.
Lancet *2*, 64
Brown J. C. and Veall N. (1953):
Maternal placental blood flow in normotensive and hypertensive women.
J. Obstet. Gynaec. Brit. Emp., *60*, 141
Buchs S. (1961):
Angeborener Hypoparathyroidismus von drei Brudern infolge Hyperparathyreoidismus der Mutter.
Schweiz. Med. Wschr. *91*, 660
Bulmer D. (1957):
The development of the human vagina.
J. Anat. *91*, 490
Burman K. D., Read J., Dimond R. C., Strum D., Wright F. D., Patow W., Earl J. M. and Wartofsky L. (1976):
Measurements of 3,3′5′-triiodothyronine (RT_3) 3,3′-L-diiodothyronine, T_3 and T_4 in human amniotic fluid and in cord and maternal serum.
J. clin. Endocrin. Metab. *43*, 1351
Burt R. L. and Davidson I. W. F. 1974):
Insulin half-life and utilization in normal pregnancy.
Obstet. Gynacol. *43*, 161
Byskov A. G. and Lintern-Moore S. (1973):
Follicle formation in the inmature mouse ovary: the role of the rete ovarii.
J. Anat. (Lond.) *116*, 217
Calderiro-Barcia R. and Posseiro J. J. (1960):
Physiology of uterine contractions.
Clin. Obstet. Gynec. 3, 386
Cardell B. S. (1953).
Hypertrophy and hyperplasia of the pancreatic islets in new-born infants.
J. Path. Bact. *66*, 335
Catt K. J., Dufau M. L. and Tsuruhara T. (1973):
Absence of intrinsic biological activity in LH and hCG subunits.
J. clin. Endocrin. Metab. *36*, 73
Cedard L., Tchobrousky C. and Guglielmina R. (1971):
Insuffisance oestrogenique paradoxale au cours d'une grossesse normale par défaut

de sulfatase placentaire.
Bull. Fed. Soc. Gynecol. Obstet. Lang. Fr. *23*, 16
Chaletzky E. (1891):
Hydatidenmole.
Thesis Univ. Bern
Channing C. P. (1970):
Influences of the in vivo and vitro hormonal environment upon luteinization of granulosa cells in tissue culture.
Recent Progr. Horm. Res. *26*, 589
Chopra I. J., Solomon D. H. and Chopra U. (1978):
Pathways of metabolism of thyroid hormones.
Rec. Progr. Horm. Res. *34*, 521
Chu L. L., MacGregor R. R., Anast C. S. et al. (1973):
Studies on the biosynthesis of rat parathyroid hormone and proparathyroid hormone: adaptation of the parathyroid gland to dietary restriction of calcium.
Endocrinology *93*, 915
Clements J. A., Reyes F. I., Winter J. S. D. and Faiman C. (1976):
Studies of human sexual development. III. Fetal pituitary and serum and amniotic fluid concentration of LH, hCG and FSH.
J. clin. Endocrin. Metab. *42*, 9
Clements J. A., Reyes F. I., Winter J. S. D. and Faiman C. (1977):
Studies on human sexual development. IV. Fetal pituitary and serum and amniotic fluid concentrations of prolactin.
J. clin. Endckrin. Metab. *44*, 408
Clements M. and Gorbman A. (1955):
Protease in amnocoetes endostyle.
Biol. Bull. *108*, 258
Cole H. S. (1975):
Problems in management of infants of diabetic mothers.
in: Camerini-Davalos R. A. and Cole H. S. (eds). Early Diabetes in Early Life. Academic Press New York
Cole R. J. (1967):
Cinematographic observation on the trophoblast and zona pellucida of the mouse blastocyst.
J. Embryol. exp. Morph. *17*, 481
Conklin J. L. (1968):
A histochemical study of mucoid cells in the pars distalis of the human hypophysis.
Anat. Rec. *160*, 59
Conklin J. L. (1968):
The development of the human fetal adenohypophysis.
Anat. Rec. *160*, 79
Coupland R. E. (1952):
The prenatal development of the abdominal para-aortic bodies in man.
J. Anat. (Lond.) *86*, 357
Coupland R. E. (1953):
On the morphology and adrenaline-noradrenaline content of chromaffin tissue.
J. Endocrin. *9*, 194
Covell W. P. (1927):
A quantitative study of the hypophysis of the human anencephalic fetus.
Amer. J. Anat. *38*, 379

Crowder R. E. (1957):
The development of the adrenal gland in man, with special reference to origin and ultimate location of cell types and evidence in favor of cell migration theory.
Contrib. Embryol. Carnegie Inst. *36*, 195

Crystle, C. D., Dubin U. H., Grannis C. F. et al. (1973):
Investigation of precursors availability in the regulation of estrogen synthesis in normal human pregnancy.
Obstet. Gynec. *42*, 718

Curry D. I., Benett L. L. and Grodsky G. M. (1968):
Requirement for calcium ion in insulin secretion by the perfused rat pancreas.
Amer. J. Physiol. *214*, 174

Dawood M. Y. and Saxena B. B. (1977):
Testosterone and dihydrotestosterone in maternal and cord blood and in amniotic fluid.
Amer. J. Obstet. Gynec. *129*, 37

Decosta E. J., Gerbie A. B., Andersen R. H. and Gallanis T. C. (1956):
Placental tumors: haemangiomas with special reference to an associated clinical syndrome.
Obstet. Gynec. *7*, 249

Denker H. W. (1972):
Furchung beim Säugetier: Differenzierung von Trophoblast — und Embryonal — knotenzellen.
Anat. Anz. *130*, 267

Deol M. S. (1973):
An experimental approach to the understanding and treatment of hereditary syndromes with congenital deafness and hypothyroidism.
J. Med. Genet. *10*, 235

Dey S. K. and Dickman Z. (1974):
Δ^5-3β-hydroxysteroid dehydrogenase activity in rat embryos on days 1 through 7 of pregnancy.
Endocrinology *95*, 321

Diczfalusy E. (1964):
Endocrine functions of the human fetoplacental unit.
Fed. Proceed. *23*, 791

Diczfalusy E. (1969):
Steroid metabolism in the foeto-placental unit.
in: The Foeto-placental Unit (Pecile A and Finzi C, eds), Amsterdam Excerpta Med. Found.

Diczfalusy E. (1974):
Endocrine function of the human fetus and placenta.
Amer. J. Obstet. Gynec. *119*, 420

Diczfalusy E. and Troen P. (1961):
Endocrine function of the human placenta.
Vitamins, Hormones *19*, 229

Di George A. M. (1968):
Congenital absence of the thymus and its immunologic consequences: concurrence with congenital hypoparathyroidism.
in: Immunologic Deficiency Disseases, Good R. A. (ed.) New York National Found.

Dobzhansky T. and Schultz J. (1934):
The distribution of sex factors in the X-chromosome of Drosophila melanogaster.
J. Genet. *28*, 249

Dorman G. H. and Sahyun P. F. (1937):
Identification and significance of spirochetes in the placenta.
Amer. J. Obstet. Gynec. *33*, 954

Dourow N. and Buyl-Strouvens M. L. (1969):
Agenesie du pancreas.
Arch. Franc. Pediatr. *26*, 641

Driscoll S. G. (1963):
Choriocarcinoma: An "incidental finding" within a term placenta.
Obstet. Gynec. *21*, 96

Drouin J. and Labrie F. (1976):
Selective effect of androgens on LH and FSH release in anterior pituitary cells
in culture.
Endocrinology *98*, 1528

Dubois M. P. (1975):
Immunoreactive somatostatin is present in discrete cells of the endocrine pancreas.
Proc. Nat. Acad. Sci USA *72*, 1340

Dufau M. L. and Villee D. B. (1969):
Aldosterone biosynthesis by the human fetal adrenal in vitro.
Biochim. Biophys. Acta *176*, 637

Duggan G. G., Dale N. E., Lyneham R. C. et al. (1974):
Calcium balance in pregnancy.
Lancet II, 926

Dungal N. (1961):
Listeriosis in four siblings.
Lancet II, 513

Dussault J. H., Hobel C. J., Distefano J. J. et al. (1972):
Triiodothyronine turnover in maternal and fetal sheep.
Endocrinology *90*, 1301

Dussault J. H., Letarte J., Guyda H. and Laberge C. (1976):
Thyroid function in neonatal hypothyroidism.
J. Pediatr. *89*, 541

Dyke van J. H. (1959):
in: Comparative Endocrinology, Gorbman A. (ed) New York, Willey

Dyková H., Jirásek J. E., Zwinger A. and Krabec Z. (1975):
The prognostic value of chorionic gonadotropin in the urine of miscarrying
women.
Čs. gynek. *40*, 417

Eberlein W. R. (1965):
Steroids and sterols in umbilical cord blood.
J. clin. Endocrin. Metab. *25*, 1101

Edwards R. G. (1973):
Studies on human conception.
Amer. J. Obstet. Gynec. *117*, 587

Enders A. C. (1965):
Formation of syncytium from cytotrophoblast in the human placenta.
Obstet. Gynec. *25*, 378

Epple A. and Lewis T. L. (1973):
Comparative histophysiology of the pancreatic islets.
Amer. Zool. *13*, 567
Epstein C. J. (1975):
Gene expression and macromolecular synthesis during preimplantation embryonic development.
Biol. Repord. *12*, 82
Euler von V. S. and Hillarp N. A. (1956):
Evidence for the presence of noradrenaline in submicroscopic structures of adrenergic axons.
Nature (Lond.) *177*, 44

Falin L. I. (1961):
The development of human hypophysis and differentiation of cells of its anterior lobe during embryonic life.
Acta Anat. *44*, 188
Falkmer S. and Östberg Y. (1976):
Production of islet hormones in invertebrates, Cyclostomes and primitive Gnathostomes.
in: The Evolution of Pancreatic Islets, Grillo T. A., Leibson L. and Epple A. (eds.).
Oxford, New York, Toronto, Sydney, Paris, Frankfurt, Pergamon Press
Feldman G. V. (1963):
Congenital toxoplasmosis.
New Engl. J. Med. *269*, 1212
Felig P. J., Wahren J., Sherroin R. and Hendler R. (1976):
Insulin, glucagon and somatostatin in normal physiology and diabetes mellitus.
Diabetes *25*, 1091
Felix W. (1912):
The development of the urogenital organs.
in: Manual of Human Embryology (Keibel A. and Mall F. P. eds.). Vol. 2
Ferguson- Smith M. A. (1966):
X-Y chromosomal interchange in the aetiology of true hermaphroditism and of XX. Klinefelter's syndrome.
Lancet *2*, 475
Ferner H. and Stockenius W. Jr. (1951):
Die Cytogenese des Inselsystems beim Menschen. Z. Zellforschr. *35*, 147
Fischel A. (1930):
Über die Entwicklung der Keimdrüsen des Menschen.
Z. Anat. *92*, 34
Fishelson L. (1970):
Protogynous sex reversal in the fish Anthias squamipinnis (Teleostei, Anthiidae) regulated by the presence or absence of a male fish.
Nature (Lond.) *227*, 90
Fisher D. A., Hobel C. J., Garza R. and Pierce C. A. (1970):
Thyroid function in the preterm fetus.
Pediatrics *46*, 208
Fisher D. A., Pyle H. R., Porter J. C. et al. (1963):
Control of water balance in the newborn.
Amer. J. Obstet. Gynec. *106*, 137
Fisher D. A., Dussault J. H., Hobel C. J. and Lam R. (1973):
Serum and thyroid gland triiodothyronine in the human fetus.
J. clin. Endocrin. Metab. *36*, 397

Fisher D. A., Dussault J. H., Sack J. and Chopra I. J. (1977):
Ontogenesis of hypothalamic-pituitary-thyroid function and metabolism in man, sheep and rat.
Rec. Progr. Horm. Res. *33*, 59

Fisher D. A. and Odell W. D. (1969):
Acute release of thyrotropin in the newborn.
J. Clin. Invest. *48*, 1670

Florian J. (1931):
Urkeimzellen bei einen 625 u langen menschlichen Embryo.
Verh. Anat. Ges. Breslau, Anat. Anz. 72. Erganzungsheft 286

Florian J. (1936):
Od prvoka k člověku (From a protozoon to man).
Melantrich, Praha

Forsyth C. O., Forbes M. and Cumings J. N. (1971):
Adrenocortical atrophy and diffuse cerebral sclerosis.
Arch. Dis. Child *46*, 273

Fox H. and Path M. C. (1968):
Morphological changes in the human placenta following fetal death.
J. Obstet. Gynec. Brit. Cwlth. *75*, 839

France J. T., Seddon R. J. and Liggins G. C. (1973):
A study of a pregnancy with low estrogen production due to placental sulphatase deficiency.
J. clin. Endocrin. Metab. *36*, 1

Franchimont P., Gaspard V., Reutes A. and Heynen G. (1972):
Polymorphism of protein and polypeptide hormones.
Clin. Endocrin. (Oxford) *1*, 315

Franchimont P. and Pasteels J. L. (1972):
Sécrétion indépendante des hormones gonadotropes et de leurs sous-unités.
C. R. Hebd. Seances Acad. Sci *275*, 1799

Franken H. (1954):
Beitrag zur Veranschaulichung von Struktur und Funktion der menschlichen Plazenta.
Zbl. Gynäk. *76*, 729

Fraser G. R. (1965):
Association of congenital deafness with goitre (Pendred's syndrome). A study of 207 families.
Ann. Hum. Genet. *28*, 201

Friesen H. (1965):
Purification of a placental factor with immunological and chemical similarity to human growth hormone.
Endocrinology *76*, 369

Friesen H. G., Fournier P. and Desjardins P. (1973):
Pituitary prolactin in pregnancy and normal and abnormal lactation.
Clin. Obstet. Gynecol. *16*, 25

Frohman L. A., Burek L. and Stachura M. E. (1972):
Characterization of growth hormone of different molecular weights in rat, dog and human pituitaries.
Endocrinology *91*, 262

Frohman L. A. and Stachura M. E. (1973):
Evidence for possible precursors in the synthesis of growth hormone by rat and

human fetal anterior pituitary in vitro.
Mt. Sinai J. Med. NY *40*, 414

Fukuchi M., Inone T., Abe H. and Kumahara Y. (1970):
Thyrotropin in human fetal pituitaries.
J. clin. Endocrin. Metab. *31*, 565

Furth E. D., Calvallio M. and Vianna B. (1967):
Familial goiter due to an organification defect in euthyroid siblings.
J. clin. Endocrin. Metab. *27*, 1137

Garel J. M., Milhand G. and Sizonenko P. C. (1965):
Thyrocalcitonine et barière placentaire chez le rat.
C. R. Acad. Sci. (Paris) *269*, 1785

George F. W. and Wilson J. D. (1978):
Conversion of androgen to estrogen by the human fetal ovary.
J. clin. Endocrin. Metab. *47*, 550

Gerloczy F. and Farkas K. (1953):
Giperparatireoidizm u novoroždennogo ot materi stradajuščej chroničeskim gipo-
paratireoidizmom.
Acta med. Acad. Sci hung. *4*, 73

German J., Simpson J. L. and Chaganti R. S. K. (1978):
Genetically determined sex-reversal in 46,XY humans.
Science *202*, 53

Genazzani A. R., Fraioli F., Hurlimann J., Fioretti P. and Felber J. P. (1975):
Immunoreactive ACTH and cortisol plasma levels during pregnancy. Detection
and partial purification of corticotropin-like placental hormone: the human
chorionic corticotropin (hCC).
Clin. Endocr. *4*, 1

Giles H. R., Lox C. D., Heine M. W. and Christian C. D. (1974):
Intrauterine fetal sex determination by radioimmunoassay of amniotic fluid
testosterone.
Gynaecol. Invest. *5*, 317

Gilmour J. R. (1937):
The embryology of the parathyroid glands, the thymus and certain associated
rudiments.
J. Path. Bact. *45*, 507

Gitlin D. and Biasucci A. (1969):
Ontogenesis of immunoreactive growth hormone, folliclestimulating hormone,
thyroid-stimulating hormone, luteinizing hormone, chorionic prolactin and chorionic gonadotropin in the human conceptus.
J. clin. Endocrin. Metab. *29*, 926

Goebelsman U., Freeman R. K., Mestman J. H. et al. (1973):
Estriol in pregnancy.
Amer. J. Obstet. Gynec. *115*, 795

Goldsmith P. C., Ross J. C., Arimura A. and Ganong W. F. (1975):
Ultrastructural localization of somatostatin in pancreatic islets of the rat.
Endocrinology *97*, 1061

Gorbman A. (1959):
Comparative Endocrinology.
New York, Willey

Gotlin R. W. and Silver H. K. (1970):
Neonatal hypoglycaemia, hyperinsulinism and absence of pancreatic alpha-cells.
Lancet II, 1346

Greenberg R. E. and Lind J. (1961):
Catecholamines in tissues of the human fetus.
Pediatrics *27*, 904

Greenberg A. H., Czernichow P., Reba R. C., Tyron J. and Blizzard R. M. (1970):
Observations on the maturation of thyroid function in early fetal life.
J. clin. Invest. *47*, 1790

Grillo T. A., Leibson L. and Epple A. (eds.) (1976):
The evolution of pancreatic islets.
Oxford, New York, Toronto, Sydney, Paris, Frankfurt, Pergamon Press

Grobstein C. (1957):
Some transmission characteristics of the tubule inducing influence on mouse meta-
nephric mesenchyme.
Exp. Cell Res. *13*, 575

Grosser O. (1927):
Frühentwicklung, Eihautbildung und Plazentation des Menschen und der Säuge-
tiere.
München, Bergmann

Gruenwald P. (1934):
Über Form und Verlauf der Keimstränge bei Embryonen der Säugetiere und des
Menschen. III. Über sekundäre Keimstränge in Hoden menschlicher Embryonen.
Z. Anat. Entwicklungsgesch. *103*, 278

Gruenwald P. (1941)
The relation of the growing Müllerian duct to the Wilffian duct and its importance
for the genesis of malformations.
Anat. Rec. *81*, 1

Grumbach M. M., Kaplan S. L., Sciarra J. J. and Burr I. M. (1968):
Chorionic growth-hormone-prolactin (CGP): secretion, disposition, biologic activity
in man and postulated function as the growth-hormone of the second half of
pregnancy.
Ann. N. Y. Acad. Sci *148*, 501

Grumbach M. M. and Kaplan S. L. (1973):
Ontogenesis of growth hormone, insulin, prolactin and gonadotropin secretion
in the human foetus.
in: Foetal neonatal physiology, Proceedings of Sir Joseph Barcroft Centenary
Sympos. Cambridge, Univ. Press, Camridge 462

Grumbach M. M. and Kaplan S. L. (1975):
Human fetal pituitary hormones and the maturation of central nervous system
regulation of anterior pituitary function.
in: Modern Perinatal Medicine (Gluck L. ed.) Chicago Yearbook Publ.

Grunt J. A. and Reynolds D. W. (1970):
Insulin, blood sugar and growth hormone levels in an anencephalic infant before
and after intravenous administration of glucose.
J. Pediatr. *76*, 112

Gurpide E., Schwers J., Welch M. T. et al. (1966):
Fetal and maternal metabolism of estradiol during pregnancy.
J. clin. Endocrin. Metab. *26*, 1355

Gustavii B. (1972):
Labour: a delayed menstruation?
Lancet II, 1149

Gustavii B. and Green K. (1972):
Release of prostaglandin F2a following injection of hypertonic saline for therapeutic abortion.
Amer. J. Obstet. Gynec. *114*, 1099

Habener J. F., Kemper B. W., Rich A. et al. (1977):
Biosynthesis of parathyroid hormone.
Rec. Progr. Horm. Res. *33*, 249

Habener J. F. and Potts J. F. Jr. (1978):
Biosynthesis of parathyroid hormone
New Engl. J. Med. *299*, 580

Hamilla G. C., Jarmain J. A. and Wynne M. D. (1961):
Fetal effect of radioactive iodine therapy in pregnant women with thyroid cancer.
Amer. J. Obstet. Gynec. *81*, 1018

Hamilton W. (1960):
Development of the human placenta in the first three month of gestation.
J. Anat. *94*, 1

Hamilton W. J. and Boyd J. D. (1966):
Specialization of syncytium of human chorion.
Brit. med. J. *1*, 1501

Hamilton W. J., MacGregor R. R., Chu L. L. H. et al. (1971):
The isolation and partial purification of a nonparathyroid hormone calcemic fraction from bovine parathyroid glands.
Endocrinology *89*, 1440

Hamilton W. J., Boyd J. D. and Mosman H. W. (1972):
Human Embryology
4th Ed. Cambridge: Heffer

Hampl R., Stárka L. and Jirásek J. E. (1973):
Testosterone and its plasma protein binding in human fetuses, newborns and mothers (in czech).
Čs. Pediatr. *28*, 546

Haour F. and Saxena B. B. (1973):
Properties of the gonadotropin receptor in bovine corpora lutea.
Proc. 21st colloquium: Protides of the Biol. Fluids (Peters H. ed.) New York, Pergamon Press

Harada A. and Hershman J. (1978):
Extraction of human chorionic thyrotropin (hCT) from the placentas: Failure to recover thyrotropic activity.
J. clin. Endocrin. Metab. *47*, 681

Hanth J. C., Parker C. R. Jr., MacDonald P. C., Porter J. C. and Johnston J. M. (1978):
A role of fetal prolactin in lung maturation.
Obstet. Gynec. *51*, 81

Hawker C., Glass J. and Rasmussen H. (1966):
Further studies on the isolation and characterization of parathyroid polypeptides.
Biochemistry *5*, 344

Hayek A., Driscoll S. G. and Warshaw J. B. (1973):
Endocrine studies in anencephaly.
J. clin. Invest. *52*, 1636

Heikkelä J. and Lukkainen T. (1971):
Urinary excretion of estriol and 15 A — hydroxyestriol in complicated pregnancies.
Amer. J. Obstet. Gynec. *110*, 509

216

Hellig H., Getteran D., Lefebre Y. and Bolté E. (1970):
Steroid production from plasma cholesterol. I. Conversion of plasma cholesterol to placental progesterone in humans.
J. clin. Endocrin. Metab. *30*, 624

Heller H. and Zaimis E. J. (1949):
The antidiuretic and oxytocic hormones in the posterior pituitary glands of newborn infants and adults.
J. Physiol. (London) *109*, 162

Hennen G., Pierce J. G. and Freychet P. (1969):
Humane chorionic thyrotropin: Further characterization and study of its secretion during pregnancy.
J. clin. Endocrin. Metab. *29*, 581

Hershman J. M. and Higgins (1978):
When mole causes thyroid dysfunction.
Contemporary Ob. Gyn. *12*, 79

Hertig A. T. (1968):
Human Trophoblast.
Springfield, 111. Thomas Publ.

Hertig A. T., Adams E. C., McKay D. G., Rock J., Mulligan W. J. and Menkin M. F. (1958):
A thirteen day ovum studied histochemically.
Amer. J. Obstet. Gynec. *76*, 1025

Hertig A. T. and Mansell H. (1956):
Tumors of the female sex organs. Part I. Hydatidiform mole and choriocarcinoma.
Atlas of Tumor Pathology, Armed Forces Inst. Path.
Washington D. C.

Hertig A. T., Rock J. and Adams E. C. (1956):
A discription of 34 human ova within the first 17 days of development.
Am. J. Anat. *98*, 435

Hertig A. T. and Sheldon (1947):
Hydatidiform mole. A pathologico-clinical correlation of 200 cases.
Amer. J. Obstet. Gynec. *53*, 1

Hillarp N. A. (1959):
Further observation on the state of the catecholamines stored in adrenal medullary granules.
Acta Physiol. Scand. *47*, 271

Hillier K., Calder A. A. and MacKenzie Z. (1975):
Prostaglandin F2A in amniotic fluid in man.
J. Endocr. *64*, 13 P

Hochstetter F. (1923):
Die Entwicklung der Zirbeldrüse. Beiträge zur Entwicklungsgeschichte des menschlichen Gehirns.
Vienna und Leipzig

Hofbauer J. (1905):
Grundzüge einer Biologie der menschlichen Plazenta mit besonderer Berücksichtigung der Fragen der fötalen Erhährung.
Vienna, Braunmüller

Holland J. F. and Hreshchryshyn (Ed) (1967):
Choriocarcinoma. VICC Monograph. Series Vol. 3.
Springer, Berlin, Heidelberg, New York

Hohndahl T. H., Johansson E. D. B. and Wide L. (1971):
The site of progestrone production in early pregnancy.
Acta Endocrinol. *67*, 353
Horký Z. (1964):
Die quantitativen Veränderungen der Vaskularisation der Zotten in der diabetischen Plazenta.
Zbl Gynäk. *86*, 1621
Horn V. and Horálek F. (1961):
Über die sogenante fibrinoide Substanz in der Plazenta.
Zbl. Allg. Path. path. Anat. *102*, 514
Hoyt W. F., Kaplan S. L., Grumbach M. M. et al. (1970):
Septo-optic dysplasia and pituitary dwarfism.
Lancet I, 893

Hsu C. T., Huang L. G. and Chen T. Y. (1962):
Metastases in benign hydatidiform mole and chorioadenoma destruens.
Amer. J. Obstet. Gynec. *84*, 1412
Huff R. L. and Eik-Nes K. B. (1966):
Metabolism in vitro of acetate and certain steroids by sex-day-old rabbit blastocysts.
J. Reprod. Fertil. *11*, 57
Huhtaniemi I., Ikonen M. and Vilko R. (1970):
Presence of testosterone and other neutral steroids in human fetal testis.
Biochem. Biophys. Res. Comm. *38*, 715
Huhtaniemi I. and Vilko R. (1970):
Quantitation of neutral steroid sulphates in the amniotic fluid of early and mid--pregnancy.
Ann. Med. Exp. Biol. Fenn. *48*, 188
Huhtaniemi I. and Vilko R. (1970):
Determination of unconjugated and sulphated neutral steroids in human fetal blood of early and mid-pregnancy.
Steroids *167*, 197
Hwang P., Guyda and Friesen H. (1971):
A radioimmunoassay for human prolactin.
Proc. Nat. Acad. Sci. USA *68*, 1902

Iklé F. A. (1964):
Dissemination von Syncytiotrophoblastzellen im mütterlichen Blut während der Gravidität.
Bull. Schweiz Akad. Med. Wiss. *20*, 62
Ikonikoff L. K. de and Cedard L. (1973):
Localization of human chorionic gonadotropic and somatomammotropic hormones by the peroxidase immunohistoenzymologic method in villi and amniotic epithelium of human placentas (from six weeks to term).
Amer. J. Obstet. Gynec. *116*, 1124
Ismail-Bergi F. and Edelman I. S. (1970):
Mechanism of thyroid calorigenesis: a role of active sodium transport.
Proc. Nat. Acad. Sci. USA *67*, 1071
Ito Y. and Higashi K. (1974):
The discovery of human placental lactogen.
Amer. J. Obstet. Gynec. *120*, 427

Iverson L. (1959):
Geographic variation in the occurrence of hydatidiform mole and choriocarcinoma.
Ann. N. Y. Acad. Sci. *80*, 178

Iwanov G. (1928):
Über die Ontogenese des chromaffinen Systems beim Menschen.
Z. Anat. Entwickl. Gesch. *84*, 238

Jagiello G., Ducayen M., Miller W., Graffeo J. and Fang J. S. (1975):
Stimulation and inhibition with LH and other hormones of female mammalian
meiosis in vitro.
J. Reprod. Fertil. *43*, 9

Jeffcoate T. N., Fliegner J. R., Russel S. H. et al. (1966):
Diagnosis of the adrenogenital syndrome before birth.
Lancet II, 553

Jirásek J. E. (1960):
Secondary proliferation of the germinal epithelium in the testes of human fetuses
(in czech).
Čs. Gynek. *5*, 57

Jirásek J. E. (1963):
Die Histotopochemie hydrolytischer Enzyme in der fetalen Schilddrüse des
Menschen.
Acta histochem. (Jena) *15*, 37

Jirásek J. E. (1965):
Die Histogenese und Histochemie der Beta-Zellen der Langerhansschen Inseln
im Pankreas menschlicher Embryonen.
Acta histochem (Jena) *22*, 62

Jirásek J. E. (1965):
Die Lokalization bzw. Beteiligung einiger Enzyme und PAS-positiver Substanzen
bei Pankreashistogenese.
Acta histochem. (Jena) *20*, 161

Jirásek J. E. (1967):
The relationship between the structure of the testis and differentiation of the
external genitalia and phenotype in man.
Ciba Found. Colloq. Endocrinol. *16*, 3

Jirásek J. E. (1969):
The development of adrenals and gonads in man.
in: Progress in Endocrinology, Excepta med. Intern. Congress Ser. No 184, 1110

Jirásek J. E. (1970):
The relationship between differentiation of the testicle, genital ducts and external
genitalia in fetal and postnatal life.
in: The human testis (Rosenberg E. R. and Paulsen C. A. eds.), New York, Plenum
Press.

Jirásek J. E. (1971):
Development of the genital system and male pseudohermaphroditism.
Johns Hopkins Univ. Press Baltimore, Maryland

Jirásek J. E. (1976):
Principles of reproductive embryology.
in: Simpson J. Disorders of sexual differentiation New York, San Francisco,
London, Academic Press 1976

Jirásek J. E. (1977):
Endokrinologie fetoplacentární jednotky.
Praha, Avicenum, Zdrav. nakl.

Jirásek J. E. (1977):
Morphogenesis of the genital system in the human.
in: Morphogenesis and Malformation of the genital system Blandau R. J. and Bergsma D. (eds.). Birth Defects Orig. Art. Ser. Vol. XIII. New York, Liss A R

Jirásek J. E. and Zwinger A. (1977):
Vývoj pochvy a hymenu.
(Development of the vagina and hymen).
Čs. Gynek. *42*, 329

Jirásek J. E. (1977):
Mechanismus regrese paramesonefrických vývodů.
(Mechanism of paramesonephric duct regression).
Čs. Gynek. *42*, 520

Jirásek J. E. (1980):
Normal development of male accessory glands.
in Male accessory sex glands, E. Spring-Mills and E.S.E. Hafes (eds) Amsterdam New York, Oxford, Elsevier

Jirásek J. E. and Lojda Z. (1964):
Ein histochemischer Beitrag zur Entwicklung der Nebennierenrinde meschlicher Embryonen und Feten.
Acta histochem. (Jena) *18*, 65

Jirásek J. E., Raboch J. and Uher J. (1968):
The relationship between the development of gonads and external genitalia in humen fetuses.
Amer. J. Obstet. Gynec. *101*, 830

Jirásek J. E., Šulcová J., Čapková A., Röhling S. and Stárka L. (1969):
Histochemical and biochemical investigation of 3β-hydroxysteroid dehydrogenase in the chorion, adrenals and gonads of human foetuses.
Endokrinologie (Dresden) *54*, 173

Jirásek J. E., Zwinger A., Dyková H. et al. (1972):
Anatomie terminálního cévního řečiště choriových klků.
(Vascular anatomy of the chorionic villi)
Čs. Gynek. *37*, 399

Jirásek J. E. and Zwinger A. (1977):
Degenerace amniového epitelu jakožto faktor limitující délku těhotenství.
(Degeneration of the amniotic epithelium as a factor limiting the length of pregnancy.)
Čs. Gynek. *42*, 254

Jirásek J. E., Zwinger A., Dyková H. et al. (1971):
Localization of chorionic gonadotropin in the fetoplacental unit.
Coll. of Abstract, Symp. on gonadotropins in endocr. disorders of hum. reprod. Smokovec p. 62

Johansson E. D. and Johansson L. E. (1071):
Progesterone levels in amniotic fluid and plasma from women. I. Levels during normal pregnancy.
Acta Obstet. Gynecol. Scand. *50*, 339

Jorgensen P., Frandsen V. A. and Svenstrup B. (1974):
Amniotic fluid oestriol concentration during the last trimester of pregnancy. Normal pregnancy.
Acta Obstet. Gynecol. Scand. (suppl.) *29*, 23

220

Josimovich J. B. (1967):
Protein hormones and gestation.
in: Comparative Aspects of Reproductive Failure, Benirschke K., (ed) New York,
Springer Verlag
Josimovich J. B. (1971):
The assessment of placental function.
J. Reprod. Med. *71*, 25
Josimovich J. B. and MacLaren J. A. (1962):
Pressence in the human placenta and term serum of a highly lactogenic substance
immunologically related to pituitary growth hormone.
Endocrinology *71*, 209
Josimovich J. B., Kosor B. and Mintz D. H. (1969):
Roles of placental lactogen in foetoplacental relations.
in: Ciba Found. Symp. on Foetal Autonomy, Wolstenholm G. E. W. (ed) London,
Churchil J. A.
Josso N. (1971):
Interspecific character of the Müllerian-inhibiting substance: Action of the human
fetal testis, ovary and adrenal on the fetal rat Müllerian duct in organ culture.
J. clin. Endocrin. Metab. *32*, 404
Josso N. (1972):
Evolution of the Müllrian-inhibiting activity of the human testis. Effect of fetal,
perinatal and postnatal human testicular tissue on the Müllarian duct of the fetal
rat in organ culture,
Biol. Neonate *20*, 368
Josso N. (1972):
Permeability of membranes to the Müllarian-inhibiting substance synthesized by
the human fetal testis in vitro. A clue to its biochemical nature.
J. clin. Endocrinol. *34*, 265
Josso N. (1973):
In vitro synthesis of Müllrian-inhibiting hormone by seminiferous tubules isolated
from the calf fetal testis.
Endocrinology *93*, 829
Josso N., Picard J. Y. and Tran D. (1977):
The anti-Müllerian hormone.
in: Morphogenesis and Malformation of the genital system (Blandau R., Bergsma D.
eds.) Birth Defects, Orig. Art. Ser. Vol. XIII p 59—84
Jost A. (1947):
Recherches sur la differentiation sexualle de l'histogénèse génitale.
Arch. Anat. Micr. Morphol. Exp. *36*, 242
Jost A. (1953):
Problems of fetal endocrinology: the gonadal and hypophyseal hormones.
Rec. Progr. Horm. Res. *8*, 379
Judd H. L., Robinson J. D., Young P. E. and Jones O. W. (1976):
Amniotic fluid testosterone levels in mid-pregnancy.
Obstet. Gynec. *48*, 690
Jungmann R. A. and Schweppe J. S. (1968):
Biosynthesis of sterols and steroids from acetate-^{14}C by human fetal ovaries.
J. clin. Endocrin. Metab. *28*, 1599
Kaplan S. L. and Grumbach M. M. (1964):
Studies of human and simian placental hormone with growth hormone-like and
prolactin-like activities.

J. clin. Endocrin. Metab. *24*, 80

Kaplan S. L. and Grumbach M. M. (1965):
Serum chorionic growth hormone prolactin and serum growth hormone in mother and fetus at term.
J. clin. Endocrin. Metab. *25*, 1370

Kaplan S. L. and Grumbach M. M. (1976):
The ontogenesis of human foetal hormones. II. Luteinizing hormone (LH) and follicle stimulating hormone (FSH).
Acta Endocrinol. (Copenhagen) *81*, 808

Kaplan S. L., Grumbach M. M. and Aubert M. L. (1976):
The ontogenesis of pituitary hormones and hypothalamic factors in the human fetus: maturation of central nervous system regulation of anterior pituitary function.
Rec. Progr. Horm. Res. 32, 161

Kaplan S. L., Grumbach M. N. and Hoyt W. F. (1970):
A syndrome of hypopituitary dwarfism, hypoplasia of optic nerves and malformation of prosencephalon. Report of 6 patients.
The Society for Pediatrics Research (abstr.)

Kaplan S. L., Grumbach M. M. and Shepard T. H. (1972):
The ontogenesis of human fetal hormones. I. Growth hormone and insulin.
J. clin. Invest. *51*, 3080

Kaplan S. L. and Hershehyshyn M. M. (1973):
Estetrol in molar pregnancies quantitated by a rapid gas chromatographic method in conjunction with estrone, estradiol-17β, estriol and pregnanediol.
Amer. J. Obstet. Gynec. *115*, 803

Kearns J. E. and Hutson W. (1963):
Tagged isomers and analogues of thyroxine (Their transmission across the human placenta and other studies).
J. Nucl. Med. *4*, 453

Keene M. F. and Hewer E. E. (1927):
Observations of the development of the human suprarenal gland.
J. Anat. *61*, 302

Keirse M. J. N. C. (1975):
Primary prostaglandins in amniotic fluid.
Amer. J. Obstet. Gynec. *129*, 474

Kingsbury B. F. (1939):
The question of a lateral thyroid in mammals with special reference to man.
Amer. J. Anat. *65*, 333

Kirchner C. (1972):
Immune histologic studies on the synthesis of a uterine-specific protein in the rabbit and its passage through the blastocyst coverings.
Fertil. Steril. *23*, 131

Kirkland R. T., Kirkland J. L., Johnson C. M., Horning M. G., Librik L. and Clayton G. W. (1973):
Congenital lipoid adrenal hyperplasia in an eight year old phenotypic female.
J. clin. Endocrin. Metab. *36*, 488

Kissane J. M. and Smith M. G. (1967):
Pathology of Infancy and Childhood.
St. Louis, Mosby

Kistner R. W. (1966):
Use of clomiphene citrate, human chorionic gonadotropin and human menopausal gonadotropin for induction of ovulation in the human female.
Fertil. Steril. *17*, 569

Klein A. H., Foley T. P., Larsen P. R. et al. (1976):
Neonatal thyroid function in congenital hypothyroidism.
J. Pediatr. *89*, 545

Klinga K., Bek E., Runnebaum B. (1978):
Maternal peripheral testosterone levels during the first half of pregnancy.
Amer. J. Obstet. Gynec. *131*, 60

Klopper A. and Biggs J. (1970):
The correlation between urinary oestriol excretion and the oestriol concentration in liquor amnii.
J. Endocrinol. *48*, 471

Koff A. K. (1933):
Development of the vagina in human fetus.
Contrib. Embryol. Carnegie Inst. Wash. *24*, 59

Kusakabe T. and Miyake T. (1964):
Thyroidal deiodination defect in three sisters with simple goiter.
J. clin. Endocrin. Metab. *24*, 456

Lamont K. G., Peréz-Palacios G., Peréz A. E. and Jaffe R. B. (1970):
Pregnenolone and pregnenolone sulphate metabolism by human fetal testes in vitro.
Steroids *16*, 127

Landau R. L. and Lugibihl K. (1967):
The effect of progesterone on the concentration of plasma aminoacids in man.
Metabolism *16*, 1114

Langhans T. (1877):
Untersuchungen über die menschliche Plazenta.
Arch. Anat. Physiol. Anat. Abt. 188

Langr F., Lomský R., Vortel V. and Jirásek J. E. (1972):
Development of glucagon-containing cells in the human foetal pancreas.
Sborn. věd. prací lék. fak. UK Hradec Králové 152 : 167-172

Lanman J. T. (1961):
The adrenal gland in the human fetus. An interpretation of its physiology and unusual developmental pattern.
Pediatrics *27*, 140

Lanman J. T. (1962):
An interpretation of human foetal adrenal structure and function.
in: Adrenal Cortex, Currie A. R. (ed.) Baltimore, Williams and Wilkins

Leblanc H. J., Anderson R. and Yen S. S. C. (1976):
Glucagon secretion in late pregnancy and the puerperium.
Amer. J. Obstet. Gynec. *125*, 708

Leblanc H., Abu- Fadil S., Lachelin C. I. and Yen S. S. C. (1977):
The effect of dopamine infusion on insulin and glucagon secretion in man.
J. clin. Endocrin. Metab. *44*, 196

Lequin R. M., Hackeng W. H. and Shopman W. (1970):
A radioimmunoassay for parathyroid hormone in man. II. Measurement of para-thyroid hormone concentration in human plasma by means of radioimmunoassay for bovine hormone.
Acta Endocrinol. *63*, 655

Levina S. E. (1965):
Morfologija gipofiza v embryogeneze čelověka.
Arkh. Anat. Gistol. Embryol. *48*, 78

Levina S. E. (1965):
Nekotoryje danyja o rozvitii nadpočečnikov i zobnoj železy v embryogeneze čelověka.
Bjull. Eksp. Biol. Med. *59*, 89

Levina S. E. (1968):
Endocrine features in development of human hypothalamus, hypophysis and placenta.
Gen. Comp. Endocrinol. *11*, 151

Li C. H. and Chung D. (1976):
Isolation and struture of an untriakonta peptide with opiate activity from camel pituitary glands.
Proc. Nat. Acad. Sc. USA *73*, 1145

Li C. H., Grumbach M. M., Kaplan S. L. and Josimovich J. B. et al. (1968):
Human chorionic somatomammotropin (hCS) proposed terminology for desig-nation of a placental hormone
Experientia *24*, 1188

Licht P., Papkoff H., Farmer S. et al. (1977):
Evolution of gonadotropin structure and function.
Rec. Prog. Horm. Res. *33*, 169

Lieberburg I. and McEven B. S. (1975):
Estradiol-17β : a metabolite of testosterone recovered in cell nuclei from limbic areas of neonatal rat brains.
Brain Res. *85*, 165

Lieberman S., Gurpide E., Lipsett M. and Salhanick H. (1977):
Steroid hormone secretions.
in: Frontiers in Reproduction and Fertility Control. Greep R. O. and Koblinsky M. A. direct. Cambridge, Massachusetts and London England the MIT Press

Liggins G. C. and Howie R. N. (1972):
A controled trial of antepartum glucocorticoid treatment for prevention of the respiratory distress syndrome in premature infants.
Pediatrics *50*, 515

Lightwood R. (1952):
Idiopathic hypercalcaemia with failure to thrive.
Arch. Dis. Childhood *27*, 302

Lipsett M. B. (1971):
17α-hydroxyprogesterone and ovarian function. IPPF research in reproduction.
Edwards R. G. ed., vol. 3, 2

Lissitzky S., Codaccioni J. L., Bismuth J. and Depieds R. (1967):
Congenital goiters with hypothyroidism and iodo-serum albumin replacing thyro-globulin.
J. clin. Endocrin. Metab. *27*, 185

Little W. A. (1960):
Placental infarction.
Obstet. Gynec. *15*, 109

Liu H. M. and Potter E. L. (1962):
Development of the human pancreas.
Arch. Pathol. *74*, 439

Lomský R., Langr F. and Vortel V. (1969):
Immunohistochemical demonstration of gastrin in mammalian islets of Langerhans.
Nature *223*, 618

Ludwig G. D. (1962):
Hyperparathyroidism in relation to pregnancy.
New Engl. J. Med. *267*, 637

Ludwig K. S. (1962):
Zur Feinstruktur der materno-fetalen Verbindung in Plazentom des Schafes
(Avis aries L).
Experentia *18*, 212

Margolis A. J. and Orcutt R. E. (1960):
Pressures in human umbilical vessels in utero.
Amer. J. Obstet. Gynec. *80*, 573

Marks A. and Samols E. (1970):
Interstinal factors in the regulation of insulin secretion.
Adv. Metab. Disord. *4*, 1

Matějka M. (1959):
Die Morphogenese der menschlichen Vagina und ihre Gesetzmässigkeiten.
Anat. Anz. *106*, 20

Matsuzuki F., Irie M. and Shizume K. (1971):
Growth hormone in human pituitary glands and cord blood.
J. clin. Endocrin. Metab. *33*, 908

*McDonald P. C., Schultz F. M., Duenhoelter G. H., Gant N. F., Jimenez J. M.,
Pritchard J. A., Porter J. C. and Johnston J. M.* (1971):
Initation of human parturition. I. Mechanism of action of arachidonic acid.
Obstet. Gynec. *44*, 629

McEven B. S. (1976):
Steroid receptors in neuroendocrine tissues: Topography, subcellular distribution
and functional implications. pp 277—304
in: Naftolin F., Ryan K. and Davids I. J. Subcellular Mechanism in Reproductive
Neuroendocrinology Elsevier, Amsterdam

McKusick V. (1976):
Mendelian inheritance in man. Catalog of autosomal dominant, autosomal recessive
and X-linked phenotypes.
The Johns Hopkins Univ. Press, Baltimore and London

MacPhee A. A., Cole F. E. and Rice B. T. (1975):
The effect of melatonin on steroidogenesis by the human ovary in vitro.
J. clin. Endocrin. Metab. *40*, 688

McQuarrie I., Bell E. T., Zimmermann B. and Wright W. S. (1950):
Deficiency of alpha cells of pancreas as possible etiological factor in familial
hypoglycogenosis.
Fed. Proc. 9, 337 (abstr.)

Midgley A. R. Jr. and Pierce G. B. Jr. (1962):
Immunohistochemical localization of human chorionic gonadotropin.
J. exp. Med. *11*, 289

Migeon J. C., Kenny F. M. and Kowarski A. (1968):
The syndrome of congenital adrenocortical unresponsivness to ACTH. Report
of six cases.
Pediatr. Res. *2*, 501

Mischell B. D. Jr., Wide L. and Gemzell C. A. (1963):
Immunological determination of human chorionic gonadotropin in serum.
J. clin. Endocrin. Metab. *23*, 125

Mishell B. R., Nakamura R. M., Barbeira J. M. and Thorneycroft I. H. (1974):
Initial detection of human chorionic gonadotropin in serum in normal gestation.
Amer. J. Obstet. Gynec. *118*, 990

Mitskewich M. S. and Levina S. E. (1965):
Investigation on the structure and gonadotropic activity of anterior pituitary in human embryogenesis.
Arch. Anat. Microsc. Morphol. Exp. *54*,

Miyai K., Azukizawa M. and Kumahara Y. (1971):
Familial isolated thyrotropin deficiency with cretenism.
New Engl. J. Med. *285*, 1043

Miyakawa I., Keda I. and Maeyama M. (1974):
Transport of ACTH across human placenta.
J. clin. Endocrin. Metab. *39*, 440

Monesi V., Molinaro M., Spalletta E. and Davoli C. (1970):
Effect of metabolic inhibitors on macromolecular synthesis and early development in the mouse embryo.
Exp. Cell. Res. *59*, 197

Money J. (1973):
Effects of prenatal androgenization and deandrogenization on behavior in human beings. pp 249—266
in: Ganong W. F. and Martini L. (eds.). Frontiers in Neuroendocrinology. Oxford Univ. Press, New York

Montelone J. A., Lee J. B., Tashijian A. H. and Cantor H. E. (1975):
Transient neonatal hypocalcaemia, hypomagnesemia and high serum parathyroid hormone with maternal hyperparathyroidism.
Ann. Int. Med. *82*, 670—672

Morgan F. J., Kammermann S. and Canfield R. E. (1972):
in: Gonadotropins Saxena Beling Ganday (eds.) New York Willey-Interscience

Morgan, C. D., Sandler M. and Panigel, M.: (1972)
Placental transfer of catecholamines in vitro and in vivo.
Am. J. Obstet. Gynec. *112*, 1068

Morison J. E. (1963):
Foetal and Neonatal Pathology London, Butterworth

Munck A. (1971):
Glucocorticoids inhibition of glucose uptake by peripheral tissue: old and new evidence, molecular mechanism and physiological significance.
Perspect. Biol. Med. *14*, 265

Murphy B. E. P., Patrick J., Denton R. L., Clark S. J., Marvin M. and Haidar R. (1975):
Cortisol in amniotic fluid during human gestation.
J. clin. Endocrin. Metab. *40*, 164

Naftolin F., Ryan K. J., Davies K. J., Reddy V. V., Flores F., Petro Z. and Kulm M. (1975):
The formation of estrogens by central neuroendocrine tissues.
Rec. Prog. Horm. Res. *31*, 295

Nagatsu T., Levitt M. and Undenfied S. (1964):
Tyrosine hydroxylase. The initial step in norepinephrine biosynthesis.
J. Biol. Chem. *239*, 2910

Nagel W. (1889):
Ueber die Entwicklung des Urogenitalsystems des Menschen.
Arch. Mikrosk. Anat. Entwicklungsmech. *34*, 269

Neri P., Tarli P., Arezzini C. et al. (1970):
Effects of pH on conformation and biological activity of human chorionic somatomammotropin (hCS).
Ann. Sclavo *12*, 663

Neubert K. (1927):
Bau und Entwicklung des menschlichen Pankreas.
Roux Arch. Festschr. Driesch. *111*, 29

Neumann S. (1897):
Das sogenannte tuberöse subchoriale Hämatom der Decidua.
Mntschr. Geburtsch. Gynäk. *6*, 17

Nichols J. (1970):
Antenatal diagnosis and treatment of the adrenogenital syndrome.
Lancet I, 83

Niercer R. D., Lammert A. C., Anderson R. and Hazard J. B. (1958):
Choriocarcinoma in mother and infant.
J. Amer. med. Assoc. *166*, 482

Niklasson E. (1970):
Familial early hypoparathyroidism associated with hypomagnesaemia.
Acta Pediatr. Scand. *59*, 715

Nitabuch R. (1887):
Beiträge zur Kenntniss der menschlichen Plazenta.
Thesis Univ. Bern

Noorden van S. and Pearse A. G. E. (1976):
The localization of immunoreactivity to insulin, glucagon and gastrin in the gut
of Amphioxus (Branchiostoma) lanceolatus.
in: The Evolution of Pancreatic Islets. Grillo T. A. I., Leibson L., Epple A. (eds.)
Oxford, New York, Toronto, Pergamon Press

Norris E. H. (1937):
The parathyroid glands and the lateral thyroid in man: their morphogenesis,
histogenesis, topographic anatomy and prenatal growth.
Carnegie Inst. Wash. Contr. Embryol. *26*, 247

Norris E. H. (1946):
Anatomical evidence of prenatal function of the human parathyroid glands.
Anat. Rec. *96*, 129

Novak E. (1950):
Pathological aspects of hydatidiform mole and choriocarcinoma.
Amer. J. Obstet. Gynec. *59*, 1355

Nussbaum M. (1880):
Zur Differenzierung des Geschlechts in Tierreich.
Arch. Mikrosk. Anat. *18*, 1

Nusynowitz M. L. and Klein M. H. (1973):
Pseudoidiopathic hypoparathyroidism. Hypoparathyroidism with ineffective parathyroid hormone.
Am. J. Med. *55*, 677

Odell W. D., Bates R. W., Riolin R. S. et al.: (1964):
Thyroid changes in choriocarcinoma.
J. clin. Endocrin. Metab. *23*, 658

Ohno S. (1967):
Sex Chromosomes and Sex-linked Genes.
Berlin, New York, Springer Verlag

Ohno S., Christian L. C., Wachtel S. S. and Koo G. C. (1976):
Hormone-like role of H-Y antigen in bovine freemartin gonad.
Nature (London) *261*, 597

Ohno S. and Gropp A. (1965):
Embryological basis for germ cell chimerism in mammals.
Cytogenetics *4*, 251

Ohno S., Tetterborn U. and Dofoku R. (1971):
Molecular biology for sex differentiation.
Hereditas *69*, 107

Oppenheimer J. H. and Surks M. (1974):
Quantitative aspects of hormone production, distribution, metabolism and activity.
Handb. Physiol. Sec. 7: Endocrinol. Vol. VII Thyroid.

Orci L., Betens D., Rufer C., Amherdt M., Ruvazolla M., Studer P., Malaisse-
-Lagae F. and Unger R. H. (1976):
Hypertrophy and hyperplasia of somatostatin-containing D-cells in diabetes.
Proc. Nat. Acad. Sci USA *73*, 1338

Orci L. and Unger R. H. (1975):
Functional subdivision of islets of Langerhans and possible role of D-cells.
Lancet II, 1243

Oordt van P. G. W. J. (1965):
Nomenclature of the hormone-producing cells in the adenohypophysis.
Gen. Comp. Endocr. *5*, 131

Osler M. (1965):
in: Leibel B. S. and Wrenshall G. A. (eds.). On the Nature and Treatment of Diabetes.
The Netherlands Exc. Med. Found.

O'Rahilly R (1973):
The embryology and anatomy of the uterus.
in: The Uterus. Norris H. J., Hertig A. T. and Abell M. R. (eds.). Baltimore, Maryland, Williams, Wilkins

O'Rahilly R. (1973):
Developmental stages in human embryos. Part A: Embryos of the first three weeks (stages 1 to 9).
Carnegie Inst. Wash. Publ. 631

Panigel M. and Anh J. N. H. (1964):
Ultrastructure des villosités placentaires humaines.
Path. et Biol. *12*, 927

Park J., Aimakhu V. E. and Jones H. W. Jr. (1975):
An etiologic and pathologic classification of male hermaphroditism.
Amer. J Obstet Gynec *123*, 505

Pasqualini J. R., Wiqvist N. and Diczfalusy E. (1966):
Biosynthesis of aldosterone by human foetuses perfused with corticosterone at mid-term.
Biochim. biophys. Acta *121*, 430

Pasteels J. L. (1963):
Recherches morphologique et expérimentales sur la sécrétion de prolactine.
Arch. Biol. (Liège) *74*, 439

Patillo R. A., Gey G. C., Delfs E. and Mattingly R. F. (1968):
In vitro identification of the trophoblastic stem cell of the human villous placenta.
Amer. J. Obstet Gynec. *100*, 582

Paul S. M. and Axelrod J. (1977):
Catecholestrogens: presence in brain and endocrine tissues.
Science *197*, 657

Pavel S. I., Dumitru I., Klepsh I. and Dorcescu M. (1973):
A gonadotropin inhibiting principle in the pineal of human fetuses: evidence for its identity with arginine vasotocin.
Neuroendocrinology *13*, 41

Pavlov C., Chard T. and Letch A. T. (1972):
Circulating levels of human chorionic somatomammotropin in late pregnancy: disappearence from the circulation after delivery, variation during labour and circadian variation.
J. Obstet. Gynaec. Brit. Cwlth. *79*, 629

Pavlova E. B., Pronina T. S. and Skebelskaya Y. B. (1968):
Histostructure of adenohypophysis of human fetuses and contents of somatotropin and adrenocorticotropic hormone.
Gen. Comp. Endocrinol. *10*, 269

Payne A. H. and Jaffe R. B. (1972):
Comparison of androgen synthesis in human fetal testis and adrenal: 3β-hydroxysteroid dehydrogenase-isomerase and 17β-steroid dehydrogenase activities.
Biochim. Bioph. Acta *279*, 202

Pearce R. M. (1903):
The development of the islands of Langerhans in the human embryo.
Amer. J. Anat. *2*, 445

Pearse A. G. E. (1952):
The cytochemistry and cytology of the normal anterior hypophysis investigated by the trichrome periodic-acid-Schiff method.
J. Path. Bact. *64*, 811

Pearse A. G. E. and Polak J. M. (1971):
Cytochemical evidence for the neural crest origin of mammalian ultimobranchial C-cells.
Histochemie *27*, 96

Pelliniemi L. J. and Niemi M. (1969):
Fine structure of the human foetal testis. I. The intersticial tissue.
Z. Zellforschr. Mikrosk. Anat. *99*, 507

Pepperell R. J., de Kretser D. M. and Burger H. G. (1975):
Studies on the metabolic clearence rate and production rate of human luteinizing hormone and on the initial half-time of its subunits in man.
J. clin. Invest. *56*, 118

Perry J. S., Heap R. B., Burton R. D. and Gadsby J. E. (1976):
Endocrinology of the blastocyst and its role in the establishment of pregnancy, in: Implantation and the Mechanism of Action of IUDs. 5th IPPF Cambridge. Workshop (Perry J. S. and Heap R. B. eds.). J. Reprod. Fertil. suppl. *25*, 85

Peters H., Himelstein-Braw and Faber M. (1976):
The normal development of the ovary in childhood.
Acta Endocrinol. (Kbh) *82*, 617

Pierce J. G., Liao T. S. Howard S. N. et al. (1971):
Studies on the structure of thyrotropin: its relationship to luteinizing hormone.
Rec. Prog. Horm. Res. *27*, 165

Pinkerton J. H., McKay D. G., Adams E. C. and Hertig A. T. (1961):
Development of the human ovary — a study using histochemical technics.
Obstet. Gynec. *18*, 152

Politzer G. (1928):
Über Zahl Lage und Beschaffenheit der Urkeimzellen eines menschlichen Embryo
mit 26—27 Ursegmentpaaren.
Z. Anat. Entwicklungsgesch. *100*, 331

Politzer G. (1933):
Die Keimbahn des Menschen.
Ztschr. Anat. *100*, 331

Politzer G. (1953):
Die Entwicklung des Wolffschen Ganges beim Menschen
Acta Anat. *18*, 343

Politzer G. and Hann F. (1935):
Über die Entwicklung der branchiogenen Organe beim Menschen.
Z. Anat. Entwickl. Gesch. *104*, 670

Porte D. Jr. (1969):
Sympathetic regulation of insulin secretion. Its relation to diabetes mellitus.
Arch. Intern. Med. *123*, 252

Potel, J.: (1958)
Die Listeriose beim Menshen.
in: Listeriosen Symposium, Roots and Stranel (eds)
Zbl. f. Veterinärmedizin

Potter E. L. (1946):
Facial characteristics of infants with bilateral renal agenesis.
Amer. J. Obstet. Gynec. *51*, 885

Potter E. L. (1975):
Pathology of the fetus and the infant.
Chicago Year Book Med. Pub.

Pronina T. S. and Sapronova A. Y. (1976):
Development of the function of endocrine pancreas in the human fetus.
in: The Evolution of Pancreatic Islets, Grillo T A I. Leibson L., Epple
A. (eds.)
Oxford, New York, Toronto, Pergamon Press.

Radwanska E., Frankenberg J. and Allen E. I. (1978):
Plasma progesterone levels in normal and abnormal early human pregnancy.
Fertil. Steril. *30*, 398

Rajfer J. and Walsh P. C. (1977):
Testicular descent.
Birth Defects Orig. Art. Ser. Vol. XIII, 107.
Morphogenesis and malformation of the genital system. Blandau R. J., Bergsma E.
(eds.) Liss A., New York

Rayford P. L., Vaitukaitis J. L. and Ross G. T. et al. (1972):
Use of specific antisera to characterise biologic activity of hCG subunit pre-
parations.
Endocrinology *91*, 144

Rees L. H., Burke C. W., Chard T., Ewans S. W. and Letworth A. T. (1975):
Possible placental origin of ACTH in normal human pregnancy.
Nature *254*, 620

Reineke E. P. (1949):
The formation of thyroxine in iodinated proteins.

Ann. N. Y. Acad. Sci. 50, 450

Reyes F. I., Boroditsky R. S., Winter J. S. D. and Faiman C. (1974):
Studies of human sexual development. II. Fetal and maternal serum gonadotropin and sex steroid concentrations.
J. clin. Endocrin. Metab. *38*, 612

Reyes F. I., Winter J. S. D. and Faiman C. (1973):
Studies of human sexual development: I. Fetal and adrenal sex steroids.
J. clin. Endocrin. Metab. *37*, 74

Rice B. F., Johanson C. A. and Sternberg W. H. (1966):
Formation of steroid hormones from acetate-I^{14}-C by a human fetal testis preparation grown in organ culture.
Steroids *7*, 79

Riddick F. A. Jr., Desai K. B., Murison P. J. and Stanburg J. B. (1969):
Familial goiter with diminished synthesis of thyroglobulin.
J. Exp. Med. *150*, 203

Rinne U. K., Kivalo E. and Talanti S. (1962):
Maturation of human hypothalamus neurosecretion.
Biol. Neonat. *4*, 351

Robinson A. G. (1965):
Isolation assay and secretion of individual human neurophysins.
J. clin. Invest. *55*, 360

Rohr K. (1899):
Die Beziehungen der mütterlichen Gefässe zu den intervillösen Räumen der reifen Plazenta speciell zur Thrombose derselben ("weisser Infarct").
Virchows Arch. path. Anat. *115*, 505

Rolschau J. (1978):
Aspects of placental pathology and growth retardation.
Acta Obstet. Gynec. Scand. suppl. 72

Romeis B. (1940):
Inner sekretorische Drüsen. II. Hypophyse.
in: v. Möllendorf's Handbuch der mikroskopische Anatomie des Menschen.
Berlin Springer-Verlag

Romer A. S. and Parsons T. S. (1977):
The vertebrate body.
Saunders W. B., Philadelphia, London, Toronto

Rosen F. and Ezrin C. (1966):
Embryology of the thyrotroph.
J. clin. Endocrin. Metab. *62*, 413

Ross G. T. (1977):
Clinical relevance of research on the structure of human chorionic gonadotropin.
Amer. J. Obstet. Gynec. *129*, 795

Rubenstein A. H., Kuzuya H. and Horowitz D. L. (1977):
Clinical significance of circulating C-peptide in diabetes mellitus and hypoglycaemic disorders.
Arch. Intern. Med. *13*, 625

Rubinstein P., Sucin-Foca N. and Nicholson F. (1977):
Genetics of juvenile diabetes mellitus. A recessive gene closely linked to HLA-D and with 50 per cent penetrance.
New Engl. J. Med. *297*, 1036

Sade J. and Rosen G. (1968):
Thyroglossal cysts and tracts.

Ann. Otol. 77, 139

Sadeghi-Najad A. and Senior B. (1974):
A familial syndrome of isolated aplasia of the anterior pituitary.
J. Pediatr. *84*, 79

Samaan N., Yen S. C. C., Friesen A. and Pearson O. H. (1966):
Serum placental lactogen levels during pregnancy and in trophoblastic disease.
J. clin. Endocrin. Metab. *26*, 1303

Samaan N., Yen S. C. C., Gonzales D. and Pearson O. H. (1968):
Metabolic effects of placental lactogen (hPL) in man.
J. clin. Endocrin. Metab. *28*, 485

Satow Y., Okamoto K., Ikeda T. et al. (1972):
Electron microscopic studies of the anterior pituitaries and adrenal cortices of normal and anencephalic human fetuses.
J. Electron. Microsc. *21*, 29

Savard K., Marsh J. M. and Rice B. F. (1965):
Gonadotropins and ovarian steroidogenesis.
Rec. Progr. Horm. Res. *21*, 285

Saxena B. B., Hasan S. H., Haour I. and Schmidt-Gollwitzer M. (1974):
Radioreceptor assay of human chorionic gonadotropins: detection of early pregnancy.
Science *184*, 793

Schaeffer L. S., Wildner M. W. and Williams R. H. (1971):
Insulin and glucagon release from human fetal pancreas slices in vitro.
Diabetes suppl. *20*, 326

Sciarra J. J., Kaplan S. L. and Grumbach M. M. (1963):
Localization of anti-human growth hormone serum with in the human placenta: evidence for a human chorionic growth-hormone-prolactin.
Nature *199*, 1005

Sciarra J. J., Tagatz G. E., Notation A. D. and Depp R. (1974):
Estriol and estetrol in amniotic fluid.
Amer. J. Obstet. Gynec. *118*, 626

Schindler A. E. (1972):
Steroide im Fruchtwasser.
Fortschr. Geburtshilfe Gynaekol. *46*, 1

Schindler A. E. and Siiteri P. K. (1968):
Isolation and quantitation of steroids from normal human amniotic fluid.
J. clin. Endocr. Metab. *28*, 1189

Schmorl G. (1893):
Pathologische-anatomische Untersuchungen über puerperal-Eklampsie.
Leipzig: Vogel

Schmorl C. G. (1905):
Über das Schicksal embolisch verscheppter Plazentarzellen.
Verhandl. deutsch. Path. Ges. *8*, 39

Scothorne R. J. (1964):
Functional capacity of fetal parathyroid glands with reference to their clinical use as homografts.
Ann. N. Y. Acad. Sci *120*, 669

Selenkow H. A., Birnbaum M. D. and Hollander C. S. (1973):
Thyroid function and dysfunction during pregnancy.
Clin. Obstet. Gynec. *16*, 66

Seppälä M., Aho I., Tissari A. and Ruoslahti E. (1972):
Radioimmunoassay of oxytocin in amniotic fluid, fetal urine and meconium during late pregnancy and delivery.
Amer. J. Obstet. Gynec. *114*, 788

Serón-Ferré M., Lawrence C. C., Siiteri P. K. and Jaffe R. B. (1978):
Steroid production by definitive and fetal zones of the human fetal adrenal gland.
J. clin. Endocrin. Metab. *47*, 603

Serra G. B., Pérez-Palacios G. and Jaffe R. B. (1970):
De novo testosterone biosynthesis in the human fetal testis.
J. clin. Endocrin. Metab. *30*, 128

Shahwan M. M., Oakey R. E. and Stitch S. R. (1969):
A new pathway of estriol biosynthesis in pregnancy.
Acta Endocr. *60*, 49

Shambaugh G. E., Kubek M. and Wilber J. (1977):
The placenta: a new locus for thyrotropin-releasing hormone (TRH).
ASCI-clinical Research

Shepard T. H., Andersen H. J. and Andersen H. (1964):
The human fetal thyroid. I. Its weight in relation to body weight, crown-rump length, foot length and estimated gestation age.
Anat. Rec. *148*, 123

Shepard T. H., Andersen H. and Andersen H. J. (1964):
Histochemical studies of the human fetal thyroid during the first half of fetal life.
Anat. Rec. *149*, 363

Shepard T. H. (1967):
Onset of function in the human fetal thyroid: biochemical and radioautographic studies from organ culture.
J. clin. Endocr. Metab. *27*, 945

Sherwood W. G., Chance G. W. and Hill D. E. (1974):
A new syndrome of pancreatic agenesis. The role of insulin and glucagon in somatic and cell growth.
Pediatr. Res. *8*, 360 (abstr.)

Shulman K. (1973):
in: Birth Defects Atlas and Compendium Bergsma D. (ed.) Baltimore Williams and Wilkins

Shutt D. A., Smith I. D. and Shearman R. P. (1974):
Oestrone. oestradiol-17β-oestriol levels in human foetal plasma during gestation and at term.
J. Endocrinol. *60*, 333

Siddall R. C. and Hartmann F. W. (1926):
Infarcts of the placenta: study of seven hundred consecutive placentas.
Amer. J. Obstet. Gynec. *12*, 683

Sibenmann R. E. (1957):
Die kongenitale Lipoidhyperplasie der Nebennierenrinde mit Nebennierenrinden- -insuffizienz.
Schweitz. Z. Path. *20*, 77

Siiteri P. K. and Wilson J. D. (1974):
Testosterone formation and metabolism during male sexual differentiation in the human embryo.
J. clin. Endocrin. Metab. *38*, 113

Siler-Khodr T. M., Morgenstern L. L. and Greenwood F. C. (1974):
Hormone synthesis and release from human fetal adenohypophysis in vitro.
J. clin. Endocrin. Metab. *39*, 891

Simon D. (1957):
La migration de cellules germinales de l'embryon de poulet vers les ébauches gonadiques: préuves expérimentales.
C. R. Seances Soc. Biol. Ses. Fil. *151*, 1576

Simpson J. L. and German J. (1970):
Pseudovaginal perineoscrotal hypospadias: genetic aspects and differentiation from other forms of male pseudohermaphroditism.
Int. J. Gynecol. Obstet. *8*, 147

Simpson J. L., Jirásek J. E., Speroff L. and Kase N. G. (1976):
Disorders of sexual differentiation.
New York, San Francisco, London, Academic Press

Skinner S. L., Lumbers E. R. and Symonds E. M. (1972):
Analysis of changes in the renin-angiotensin system during pregnancy.
Clin. Sci. *42*, 479

Skou J. C. (1965):
Enzymatic basis for active transport of Na+ and K+ across cell membranes.
Physiol. Rev. *45*, 598

Smart P. J. G. (1962):
Some observation on the vascular morphology of the foetal side of the human placenta.
J. Obstet. Gynaec. Brit. Cwlth. *69*, 929

Smith C. A. (1959):
in: The Physiology of the Newborn Infant, 3rd ed. Springfield 111. Thomas

Smith D. W. (1976):
Recognizable Patterns of Human Malformations.
Saunders

Spellacy W. N. (1974):
Distribution of human placental lactogen in the last half of normal and complicated pregnancies.
Amer. J. Obstet. Gynec. *120*, 219

Spellacy W. N., Buhi W. C., Bradley B. and Holsinger K. K. (1973):
Maternal, fetal and amniotic fluid levels of glucose, insulin and growth hormone.
Obstet. Gynec. *41*, 323

Stanbury J. B. (1963):
The metabolic errors in certain types of familial goiter.
Rec. Progr. Horm. Res. *19*, 547

Stanbury J. B. (1972):
Familial goiter.
in: Stanbury J. B., Wyngaarden J. B. and Frederickson D. S. (eds.)
The Metabolic Basis of Inherited Disease. New York, McGraw-Hill

Stanbury J. B. and Chapman E. M. (1960):
Congenital hypothyroidism with goiter: absence of an iodine-concentrating mechanism.
Lancet I, 1162

Stanbury J. B., Rocmans P., Buhler V. K. and Ochi Y. (1968):
Congenital hypothyroidism with impaired thyroid response to thyrotropin.
New Engl. J. Med. *279*, 1132

Stern L., Grunberg R. E. and Lind J. (1961):
Catecholamine excretion in the newborn period: effect of short periods of induced hypoxia.
Acta Pediat. *50*, 497

Stern L., Lees M. H. and Leduc J. (1965):
Environmental temperature, oxygen consumption and catecholamine excretion in newborn infants.
Pediatricts *36*, 367

Stern L., Lind L. and Kaplan B. (1961):
Direct human foetal electrocardiography (with studies of the effects of adrenalin, atropine, clamping of the umbilical cord and placental separation on the foetal ECG).
Biol. Neonat. *3*, 49

Stieve H. (1930):
Männliche Genitalorgane.
in: Handbuch der mikroskopischen Anatomie des Menschen (W. von Möllendrof ed.) Vol. 7, Berlin, New York, Springer-Verlag

Stock R. J., Josimovich J. B. Kosor B., Klopper A. and Wilson G. R. (1971):
The effect of chorionic gonadotropin and chorionic somatomammotropin on steroidogenesis in the corpus luteum.
J. Obstet. Gynaec. Brit. Cwlth. *78*, 549

Strakosch W. (1956):
Über Chorionangiome.
Geburtsch. u. Frauenheilk. *16*, 485

Strauss F., Benirschke K. and Driscoll S. (1967):
Pathology of the Placenta.
in: Handbuch der speziellen pathologischen Anatomie und Histologie. Lubarsch O., Henke F., Rössle R. and Uehlinger (eds.) Berlin Springer-Verlag

Strott C. A., Yoshimi T., Ross G. T. and Lipsett M. B. (1969):
Ovarian pathology: relationship between plasma LH and steroidogenesis by the follicle and corpus luteum, effect of hCG.
J. clin. Endocrin. Metab. *29*, 1157

Sugiyama S., Taki A., Machida Y. and Furihata T. (1959):
The significance and rate of the ultimobranchial body in man in relation to the development of the thyroid gland.
Okajimes Folia anat. jap. *32*, 329

Šulcová J., Jirásek J. E. and Stárka L. (1973):
Transformation of testosterone into dihydrotestosterone by the primordia of human genitalia and by the fetal suprascapular skin.
Steroids Lipids Res. *4*, 129

Sulimovici S. and Lunenfeld B. (1972):
Effect of cyclic 3,5'-adenosine monophosphate on gonadal diphosphopyridine and triphosphopyridine nucleotide linked dehydrogenases.
in: Gonadotropins. Saxena B. B., Beling C. G., Gandy H. M. (eds.) Willey-Interscience, New York

Swaneck G. E., Chu L. L. H. and Edelman I. S. (1970):
Stereospecific binding of aldosterone to renal chromatin.
J. Biol. Chem. *245*, 5382

Symonds E. M., Standley M. A. and Skinner S. L. (1968):
Production of renin by in vitro cultures of human chorion and uterine muscle.
Nature *217*, 1152

Szentagothai J., Flerko B., Mess B. and Halasz B. (1968):
Hypothalamic control of the anterior pituitary.
3rd ed. Akademiai Kiado Budapest

Talegdy G., Weeks J. W., Wiqvist N. and Diczfalusy E. (1969):
Sterol and steroid synthesis by human fetuses perfused with acetate and cholesterol
at midgestation.
Acta Endocrin. *61* suppl. 138, 54

Tata J. R. and Widnell C. C. (1963):
Ribonucleic acid synthesis during the early action of thyroid hormones.
Biochem. J. *98*, 604

Thompson C. R. and Hansen L. M. (1970):
Pergonal (menotropins): a summary of clinical experience in the inductionfo
ovulation and pregnancy.
Fertil. Steril. *21*, 844

Thompson J. D. (1975):
Gastrointestinal Hormones.
Austin and London, U. of Texas Press

Tomkins G. M. and Martin D. W. Jr. (1970):
Hormones and gene expression.
Ann. Rev. Genet. *4*, 91

Townsley J. D., Gartman L. J. and Crystle C. D. (1973):
Maternal serum 17β-estradiol levels in normal and complicated pregnancies.
Amer. J. Obstet. Gynec. *115*, 830

Tribe M. and Brambell F. W. R. (1932):
The origin and migration of the primordial germ cells of Sphenodon punctatus.
Q. J. Microsc. Sci. *75*, 251

Troen P., Nelson B., Wiqvist N. and Diczfalusy E. (1961):
Pattern of oestriol conjugates in human cord blood, amniotic fluid and urine
of newborns.
Acta Endocrinol. *38*, 361

Tyson J. E., Hwang P., Guyda H. and Friesen H. G. (1972):
Studies of prolactin secretion in human pregnancy.
Amer. J. Obstet. Gynec. *113*, 14

Uher J., Jirásek J. E. and Šima A. (1963):
Histochemische Studie von Blasenmole und Plazenta eines fünf Monate alten
Fetus.
Zbl. Gynäk. *85*, 477

Unger R. H. (1976):
Diabetes and the alpha cell.
Diabetes *25*, 136

Uotilla U. N. (1940):
The early embryological development of the fetal and permanent adrenal cortex
in man.
Anat. Rec. *76*, 183

Vacek Z. (1960):
β-glucuronidase, alkaline phosphatase and non-specific esterase in the adrenal
gland of human embryos.
Acta histoch. (Jena) *10*, 248

Vaitukaitis J. L., Ross G. T., Braunstein G. D. and Rayford P. L. (1976):
Gonadotropins and their subunits: basic and clinical studies.
Rec. Progr. Horm. Res. *32*, 289

Vaitukaitis J. L., Ross G. T., Reichert L. E. Jr. and Ward D. N. (1972):
Immunologic basis for within and between species cross-reactivity of luteinizing
hormone.
Endocrinology *91*, 1337

Valenta L., Bode H. H., Vickery A. L. and Mallof F. (1971):
Lack of thyroid peroxidase activity: a cause of congenital goitrous hypothyroidism.
J. clin. Invest *50*, 94 A

Vilas E. (1933):
Über die Entwicklung des Müllerischen Hügels und des Hymen beim Menschen.
Z. Anat. Entwicklungsgesch. *101*, 752

Villee C. A. and Loring J. M. (1969):
The synthesis and cleavage of steroid sulphates in the human fetus and placenta.
in: The Foeto-Placental unit (Pecile A., Finzi C. eds.) Excerpta Med. Found.
Amsterdam, Netherlands 182

Villee D. B. (1966):
The role of progesterone in the development of adrenal enzymes.
Inter. Congr. Ser. III. Proc. of the 2nd Intern. Congr. on Hormonal Steroids
Milan, Italy, Amsterdam, Netherlands. Exc. Med. Found

Villee D. B. (1972):
The development of steroidogenesis.
Amer. J. Med. *53*, 533

Villee D. B. and Driscoll S. G. (1965):
Pregnenolone and progesterone metabolism in human adrenals from twin female
fetuses.
Endocrinology *77*, 602

Villee D. B., Engel L. L., Loring J. M. and Villee C. A.
Steroid hydroxylation in human fetal adrenals: formation of 16α-hydroxypro-
gesterone, 17-hydroxyprogesterone and deoxycorticosterone.
Endocrinology *69*, 354

Vojta M. and Jirásek J. E. (1965):
Probleme der molaren Degeneration des Chorion.
Zbl. Gynäk. *87*, 1215

Wachtel S. S., Ohno S., Koo G. C. and Boyse E. A. (1975):
Possible role for H-Y antigen in the primary determination of sex.
Nature (London) *257*, 235

Waidel E. (1960):
Zur Histochemie der fetalen Adenohypophyse.
Arch. f. Gynäk. *194*, 39

Waldeyer W. (1870):
Eirstock und Ei.
Leipzig, Engelmann

Wales R. G. (1975):
Maturation of the mammalian embryo. Biochemical aspects.
Biol. Reprod. *12*, 66

Warne G. L., Faiman C., Reyes F. I. and Winter J. S. D. (1977):
Studies on human sexual development. Concentrations of testosterone, 17-hydroxy-
progesterone and progesterone in human amniotic fluid throughout gestation.
J. clin. Endocrin. Metab. *44*, 934

Warne G. L., Reyes F. I., Faiman C. and Winter J. S. D. (1978):
Studies on human sexual development. VI. Concentrations of unconjugated dehydroepiandrosterone, estradiol and estriol in amniotic fluid throught gestation.
J. clin. Endocrin. Metab. *47*, 1363

Warthin A. S. (1907):
Tuberculosis of the placenta.
J. infect. Dis. *4*, 347

Weismann A. (1885):
Die Continuität des Keimplasmaa als Grundlage einer Theorie der Vererbung.
Jena, Fischer

Weller G. L. Jr. (1933):
Development of the thyroid, parathyroid and thymus glands in man.
Contrib. Embryol. Carnegie Inst. Wash. *24*, 94

Wiedemann H. R. (1969):
Das EMG-Syndrom: Exomphalos, Makroglossie, Gigantismus und Kohlenhyd-ratstoffwechselstörung.
J. Kinderheilk. *106*, 171

Wilkin P. (1954):
Contribution a l'étude de la circulation placentaire d'origine foetale.
Gynéc. et Obstet. *53*, 239

Wilkin P. (1958):
Le placenta humain.
Snoeck (ed.), Paris, Masson

Wilkin P. (1965):
Pathologie du Placenta.
Masson, Paris

Williams F. T. and Scriver C. R. (1973):
Pseudohypoparathyroidism.
in: Birth Defects, Atlas and Compendium. Bergsma D. (ed.) Baltimore, Williams and Wilkins Co.

Willis R. A. (1958):
The Borderland of Embryology and Pathology.
London, Butterworth

Wilson R., Bird C. E., Wiqvist N. et al. (1966):
Metabolism of progesterone by the perfused adrenalectomized human fetus.
J. clin. Endocrin. Metab. *26*, 1155

Winick M. and McCrosy W. W. (1968):
Renal differentiation. A model for the study of development.
in: Birth Defects, Orig. Art. Ser. Vol. IV, Bergsma D. (ed.)

Winters A. J., Colston C., MacDonald P. C. and Porter J. C. (1975):
Fetal plasma prolactin levels.
J. clin. Endocrin. Metab. *41*, 626

Winters A. J., Eskay R. L. and Porter J. D. (1974):
Concentration and distribution of TRH and LRH in the human fetal brain.
J. clin. Endocrin. Metab. *39*, 960

Winters A. J., Oliver C., Colston C., MacDonald P. C. and Porter J. C. (1974):
Plasma ACTH levels in the human fetus and neonate as related to age and parturition.
J. clin. Endocrin. Metab. *39*, 269

Winters A. J., Porter J. C. and MacDonald P. C. (1974):
ACTH in human umblical cord blood.
Gynecol. Invest. *5*, 33

Witschi E. (1929):
Sex reversal in female tadpoles of Rana sylvatica following the application of high temperature.
J. Exper. Zool. Philadelphia *52*, 267

Witschi E. (1948):
Migration of the germ cells from the yolk-sac to the primitive gonadal folds.
Contrib. Embryol. Carnegie Inst. Wash. *32*, 67

Woodland H. R. and Graham C. F. (1969):
RNA synthesis during early development of the mouse.
Nature (London) *221*, 327

Wurtman R. J. and Axelrod J. (1965):
Adrenaline synthesis: control by the pituitary gland and adrenal glucocorticoids.
Science *150*, 1464

Yen S. S. C. (1973):
Endocrine regulation of metabolic homeostasis during pregnancy.
Clin. Obstet. Gynecol. *16*, 130

Yen S. S. C., Lierena O., Little B. et al. (1968):
Disappearence rates of endogenous luteinizing hormone and chorionic gonadotropin in man.
J. clin. Endocrin. Metab. *28*, 1763

Yen S. S. C., Pearson O. H. and Rankin J. S. (1968):
Radioimmunoassay of serum chorionic gonadotropin and placental lactogen in trophoblastic disease.
Obstet. Gynec. *32*, 86

Yen S. S. C., Samaan N. and Pearson O. H. (1967):
Growth hormone levels in pregnancy.
J. clin. Endocrin. Metab. *27*, 1341

Yen S. S. C., Siler T. M. and DeVane G. W. (1974):
Effect of somatostatin in patients with acromegaly: suppression of growth hormone, prolactin, insulin and glucose levels.
New Engl. J. Med. *290*, 935

Yen S. S. C., Siler T. M., DeVane G. W. and Rivier J. (1973):
Biological effects of somatostatin in normal and acromegalic subjects.
in: Raiti S. (ed.) Advances in human growth hormone research.
U. S. Govt. Printing Office, Baltimore Med. 609

Yen S. S. C., Tsai C. C. and Vela P. (1971):
Gestational diabetogenesis: Quantitative analysis of glucose-insulin interrelationship between normal pregnancy and pregnancy with gestational diabetes.
Amer. J. Obstet. Gynec. *11*, 792

Zachmann M., Völlmin J. A., Hamilton W. and Prader A. (1972):
Steroid 17,20-desmolase deficiency: a new cause of male pseudohermaphroditism.
Clin. Endocrinol. *1*, 369

Zuspan F. and Abott M. (1970):
Identification of a pressor substance in amniotic fluid.
I. Role of epinephrine and norepinephrine.
Amer. J. Obstet. Gynec. *107*, 664

Zuspan F., Behrman R. and Paton J.
Amniotic fluid, epinephrine and norepinephrine.
Amer. J. Obstet. Gynec. *118*, 837

SUBJECT INDEX

243

244